Folklore and Society

Series Editors

Roger Abrahams
Bruce Jackson
Marta Weigle

*A list of books in the series appears
at the back of this book.*

Steppin' *on the* Blues

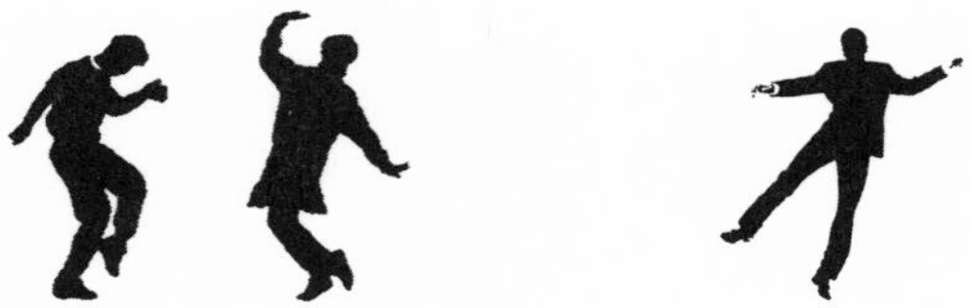

The Visible

Rhythms of

African American

Dance

Steppin'

 ON THE *Blues*

Jacqui Malone

University of Illinois Press   Urbana and Chicago

© 1996 by the Board of Trustees of the University of Illinois
Manufactured in the United States of America
1 2 3 4 5 C P 5 4 3 2

This book is printed on acid-free paper.

Library of Congress Cataloging-in-Publication Data

Malone, Jacqui.
  Steppin' on the blues : the visible rhythms of African American
dance /Jacqui Malone.
      p.   cm.
  Includes bibliographical references and index.
  ISBN 0-252-02211-4. — ISBN 0-252-06508-5 (pbk.)
  1. Afro-American dance—History. I. Title.
GV1624.7.A34M35   1996
793.3'1973—dc20   95-4413
                                                              CIP

For my parents

Maggie Royster Malone and Fred Washington Malone

Contents

Acknowledgments

My ideas for this book began to form while taking courses with the dance historian and critic Sally Sommer. For her encouragement, inspiration, and intellectual leadership I am deeply grateful. To Marshall Stearns and Jean Stearns I owe a special debt. Their fundamental contributions to the field of American vernacular dance have smoothed my path and have been an ongoing source of inspiration.

I wish to extend warm thanks to the following friends and colleagues who provided knowledge and support over the last six years: William Ferris, C. Daniel Dawson, John F. Szwed, Robert Farris Thompson, K. Kia Bunseki Fu-Kiau, Albert Murray, Richard Newman, Erness Brody, Nathan Brody, Jill Williams, Leroy Williams, Marion Coles, Buster Brown, Janice Monsanto-Koslosky, Jennifer Brody, Al Smith, Beverly Bruce, Richard Slotkin, Deborah Willis, Ernie Smith, James Bartow, Suchi Branfman, Susan Matthews, Hank Smith, Shirley Rushing, Mary Gordon, Arthur Cash, Charmaine Warren, and Delilah Jackson.

Others who helped in a variety of ways are Sheila Biddle, Eileen Southern, LeRoy Myers, Louie Bellson, Honi Coles, Sali Ann Kriegsman, Wynton Marsalis, Norma Miller, Frankie Manning, Rob Gibson, LaVaughan Robinson, John Bredar, Bessie Dudley, Melvin Dixon, John Gray, Frank Driggs, Eleanor Harris, Louise Roberts, Steve Good, Donna Good, Jean Hunnicutt, Alan Colon, Robert P. Crease, Monifa Tippitt, Deborah Wolfe, Larry Schulz, Christopher Porché West, Michael P. Smith, Susan Harris, Sterling Stuckey, St. Clair Bourne, and Richard Saylor.

The Schomburg Center for Research in Black Culture, New York Public Library, provided a Scholar-in-Residence Fellowship that supplied the time and financial support to complete large sections of this book. I am particularly indebted to Howard Dodson, chief of the Schomburg, Arnold Rampersad, director of the Scholars-in-Residence Program, and Diana Lachatanere, Aisha al-Adawiya, Alice Adamczyk, Genette McLaurin, Betty Odabashian, Jim Huffman, Mary Yearwood, and Gail Anderson.

For their professionalism and kindness I wish to thank the staffs of the William Ransom Hogan Jazz Archive at Tulane University, the Center for the Study of Southern Culture and the Living Blues Archive at the University of Mississippi, the Caribbean Cultural Center in New York City, the Performing Arts Research Center at Lincoln Center, the Jazz Oral History Program at the Smithsonian Institution, the Institute for Jazz Studies at Rutgers University, the Louisiana State Museum, and the Jean Lafitte National Historical Park and Preserve Library in New Orleans.

Special thanks to Clifford L. Muse Jr. at the Moorland-Spingarn Research Center, Howard University; Andrew Simons and Brenda Square at the Amistad Research Center, Tulane University; Bob Scott and Beth Juhl at Butler Library, Columbia University; James N. Eaton at the Black Archives Research Center and Museum, Florida A&M University; Pat Willis at the Beinecke Rare Book and Manuscript Library, Yale University; and Janice Jones at the National Headquarters Office of Kappa Alpha Psi Fraternity, Inc., Philadelphia, Pennsylvania.

To Queens College, which supported this project with a leave of absence, and to my colleagues in the Department of Drama, Theater, and Dance, I offer my thanks. For its generous support, I am pleased to acknowledge the Research Foundation of the City University of New York.

Much of the original research for *Steppin' on the Blues* required field trips to several cities. During visits to Florida A&M University in Tallahassee I profited richly from the generous assistance of the following persons: Julian E. White, William P. Foster, Julian Adderley Sr., Beverly A. Barber, and Tony Whitehurst. Follow-up interviews with Thomas Lyle, Nathan B. Young, Frank Pinder II, Nat Adderley, and Leander Kirksey helped round out the history of the Marching 100. Special thanks to LaVern Moore and Oscar Moore, whose generous hospitality made my visits to Tallahassee both pleasurable and enriching.

To my official jazz dance consultant, Cholly Atkins, and his wonderful wife, Maye Atkinson, I am profoundly grateful. During visits to Las Vegas they offered warm hospitality, insights, and words of support. I am also indebted to the O'Jays: Sammy Strain, Eddie Levert Sr., and Walter Williams. They not only agreed to extensive interviews but they also welcomed me to several vocal choreography rehearsals. Merald "Bubba" Knight of Glady Knight and the Pips graciously talked with me at length about his experiences with Cholly Atkins. For interviews, I also wish to thank Melvin Franklin, Otis Williams, Richard Street, and Ron Tyson of the Temptations.

At Howard University in Washington, D.C., students and staff members responded with warmth and patience to my endless questions about the evolution of stepping on campus. I am pleased to thank administrators Vincent Johns, Belinda Watkins, and Raymond Archer and step masters Valerie Holiday, Paul Woodruff, Andrew Johnstone, Cedrice Davis, Damon Patterson, and Ron Paige. Ethel O'Meally, Joseph Latta, and my good friend Judi Moore Latta provided assistance and housing during several trips to Washington. Many thanks for their hospitality and support.

In New Orleans, Cyril Crocker took me into his home, introduced me to the city, and gave generously of his time and knowledge. For his extraordinary kindness, I extend a special thank you. To those persons in New Orleans who made time for interviews and conversations, I offer my gratitude: Michael White, Danny Barker, Gregory Stafford, Nathaniel Gray, Norman Dixon, Kenneth Leary, Chief Allison Montana, Jules Cahn, Chandra McCormick, Keith Calhoun, Kalamu Ya Salaam, Tom Dent, and Donald M. Marquis.

For teaching me to analyze dance, I am profoundly indebted to the choreographer Eleo Pomare. To Rufus Gant, my high school tennis coach, I extend warm gratitude for those early lessons in steadfastness.

I salute my editor, Karen Hewitt, for her care, patience, and strong belief in the project, and my copyeditor, Becky Standard, who helped polish and shape the manuscript with great sensitivity and thoroughness. I am also deeply grateful to Roger D. Abrahams. His wise counsel and penetrating questions made this a better book than it otherwise would have been.

Above all, I wish to thank my sisters, Barbara Halsey and Linda Malone-Colon; my wonderful parents, Maggie and Fred Malone, who supported me in countless ways; my sons, Douglass and Gabriel, who sacrificed the most while *Steppin' on the Blues* was being written; and my partner and friend, Robert G. O'Meally, who read these chapters many times, in many forms.

Introduction

Albert Murray calls the African American public dance a ritual of purification, affirmation, and celebration. It helps drive the blues away and provides rich opportunities to symbolically challenge societal hierarchies by offering powers and freedoms that are impossible in ordinary life. At a dance, anyone with the right moves may become king or queen of the floor. It is within this ritual context—and other similarly charged ones—that social vernacular dance is extraordinarily significant and influential. These public dance settings inspire new social dances and give longevity to old ones. Beyond this, the steps and styles they generate provide a mighty storehouse of materials for choreographers of vernacular dance in performance and thereby influence all of American culture.

Steppin' on the Blues: The Visible Rhythms of African American Dance is an attempt to understand the cultural history of a movement system—African American vernacular dance—and its accompanying meanings. I analyze the pervasiveness of dance in African American culture and focus on the Africanisms that have helped the capacity of black American dance to remain vital, dynamic, and distinctive. Through a close look at the evolution and recycling of vernacular dance in three contemporary African American institutions—vocal harmony groups, black college and university marching bands, and black sororities and fraternities—I examine intricately choreographed dance that is derived from black social dance.

The styles perfected by the dancers in these institutions developed through the coming together, on American soil, of central and western African dance with European dance. Because the evolution of these dances paralleled, influenced, and was influenced by the growth of black American music, especially jazz, I also analyze the interrelatedness of instrumental music, song, and dance in African American culture.

Throughout this book, the term *vernacular* refers to dance performed to the rhythms of African American music: dance that makes those rhythms visible. This is America's preeminent vernacular dance. It derives not from the "academy," but from the farms and plantations of the South, slave festivals of the North, levees, urban streets, dance halls, theaters, and cabarets. It is constantly changing. The changes, however, always reflect an evolving tradition and a vital process of cultural production. In *Going to the Territory*, Ralph Ellison defines the vernacular in a way that I find quite useful:

> I see the vernacular as a dynamic *process* in which the most refined styles from the past are continually merged with the play-it-by-eye-and-by-ear improvisations which we invent in our efforts to control our environment and entertain ourselves. And this not only in language and literature, but in architecture and cuisine, in music, costume, and dance, and in tools and technology. In it the styles and techniques of the past are adjusted to the needs of the present, and in its integrative action the high styles of the past are democratized. . . . Wherever we find the vernacular process operating we also find individuals who act as transmitters between it and earlier styles, tastes, and techniques. In the United States all social barriers are vulnerable to cultural styles.[1]

Vernacular dance gave birth to several international dance crazes, including the cakewalk, the Charleston, and the lindy hop. Its hallmarks are improvisation and spontaneity, propulsive rhythm, call-and-response patterns, self-expression, elegance, and control. Zora Neale Hurston has invented the most telling phrases to describe the quality of this dance style: "compelling insinuation" and "dynamic suggestion."[2]

American dance historians have traditionally fixed their attention on concert or theater dance. In doing so, they have made the capital mistake of ignoring American vernacular dance, one of this country's most important contributions to world culture. Since Marshall Stearns's and Jean Stearns's pioneering *Jazz Dance*, published in 1968, very few books have discussed African American vernacular dance in a comprehensive way. Lynne Fauley Emery's *Black Dance from 1619 to Today* is a valuable contribution to the field of dance scholarship, as is Katrina Hazzard-Gordon's *Jookin'*, which discusses the development of black social dance in America.

It is significant that American scholars in disciplines other than dance have done much of the groundbreaking analyses in this area of study. For example, the writings of the art historian Robert Farris Thompson provide a brilliant framework for discussing the roots of black vernacular dance in traditional African cultures and how this dance fits into the larger context of dances of the African diaspora. Albert Murray's *Stomping the Blues* establishes a structure and a language for discussing the relationship between jazz dance and jazz music. Roger Abrahams's *Singing the Master* and Sterling Stuckey's *Slave Culture* and *Going through the Storm* include the most insightful contemporary analyses of dance performed by slaves. However, no recently published books thoroughly explore contemporary choreographed vernacular dance in performance.

By focusing on African American institutions that have kept this form alive, recycled it, and, most importantly, linked it to a tradition, I explore some of the venues that have allowed vernacular dance to continue to thrive. The current lively existence of black fraternities and sororities, vocal groups, and black college marching bands has helped ensure the many revivals, revisions, and reinterpretations of classic American vernacular dances.

I begin by examining the roots of vernacular dance in western and central African traditional cultures and demonstrating how these traditions were continued in African American culture. I then set the stage for the evolution of vocal choreography by charting vernacular dance in performance from slavery through 1950. During this period African American musicians, singers, and dancers trained and performed in many of the same arenas. They inspired each other and pushed the evolution of their art forms along through improvisation, competition, and hard work. A close examination of the African American artist in the evolution of American theatrical history reveals that there is a long and enduring tradition of dancing singers and dancing musicians. The dancing singers of black vocal groups and the dancing musicians of black college and university marching bands have added richly to this tradition.

Chapter 7 documents the work of Cholly Atkins, the father of vocal choreography and a member of the classic tap duo Coles and Atkins. With the decline of tap dancing, Atkins easily made the transition from tap to rhythm and blues and became staff choreographer at Motown Records. From this vantage point, he trained Motown's recording artists to perform choreographed visualizations that fit hand-in-glove with the new music.

In the next two chapters I focus on Florida A&M University's 329-piece marching/dancing band. I place the band within a broad cultural and historical brass band context and discuss its evolution in relation to the development of America's military bands, minstrel bands, and New Orleans marching bands. The FAMU band, with its jazz-spirited steps, is a primary carrier of African American cultural traditions in gesture, music, and dance.

Fraternal and sororal organizations have long served as vehicles for developing and preserving vernacular dance. From the colorful parades of the True Reformers and the eye-catching drill teams of the Elks to the ebullient second-line dancing of New Orleans' black social aid and pleasure clubs, black vernacular movement has enriched a broad spectrum of African American institutions. According to the historian Robert C. Toll, black marching and social club steppers appeared in the productions of Edward Harrigan and Tony Hart as early as 1877.[3] The biography of the black Reconstruction leader P. B. S. Pinchback lists numerous social-political clubs and benevolent societies that served as springboards for black street bands in New Orleans during the 1880s. Their major activities included dance on a large scale.

Dance, music, and song play a major role in western and central African voluntary associations and secret societies. It was inevitable that these cultural forms would find their place in similar black American organizations. By the 1960s, dancing and singing had become an important part of the rituals of African American Greek-letter fraternities and sororities at colleges across the nation. Out of the gradual evolution of rhythmical marching and dance, "stepping" emerged in the last decades of the twentieth century. Competitive stepping performances, called "step shows," feature verbal play, singing, and vigorous polyrhythmic body movement.

The final chapter explores the cultural roots of stepping and its function and organizational structure at Howard University, the birthplace of more than half of the eight major African American Greek-letter groups. The confluence of dance, music, and song in the step shows of these organizations mirrors the importance and linkage of these artistic forms in western and central African voluntary associations and initiation rites.

The widespread activities of African American sorority and fraternity stepping teams, black vocal groups, and historically black college bands have become extremely important in asserting and maintaining an African American sense of community across class and regional lines. Black dance breaks down barriers of gender, age, sex, region, and class.

Many scholars of American culture have traditionally failed to acknowledge how intragroup diversity influences vernacular activity. Therefore, forms of vernacular creativity that come out of black middle-class milieux are often not recognized as representative modes.[4] In his ethnographic study *The World from Brown's Lounge*, Michael J. Bell shows how the patrons of a Philadelphia black middle-class bar introduce art into their everyday lives through African American forms of verbal play. Bell points out that by ignoring the activities of working- and middle-class groups, scholars of African American studies have "unnecessarily limited public understanding of how extensive and pervasive are the patterns that their researches have uncovered."[5] This has been especially true, writes the folklorist John W. Roberts, of vernacular activity that has evolved in black social clubs, sororities, fraternities, lodges, and various religious denominations. Their rituals and other cultural expressions have been ignored "in the effort to imagine an African American *folk* in a traditional sense."[6]

Through rituals involving dance, music, song, and language, African Americans continue to find celebratory ways to "evoke the spirit" and at the same time perpetuate common values, reaffirm community, and re-order society. Competitive interaction[7] is the driving force that keeps African American dance, music, and song in the avant-garde worldwide. We see it, for example, in the jam sessions of jazz musicians, cutting sessions of tap dancers, challenge matches of break dancers, colorful parades of black social aid and pleasure clubs, and the "sing-offs" of blues shouters of the twenties, gospel quartets of the thirties and forties, and doo wop vocalists of the fifties. Through the competitive interaction of such verbal dueling strategies as playing the dozens, woofing, sounding, and signifying, African Americans have revitalized and reenergized American language.[8] When the bands of historically black colleges gather at Grambling University for the "Battle of the Bands" or the Howard University step teams meet for their annual homecoming "throwdown," they are adding to a long tradition of combative interplay that was brought to North America from traditional sub-Saharan cultures.

Such African American festive events provide occasions to experience kinesthetic and verbal "ways of moving together"[9] that spur the participants on to greater artistic heights while simultaneously creating a spirit of kin-ship and solidarity. Roger Abrahams's eloquent statement addresses this point:

> Cutting, jamming, and breaking, marching, and shouting mean getting up against and competing through artful imitation, going beyond the last performer in his or her own terms. We tend to think of shouting, for instance, in the standard English sense of referring to noisemaking, but it means the holy way of moving the whole congregation, whether through vocal or movement vocabulary. . . . Through moving together while playing apart, the entire universe is animated for the moment, as

the spirit descends on the group, even when the spirit can't be called holy. *This* is the center of the aesthetic of the cool, I promise, not just in America but throughout the Black New World and much of subsaharan Africa.[10]

"Battles of aesthetic virtuosity" are central to West Indian tea meetings, Haitian Rara bands, Brazilian capoeira (brought to that country by Angolan slaves), the culture clubs of South African townships, the calypso bands of Trinidad, dance clubs of western Africa's Anlo Ewe, the Jonkonnu bands of Jamaica, the Mardi Gras Indians of New Orleans, and many festivals in the United States, the Caribbean, and South America.

Peter Abrahams's *Tell Freedom*, a 1954 account of his childhood in Johannesburg, includes a vivid example of cutting among parading groups of young males:

> There were six coon teams in Vrededorp that year. Each team tried to outdo the others in uniform, dancing, and singing. A team was made up of between twenty and thirty men and boys. Their uniforms were of the brightest and shiniest silk materials. And each team wore a different combination of colours. . . . A whistle blew. The team set off, down the centre of the street. The leader twirled his stick. Those behind him danced. . . . And sometimes, when two teams met, there was a battle of dancing for the right of way. The teams would stop, facing each other. And the two leaders would dance against each other. That was a sight! They whirled and leaped; made intricate patterns with their sticks; danced on their brightly coloured handkerchiefs, on their bellies, on their hands. Right of way went to the victor. The vanquished made a passage and played the victors through. And oh, how the victorious leader danced through that human passage![11]

Among the Saramaka of central Suriname, folktales (*kóntu*) performed at funeral celebrations are interrupted periodically with short stories that often include song, speech, mime, and dance. The term used to describe the process of interrupting is *kóti* ("to cut [into, across, off]"). The aesthetic success of an evening of tale-telling depends explicitly on listeners' cutting into longer narratives with brief "tale nuggets."[12]

The dynamic performances of African American sorority and fraternity stepping teams, vocal groups, and historically black college and university bands reflect cultural patterns that can be found in many African-based cultures. They must be seen, not as isolated phenomena, but as part of the continuum of black diaspora creativity.

The main point I wish to make in *Steppin' on the Blues* is that African

American vernacular dance has profound meaning beyond its apparent aesthetic magnetism. It represents an art style. Albert Murray reminds us that "the creation of an art style is . . . a major cultural achievement. In fact, it is perhaps the highest as well as the most comprehensive fulfillment of culture; for an art style, after all, reflects nothing so much as the ultimate synthesis and refinement of a life style."[13] African American vernacular dance embodies African American values. It reflects a way of looking at the world and provides a means of survival.

Chapter One

"*Gimme de Kneebone Bent*": *Music and Dance in Africa*

Music is a challenge to human destiny; a refusal to accept the tran-
sience of this life; and an attempt to transform the finality of death into
another kind of living.
— Francis Bebey, *African Music: A People's Art*

Dance with bended knees, lest you be taken for a corpse.
— Kongo Proverb

In many African languages there is no word to define music. Its pervasiveness in the lives of sub-Saharan Africans makes the use of the
term superfluous. Music provides enjoyment and allows people to celebrate festivals and funerals; to compete with one another; to recite history, proverbs, and poetry; and to encounter gods. It teaches social patterns
and values and helps people to work, to grow up, and to praise or criti-
cize the behavior of community members.

The Zairian scholar K. Kia Bunseki Fu-Kiau calls Africa the "dancing
continent" where music is "the expression of life, peace, and harmony."
Drumming, singing, and dancing create songs of peace, inner strength,
and power. Among the Fajulu, even the origin of humankind is inextri-
cably linked with dance and music. They believe that in the beginning
there were two worlds and the people of both used drum messages to in-
vite one another to dance parties.[1]

In any discussion of this vast continent's dance and music, it is appropriate to speak of *African musics* and *African dances* because of the many
cultural differences in musical and movement styles. Africa's musical styles
are as diverse as its peoples; and this diversity is at the heart of the conti-

nent's tremendous richness in the arts. Yet, comparative studies of various traditional African cultures show that some commonalities do exist. They grow out of a shared conceptual approach to the arts. The people of black Africa have related ways of experiencing, creating, learning, and evaluating dance and music. The African musicologist J. H. Kwabena Nketia explains that there is a system of distinct but related traditions that have similar or overlapping styles and practices. These traditions share many of the same elements of context, basic procedure, and internal pattern. The commonalities that link traditional African cultures can serve as a basis for understanding the aesthetic values that help shape African American artistic forms.[2]

Most European conceptions of art would separate music from dance and both music and dance from the social situations that produced them. Most traditional African conceptions, on the other hand, couple music with one or more other art forms, including dance. And most Africans experience music as part of a multidimensional social event that may take place in a village square, a town plaza, a courtyard, a dance plaza, a marketplace, a street corner where groups normally meet for singing and dancing, or a sacred place selected for a particular rite. Invariably audience members participate verbally and through physical movement. Indeed, societal values encourage this kind of participation because it allows members of the community to interact socially in musical situations. Moreover, articulating the beat through motor response heightens one's enjoyment of the music and makes one feel more involved in the musical event.[3]

Restrained contemplative behavior is not expected, nor is it assigned any particular value in this setting. Participants are encouraged to shout appreciation or disapproval if the performance does not meet the artistic standards of the community. The two most prominent features of a traditional dance plaza in action are vitality and dynamism. Performers must give of themselves totally to such occasions, with some dance events continuing for hours or even days without loss of energy. Even when the dances are old, they retain a freshness and a capacity to renew experience that never fails to draw large audiences.[4]

In *African Rhythm and African Sensibility* John Miller Chernoff maintains that people in Africa "do not so much observe rituals in their lives as *they ritualize their lives.*"[5] Through a typical day, one moves, in traditional African societies, from one ritualized activity to another and then another. And the ethical and philosophical values of such societies are generally articulated in the art (inevitably connected with ritual) pro-

duced by that society. According to Nketia, "a village that has no organized music or neglects community singing, drumming, or dancing is
said to be dead."[6] Fu-Kiau, initiated in the Bakongo culture of central
Africa, asserts:

> Kongo people drum, sing, and dance to raise their families with the bal-
> ance provided by the sound of music. They drum, sing, and dance to
> moan their dead; they drum sing and dance to strengthen their institu-
> tions. Furthermore [they] drum, sing, and dance because life itself is a
> perpetual melody. They produce music and enjoy it to be [at] peace with
> themselves, . . . nature, and with the universe as well. Drumming, sing-
> ing, and dancing is a powerful spiritual "MEDICIN/N'KISI" that helps
> one to excel at work, at war, even under oppression. . . . There is a be-
> lief among the Bantu people, especially among the Bakongo, that phys-
> ical health is, first of all, an inner matter. The matter of kinenga [or]
> balance is the key to self-healing power.[7]

Instrumental music, dance, song, literature, and the visual arts are essential to life in traditional African societies. Since antiquity, African visual art has been integrated with the cosmology and values of society. The
art historian Robert Farris Thompson has written brilliantly about the relationship between dance and African art history. According to Thompson, "Africa . . . introduces a different art history, a history of *danced* art."[8]
African sculptural figures often represent bodily shapes and gestures that
are meaningful within specific African cultures. Traditional western African sculptors seem less interested in precise anatomical representation
than in the more subtle processes of implied bodily motion. Members of
many traditional societies believe that when they assume certain stances
or when they dance, they are reenacting ancestral patterns that have been
in existence for centuries; that indeed, through their African art in motion, they are regenerating all their ancestors back to the beginning of time.
A Kongo taxi driver told Thompson, "Our ancestors gave us these dances, we cannot forget them." In Dahomey he was told, "It is our blood that
is dancing." Thompson concludes, "The pleasure taken in viewing vitally inflected sculpture or the dance therefore stems, in part, from sensations
of participation in an alternative, ancient, far superior universe." According to this analysis, dancers themselves become a magnificent form of
sculptural art. Through the dance, sculpture is recreated for public view.
Africans brought to North America were no doubt affirming their ancestral values when they sang a slave song that urged dancers to "gimme de
kneebone bent." To many western and central Africans, flexed joints rep-

resented life and energy, while straightened hips, elbows, and knees epitomized rigidity and death. "The bent kneebone symbolized the ability to 'get down.'"[9]

Many African musics are derived from language, and many of the continent's more than seven hundred distinct languages are tonal. There is a sense in which music and language are synonymous since music grows out of the rhythmic onomatopoeia as well as the intonations of speech. "The musicality of many *Bantu* words is so precise that they can be transcribed on a stave."[10]

African drummers play melody as well as rhythm and they can tune their drums to speak linguistically specific sounds based on the player's language, so that the music itself constitutes a sounded text. In order to make their drums "talk," these musicians must have an extremely acute sense of pitch. Rhythmic repetition is so important in this context because it helps the drummers to clarify what they are saying. This linguistic aspect of the drumming makes for new rhythms (corresponding to new statements being drummed), but it also limits improvisation because the rhythms must be very specific to make good sense as language. Still, drum conversations (which, again, never proceeded wholly apart from the dance) can be full of intricacy, drive, and competitive wit:

> Ewe drummers sometimes engage in competitions, hurtling insults at each other on their drums or trying to duplicate each other's improvisations and body movements. Often, when Gideon was going to be around, other drummers would not even appear: they were afraid to go up against [him]. Gideon could always invent witty remarks which could be clearly understood, which involved extremely subtle beating, and which always fit perfectly into the rhythms of the ensemble. He stumped everybody, and when he wanted to, he completely stupefied them. (Gideon could play three drums while he rolled backwards into a head-and-shoulder stand, clapping his feet together and singing at the same time.)[11]

In the kingdom of the Kongo, an ancient Bantu-speaking nation, gesture constituted a language: "From words to the rhythms of music and the dance there was no discontinuity in the traditional society of the Kongo; they were all language, whether of sound or gesture."[12] In many parts of Africa, dance serves as an artistic means of communication that can transmit thoughts through the choice of specific postures, facial expressions, and movements. Through the subtlety of their movement, dancers can address social and religious issues; and they can express gratitude, friendship, and hostility. An Akan dancer who points the right hand skyward is saying, "I look to God." Placing the right forefinger lightly against the head means, "It is a matter for my head, something I should think seriously about, something that I must solve for myself." Placing the right forefinger below the right eye signifies, "I have nothing to say, but see how things will go." A dancer who rolls both hands inward while stretching the right arm with the final musical beats is saying, "If you bind me with cords, I shall break them into pieces."[13]

Although some African cultures do feature music purely for listening pleasure, music that accompanies dance, or dance-beat-oriented music, is much more prevalent. In such dance-and-music settings, the choices of instrumentation, types of music played, and variety of movement—and how the three are related—vary greatly depending upon the occasion and the culture. The music for dance might be provided by a single drum, a drum ensemble, or various groupings of trumpets, flutes, chordophones, drums, and xylophones. Some drum ensembles play in combination with voices.[14]

As for the dance, different groups emphasize different parts of the body. The Anlo-Ewe and Lobi of Ghana emphasize the upper body, while the Kalabari of Nigeria give a subtle accent to the hips. The Akan of Ghana use the hands and feet in specific ways. Strong contraction-release movements of the pelvis and upper torso characterize both female and male dancing in Agbor. Such movements as leaping, tumbling, shaking, stooping, stamping, squatting, and lifting might be included as elements of the dance. With the exception of processions or other occasions where there is mass movement, free dancing, or individual performance, most events in traditional African cultures feature dances in lines and circles. Dance teams also employ semicircles and serpentine formations, and small groups use other spatial arrangements.[15]

While dancers are most responsive to rhythm, the expressive quality of their performance is also influenced by systems of tonal organization, which include modes and scales. But most often rhythm is articulated in basic dance movements. The rhythm of melodic or nonmelodic instruments and song rhythms defined for dance movement determine which movement sequences are chosen and how they are grouped. Movement sequences, organized linearly or multilinearly, can be simple or extremely complex: "In European dance the emphasis is on the performer moving from one distinct spatial position to the next, whereas dancers in Africa often move through a subtle complex of spatial gradings with the emphasis on the rhythmo-dynamic aspects of the movement and the closely knit relationship between movement and music."[16]

Prechoreographed or prearranged dances are tied to specific rhythms, while those that emphasize individual expression provide musicians with opportunities for more creative freedom. Individual dance allows for maximum improvisation and communication with the master drummer under established rules of etiquette that both participants must follow. When a dancer enters the circle, the relationship between the master drummer and an individual dancer must be one of mutual respect and creative inspiration. The improvisation is often led by the drummer, but there are instances when the dancer leads or there is a mutual exchange of initiative.[17]

The Ewe master drummer is chiefly concerned with propulsion and levitation. High staccato tones call for airborne or upward movement and deep tones are associated with earthbound movement. As S. D. Cudjoe explains, the master drummer

> grounds and lifts the dancer's foot a fraction ahead of the dancer's corresponding movements. . . . The real art of master-drumming does not consist merely in playing beautiful contrasting themes, but in the drummer's ability to introject his themes before the dancer shows obvious signs of waning vigor. A true master must time his utterances to replenish the dancer's physical and aesthetic energy at the right psychological moment. It is this magical sense of timing which wings the Ewe dancer into seemingly tireless motion. It is this, and not the so-called hypnotic influence of the drum, which turns the best of Ewe dancing into mobile sculpture.[18]

Through rhythmical phrases played on the drum, the Yoruba master drummer calls out the steps and patterns in religious ceremonies. In these settings, the dancing is symbolic and ordered and timing and body placement must be exact. Here the musician is the dancer is the musician. Among the Frafra in northern Ghana, the participants in the galgo dance sing, drum, and perform acrobatics. In western Africa, a good drummer is a good dancer and a good dancer is a good drummer, "although the degree of specialty and professionalism varies with each individual."[19]

For certain Akan dances, the master drummer—communicating both verbally and musically—gives directions to the dancer: "Move outwards, move towards us; take it easy; do it gracefully." In Akan societies, finishing the dance properly is of the utmost importance:

When at an appropriate moment the dancer stretches his hands side-
ways, jumps up and crosses his legs in the landing, the master drummer begins the piece proper followed by the rest [of the drummers], for
the crossing of the legs is the sign that the dancer is ready to dance vigorously. From this point the dancer must follow the drumming closely
for the cue to end the dance in a posture or appropriate gesture carefully timed to the end beats. The timing of the end gesture is very important, for it is one of the fine points in the collaboration between
drummers and dancers to which every spectator looks forward. If a dancer misplaces it, he exposes himself to ridicule and booing.[20]

A good dancer is one who converses with music, clearly hears and feels
the beat, and is capable of using different parts of the body to create visualizations of the rhythms. Dancers who move well and follow the beat
closely make improvisation easier for the drummers because their movements are usually clearer. "Without dancers, many drummers cannot bring
forth a wide range of variations, and in this regard we can suggest that
dance probably played one of the important inspirational roles in the early
development of jazz."[21]

Again, the close relationship between African musics and African dances is vital and cannot be overemphasized. Thompson has identified five traits
of western African music that are also present in the dance: dominance of
a percussive concept of performance, multiple meter, apart playing and
dancing, call and response, and songs of allusion/dances of derision. Dominance of a percussive concept of performance defines the way musicians
play their instruments and the way dancers move their bodies. Although at
times the movements of western African dances can be rounded and flowing, they tend to be vigorous and sharp. Much the same can be said of the
musical practices of black slaves in the United States. W. C. Handy heard
his grandfather's accounts of music making during slavery: "A boy would
stand behind the fiddler with a pair of knitting needles in his hand. From
this position the youngster would reach around the fiddler's left shoulder
and beat on the strings in the manner of a snare drummer." Albert Murray
has described the jazz dancer as a percussive instrument in dialogue with
musicians who play their instruments in a percussive manner: "A jazz musician exploits the percussive sound of the trumpet; a piano becomes a drum,
a bass fiddle becomes a drum, all the instruments are [drums], way down
under. That's the African-derived influence."[22]

"Multiple meter" refers to the use of cross rhythms. Musicians create
tension in the music by playing several different rhythms at the same time.

Dancers articulate some of the rhythms in different parts of their bodies, but it is extremely important that they maintain clarity. Peggy Harper's study of dance styles in Nigeria reveals that dancers there commonly combine at least two rhythms in their movement; the simultaneous blending of three rhythms can be seen among highly skilled dancers, and, on rare occasions, the articulation of as many as four distinct rhythms may be seen.[23]

Early chroniclers of sub-Saharan dance consistently commented on the absence of closed couple dancing. Dancing apart allows for a better dialogue with the music. "To dance with arms enlaced around the partner, in the manner of pre-jazz Western ballrooms, lessens the opportunity to converse," according to Thompson. The hands and arms are not free to communicate the rhythms of the music. Closed couple dancing was thought to be immoral in many traditional African societies. The Ugandan poet Okot p'Bitek's *Song of Lawino* articulates this belief:

> It is true, Ocol
> I cannot dance the ballroom
>   dance.
> Being held so tightly
> I feel ashamed,
> Being held so tightly in public
> I cannot do it
> It looks shameful to me!
>
> I am completely ignorant
> Of the dances of foreigners
> And I do not like it.
> Holding each other
> Tightly, tightly
> In public,
> I cannot.[24]

Thompson's category of "apart playing" for musicians refers to the practice of drumming different overlapping rhythms at the same time, with each rhythm contributing to the polymetric whole. Through improvisation, the master drummer makes radical departures from the drum choir. Thompson observes that western African musicians respond to the music while playing by moving their bodies, especially the trunk and head, in response to the rhythms they are playing. This is vastly different from a European symphonic orchestra, in which the bodies of the musicians are relatively motionless.[25]

Call and response "is a special form of antiphony, wherein a caller alternates his lines with the regularly timed responses of a chorus; it is the formal structure of indigenous singing. . . . The caller frequently overlaps or interrupts the chorus." Dances are often built around a call-and-response performance structure. The Bakongo of central Africa practice the use of this form. Movement always includes two persons or two groups of people: "a solo dancer in front of a group, or an individual before another in a group, or an individual before another in a couple, or two groups placed in front of the other. They perform periodic movements that are like questions and responses."[26] This dynamic process of questioning and answering, calling and responding, proved central to Africans in the Americas.

The most widely used musical instrument among African peoples is the human voice. But European standards of beautiful vocalization are not applicable. The use of songs as speech utterances is quite common. Vocal grunts, rapid text delivery, whispers, and special interjections or explosive sounds are not unusual. Speech and song are often present within the same piece. A good singer among the Akan must have a strong voice, good concentration, a command of language, excellent memory, the ability to improvise texts and adapt tunes to new words, and the skills to extemporaneously fit tunes to words. Respected singers must be able to act and express the depth of their musical feeling outwardly or articulate the beat bodily through movement. They should also be skilled at encouraging others to participate at the right moments; soloists who are performing without a supporting chorus are expected to inspire listeners to sing a refrain or chorus periodically.[27]

Vocal music is particularly powerful in oral cultures as a means of recording traditions and delivering social commentary. Songs of insult, topical songs, and songs of incitement are present in many traditional cultures. The ability of skilled singers to make spontaneous additions to songs and recreate lines is valued. Songs of allusion serve as vehicles of social control. Satire is used to preserve indigenous values and wisdom. Chernoff observes that "people in Africa spend a lot of time laughing at the irony of misguided efforts and the distortions of participation. Yet in its way too, their sense of humor continues to show their concern for community: they have a preference for satire, and even the most satirical imitation is displayed to encourage better participation." People who have stepped outside the bounds of approved social behavior face the risk of being reprimanded publicly through song.[28]

According to Thompson, dances of derision are legion among African peoples. Pride and pretension are targeted by dancers as well as singers. So powerful was this practice in what has become the Republic of Zambia that colonial authorities found it necessary to pass a law against participating in dances of derision: "No person may organize or take part in any dance which is calculated to hold up to ridicule or to bring into contempt any person, religion, or duly constituted authority." In contemporary Ghanaian nightclubs, those showing off on the dance floor might be satirized and imitated by other dancers, but an awkward dancer who cannot do better will not suffer the same treatment. Observers might simply say, "A bad dance does not kill the Earth."[29]

For their part, African Americans have a long history of derision dancing. Indeed, the roots of America's first international dance craze, the cakewalk, are grounded in black parody. In 1901, a former slave told the actor Leigh Whipper: "Us slaves watched white folks' parties where the guests danced a minuet and then paraded in a grand march, with the ladies and gentlemen going different ways and then meeting again, arm in arm, and marching down the center together. Then we'd do it, too, *but we used to mock 'em* every step. Sometimes the white folks noticed it, but they seemed to like it; I guess they thought we couldn't dance any better." While the slaves were doing a takeoff on the "grand manners" of their owners, everyone gathered to watch the fun—even those who were being mocked. As Marshall Stearns and Jean Stearns, the authors of *Jazz Dance*, put it, "the Negro was frequently embroidering upon the mask of what was expected—making oblique fun of white folks." And the practice of derisive dance has stood the test of time in the Americas: Thompson has observed it among contemporary Puerto Rican dancers in New York City dance halls.[30]

These five traits of dance combine in different African cultures to provide unique styles. Chernoff was once told by a group of Ghanaians that the people of Zaire and Congo were "very cool in their ways" and "really good-timers." Personal coolness is an important hallmark of good style. Thompson has coined this phrase for such a set of values and attitudes: "an aesthetic of the cool." *Coolness* in this context has to do with control, transcendental balance, and directing one's energy with a clear purpose in mind. Thompson has identified this concept in the languages of thirty-five western and central African cultures. The Gola of Liberia define coolness in this way: "Ability to be nonchalant at the right moment . . . to reveal no emotion in situations where excitement and sentimentality are acceptable—in other words, to act as though one's mind were in another world. It is particularly admirable to do difficult tasks with an air of ease and silent disdain. Women are admired for a surly detached expression, and somnambulistic movement and attitude during the dance or other performance is considered very attractive." Thus, coolness is a metaphor for right living and diplomacy; it is "an all-embracing positive attribute which combines notions of composure, silence, vitality, healing, and social purification."[31]

At a traditional western or central African musical event, coolness can be exhibited through the way dancers, musicians, and other participants carry themselves. The behavior of people in a musical setting reflects the values they try to exercise in their day-to-day relationships with each other. Self-abandonment and frenzy have no place in this environment. A social event is an occasion to show character, to become ancestral, to exhibit control, composure, and good taste. Good dancers cool their faces when they enter the ring. Flamboyant behavior and virtuosity for virtuosity's sake are frowned upon. The canons of good behavior insist that dancers become completely engrossed in what they are doing and avoid "throwing glances" at the audience. Musicians are expected to operate effectively within the polymetric whole and not improvise randomly. They must be responsive to the social occasion and work to make it as meaningful as possible. Chernoff says it best: "In raising certain cultural themes to the level of institutional processes, music informs character and provides continuity with traditional values."[32]

Thompson has identified coolness in the walks of young, urban African American males, where it remains a way of asserting strength, although the African spiritual meaning has been lost. Indeed the "mask" of coolness emerges in African American culture, where it is greatly sought and highly prized.[33]

These codes of behavior, including coolness, offer avenues of criticism. In traditional African cultures, criticism of art is mainly verbal, and because meaning is at the core of all music and dance, there is great concern that artistic forms be understood within specific cultural contexts. Nketia recalls doing research among the Akan:

> When I was working among the Akan of Ghana—and I happen to be one myself—frequently someone would come to me and ask me: Do you understand what the performers are doing? Are you following it? Do you understand the song? Do you understand what the drums are *saying?* Do you know why this piece is being played? They were all

anxious to make me aware of the fact that there were other "areas of meaning" besides the sounds of drums and voices. There were things happening in the musical situation which they considered relevant. There were associations of all kinds with the musical event which they considered a part of its meaning. There were norms of behavior in musical situations which required some notice.[34]

Some of the most insightful documentation on dance criticism south of the Sahara has been done by Thompson. Between 1964 and 1973, he videotaped dancers and interviewed experts and local observers of several cultures in western and central Africa: Fon, Popo, and Yoruba of Dahomey, Abakpa and Yoruba of Nigeria, Ejagham and Banyang of Cameroon, Kongo of Zaire, and Dan of Liberia. Interviewees in each country discussed such performance elements as dress, finish, timing, style, and thematic balance. Thompson asked participants about their own dance styles and about videotapes of dances from other African cultures. His findings have significant implications for analyzing African American dance styles and gestures. The following comments are particularly meaningful:

Luba say: one must move one's hips in as supple a manner as possible. (Kongo)

You should not align the limbs in too straight a manner. (Kongo)

You should dance bending deep. (Kongo)

It pleases me because she dances with her thighs straight and parallel. (Yoruba)

Stiffness is bad in standing, in bodily beauty. (Dan)

The good dancer is the dancer who dances like a body without bones. (Dan)

One dances with the hands, with the legs, and by twisting the buttocks side to side. (Yoruba)

I like the color, the dress, the style; they show the sign of the music as they dance. (Ejagham)

The feet say what the drum says. (Yoruba)

Keep your elbows and hips close-in to the body; you must move your entire body, vibrate the whole, but you must keep the movement self-contained, not go too far out with gestures and thrusts of the arms and legs. (Kongo)

> There is no mistaking a completely beautiful person who walks and talks
> and acts and looks beautifully. We teach the composing of the face, the
> right way of walking, the right proportion of standing, and the right way
> of acting with the body when making conversation. (Dan)[35]

In these critical sessions in the field led by Thompson, the bodily movements of young people were often subjected to close scrutiny by adults.
Thompson asked one informant about dance criticism during his childhood: "My grandparents watched me beginning to dance in the village
square. They watched and then told me: you don't have enough gestures,
(ko tam koyepete te seno), your feet are heavy (mboli bur), make your arms
supple (ntin), keep your feet rapid (mbiol ntina)."[36]

Children in traditional African societies are constantly surrounded by
instrumental music, song, and dance. Their musical training is a lifelong
process that begins at birth with cradle songs and prepares them for participation in all aspects of adult life. On the backs of their relatives, they
experience the rhythms associated with work. At festivals and other social
events, their relatives dance with them on their backs until they are old
enough to join the activities for themselves. Rhythmical facility is built into
their everyday lives, so that, for example, the children experience the
sounding of three beats against two beats and are thereby aided in the
development of a "two-dimensional attitude to rhythm." Children are
encouraged to begin tapping out rhythms as soon as an adequate degree
of arm control is developed. At the age of three or four, they begin making their own instruments.[37]

Throughout western and central Africa, music is a prominent feature
of children's play. The youngest members of Ewe societies learn games
that develop a feeling for multiple rhythms. One such game is played after swimming and involves sitting in the sand and beating 6/4 against 4/4.
Through open air dances and stories they absorb much about their culture at a very early age. Children in Yoruba cultures know the basic elements of festival dances by the age of five; at six they can usually participate accurately with adolescents in songs and dance patterns.[38]

Musical training is largely a matter of apprenticeship since "exposure
to musical situations and participation are emphasized more than formal
teaching." Children destined to become professional musicians are encouraged to begin studying very early. Although exceptions are made for highly
gifted individuals, Yoruban master drummers are usually born into drumming families and their training never officially ends, for they are constant-

ly being challenged by older drummers and constantly challenging younger drummers. Their artistry is reflected in their ability to move members of the community and to touch their hearts; technical perfection on all instruments in the drum choir is assumed. The Yoruban master drummer "is a composer, the ensemble conductor, a poet, a historian, a repository of religious knowledge, a philosopher, the coordinator of dance and song in some music, and a psychologist par excellence."[39]

The importance of instrumental music, song, and dance in traditional African life cannot be overstressed. Music making is a communitywide experience that lends continuity to musical traditions and is based on individual and group efforts. Nketia confirms that "it is the creative individual who builds up the repertoire or re-creates it, but those who learn it and perform it on social occasions sustain the tradition and make it a part of the common heritage."[40] Africans' strong attitudes toward music and dance—and of the vital links between them—set the stage for the dancing and music-making cultures to come in North and South America.

"Keep to the Rhythm and You'll Keep to Life": Meaning and Style in African American Vernacular Dance

Listen Ocol, my old friend
The ways of your ancestors
Are good,
Their customs are solid
And not hollow
They are not thin, not easily breakable
They cannot be blown away
By the winds
Because their roots reach deep into the soil.
—Okot p'Bitek, *Song of Lawino, Song of Ocol*

To us life with its rhythms and cycles is dance and dance is life.
—A. M. Opoku, "Thoughts from the School of Music and Drama"

Through art we celebrate life. As Albert Murray says, "Our highest qualities come from art; that's how we know who we are, what we want, what we want to do."[1] The attainment of wholeness, rather than the amassing of power, is what ultimately makes people happy, and the goal of art is to help achieve that wholeness by providing humanity with basic "equipment for living."[2] Among African Americans that equipment is partially rooted in a vital and dynamic cultural style.

African American vernacular dance, like jazz music, mirrors the values and worldview of its creators. Even in the face of tremendous adversity, it evinces an affirmation and celebration of life. Furthermore, African

American dance serves some of the same purposes as traditional dances in western and central African cultures: on both continents black dance is a source of energy, joy, and inspiration; a spiritual antidote to oppression; and a way to lighten work, teach social values, and strengthen institutions. It also teaches the unity of mind and body and regenerates mental and physical power. The role of dance as a regenerative force is echoed in the words of Bessie Jones of the Georgia Sea Islands: "We'd sing different songs, and then we'd dance a while to rest ourselves."[3]

Much has been written about the role of music and folklore among black people in the United States, but the meaning and the pervasiveness of dance have been sorely neglected despite the fact that dance touches almost every aspect of African American life. As Melville Herskovits tells us, "The dance itself has in characteristic form carried over into the New World to a greater degree than almost any other trait of African culture[s]." Since the publication of Herskovits's groundbreaking work, *The Myth of the Negro Past*, the identification of African continuances in African American culture has been a source of much debate among American studies scholars. Fortunately, the discourse has evolved beyond a search for specific elements to the recognition of shared cultural processes of creativity, based on the notion that "art moves within people" and that cultural continuity is never completely broken.[4] The composer and scholar Olly Wilson suggests that African and African American music and dance share similar "ways of doing things, although the specific qualities of the something that is done varies with time and place and is also influenced by a number of elements outside the tradition."[5] Recognition of the strong relationship between the dances of traditional African cultures and the dances of black Americans is now a commonplace among students and scholars of American history, music, and dance.

Although visual source materials are not available to trace with accuracy the evolution of African American dances in the United States during the seventeenth, eighteenth, and nineteenth centuries, certain movement patterns, gestures, attitudes, and stylizations present in the body language of contemporary black Americans are assertive proof of African influences. African Americans "refine all movement in the direction of dance-beat elegance. Their work movements become dance movements and so do their play movements; and so, indeed, do all the movements they use every day, including the way they walk, stand, turn, wave, shake hands, reach, or make any gesture at all."[6]

Because movement behavior has a tendency to be conservative, the stylistic features of movement and dance represent a significant area of "historical inertia."[7] Hence, the dance movements and body language embedded in the muscle memory of captives from western and central Africa provided a deep and enduring wellspring of creativity for black Americans.

Five percent of the approximately twelve million slaves taken from Africa were transported to North America. Colonial populations, especially in the south, had heavy concentrations of Africans. By 1720, South Carolina, the port of entry for most slaves, was dominated by western Africans. There were twelve thousand black inhabitants and nine thousand Europeans. Seventy percent of the slaves brought to Charleston between 1735 and 1740 were transported from Angola; and at the onset of the American Revolution, South Carolina was over 50 percent black. During North America's peak years of importation, 1741 to 1810, slaves were exported in large numbers from central Africa's Bantu-speaking areas.[8]

Peter Wood has written insightfully about the presence of Africans in colonial South Carolina. His findings reveal that "the Bakongo culture of the Congo River area was well represented in South Carolina's early black majority." The Bakongo are descendants of an ancient classical civilization, Kongo, that included modern Bas-Zaïre and neighboring lands in modern Cabinda, Gabon, Congo-Brazzaville, and northern Angola. During the Atlantic slave trade,

> thousands of persons were abducted from this culturally rich area. And as opposed to a prevalent view of Africans—as belonging to different "tribes," speaking different "dialects," thrown together in the holds of slave ships, and hopelessly alienated, one from the other—Africans from Kongo and Angola shared fundamental beliefs and languages. When they met on the plantations and in the cities of the western hemisphere, they fostered their heritage. Kongo civilization and art were not obliterated in the New World: they resurfaced in the coming together here and there, of numerous slaves from Kongo and Angola.[9]

In the kingdom of the Kongo, dancing was rarely done for pleasure alone; it usually functioned within ritual dramas. The sacred implications of dancing made it a primary part of initiation ceremonies; indeed, all other important Kongo rites involved dance because spiritual power itself could not be summoned without the influence of designated ceremonial dances. Kongo-Angolan culture "has inspired the whole planet to dance," writes C. Daniel Dawson. "In the Americas everyone practices some aspects of these Central African traditions in their daily lives, but without recognizing these activities as having a Kongo-Angola origin. For example, rumba, tango and samba, to name just three dances, are viewed in their respective countries as national dances. In reality, these dances should be understood as Central African movement forms shared with the world through their countries." Pelvic thrusts and circular pelvic movements known as the "Congo grind" in American jazz dance parlance probably have a Kongo-Angola origin.[10]

Bantu-speaking peoples constituted the largest culturally related group brought to North America: 41 percent of those arriving between 1701 and 1810. During that same period, western Africans comprised 59 percent of the newly arrived slaves, but their languages were less related. New Orleans, in particular, was a stronghold of Kongo-Angolan culture.[11]

From that culture came music, literature, art, drama, religion, philosophy, social morality, and speech. ("Bantu speech has a proven ability to move into a culture, to absorb it, and to change its language.")[12] Many western and central African adaptations have become thoroughly woven into the fabric of American culture, while their origins have been unwittingly or deliberately obscured.

Resilience toward new experience is a deeply ingrained tradition in many African societies. The Africanist Georges Balandier makes this observation about Kongo culture: "In the Kongo a way of life managed to survive where towns fell in ruins and powers collapsed. This way of life made it possible to make a new start without being disloyal to tradition, without forgetting a style of existence which remained a precious possession inherited from the ancestors. The setting and the institutions might change; the Mukongo slowly altered the habits that governed his daily life. Innovations did not worry him, as long as they did not disturb the ancient fabric of his days." Among western African peoples it was not unusual for the conquerors and the conquered to adopt each other's gods.[13]

The ability to disregard outer form yet retain inner values led to the persistent reworking of African musics and dances even in new and difficult settings. The attitude of people in traditional African cultures toward what is new and foreign endowed North American slaves with a psychological resilience that proved to be their mainstay in facing difficulties in their new lands. The historian Lawrence W. Levine maintains that "culture is not a fixed condition but a process: the product of interaction between the past and present. Its toughness and resiliency are determined not by a culture's ability to withstand change, which indeed may be a sign of stagnation not life, but by its ability to react creatively and responsively to the realities of a new situation."[14]

Murray calls black Americans' cultural mechanism for surviving the adverse circumstances in the United States a "riff-style life style." "We swing because we survived by being flexible and resilient." Murray adds, "riff-style flexibility and an open disposition towards the vernacular underlie the incomparable endurance of black soulfulness or humanity."[15]

Much of what looks like mere entertainment to someone unfamiliar with black idiomatic expression has spiritual significance for persons grounded in African American culture. Although their rituals do not necessarily have the specific religious meanings of rites that were practiced by their ancestors, black Americans nonetheless *ritualize their lives.*[16]

Murray, who has written extensively about the ritual significance of the public jazz dance or the "Saturday night function," sees the dance hall as a temple where rituals of purification, affirmation, and celebration are held. It is a place where the "blues idiom" dancer disperses hard times or adversity as she or he *stomps the blues.* At the Saturday night function, the music and the dance serve as a potent counterstatement to blue moods; and the dancer's response to the music is actually a lesson in how to live. "The blues-idiom dancer like the solo instrumentalist turns disjunctures into continuities [and] is not disconcerted by intrusions, lapses, shifts in rhythm, intensification of tempo, for instance; but is inspired by them to higher and richer levels of improvisation." "What the customary blues-idiom dance movement reflects is a disposition to encounter obstacle after obstacle as a matter of course." Dance-beat improvisation is "so much a part of many people's equipment for living that they hardly ever think about it as such anymore."[17]

Most black Americans learn vernacular dance within the context of their culture. Children are taught to hear and feel the beat at a very young age, and they grow up listening and moving to music. It is not uncommon to witness very young children performing the most current social dances. Traditional African American children's games revolve around dance, and its influence can be seen in almost all physical activities. Song and dance are an integral part of storytelling, for example. Cheerleading becomes dance, double-dutch rope jumping becomes dance, and so do the agile exertions of teenage athletes.[18]

Play serves as training for performance. It teaches us the rules of the game and of a culture. Through interaction, we learn fair play. That is, we learn the ethics of a culture and we learn to identify good play, which is similar to learning how to recognize good performance. The determining factors have to do with personal creativity, styling, and aesthetics. Thus play becomes performance.[19]

In an essay entitled "Remembering Richard Wright," Ralph Ellison comments that although Wright possessed the confidence of a jazz man, he knew little about jazz and "didn't even know how to dance. Which is to say that he didn't possess the full range of Afro-American culture."[20] Black youth and adults generally don't take classes to learn social dance — their academies are dance halls, house parties, social clubs, and the streets. In fact, formal dance studios are usually years behind the real source of America's major social dances: the black community. The tap dancer Charles "Honi" Coles concurs: "In my neighborhood in Philadelphia, the only form of recreation was dancing. Everyone I knew could dance. We used to dance on street corners at night, and then we'd start going to the various neighborhood houses and amateur contests. . . . I [didn't] know anyone who went to school to learn show business or dancing. You learned it . . . as you were exposed to it." Training in this context is a matter of conditioning. It is informal, but it is training nevertheless. Because the training is so subtle, the outcome often seems like second nature.[21]

Black idiomatic dancers have always found the European tradition of dance manuals and dancing masters inadequate for their approach to creating and learning movement, just as jazz musicians have found the European musical notation system not totally adequate for their purposes. European dances lack the freedom of expression that is inherent in vernacular dance. The rigidly codified dances that were studied so systematically by planters in colonial America served as a point of departure for North American slaves, who took what they could use from the dance traditions of Europeans, but retained their own African-derived style, steps, and rhythmical sense.

A tendency to "dance the song" in traditional African cultures was preserved in the secular and sacred expression of U.S. slaves. Spirituals were always sung with some degree of body motion. A black plantation preacher testifies: "The way in which we worshiped is almost indescribable. The singing was accompanied by a certain ecstasy of motion, clapping of hands, tossing of heads, which would continue without cessation about half an hour; one would lead off in a kind of recitative style, others joining in the chorus. The old house partook of the ecstasy; it rang with their jubilant shouts, and shook in all its joints." To thoroughly understand these slave songs one must imagine them as performed. For they were not just sung at worship services and in the field but they were also danced in the ring shout. A band of shouters dramatized the lyrics through movement. The elements involved in performing the African American ring shout, as practiced during slavery, represented dramatic continuances of western and central African expressive culture.[22]

U.S. slave literature is replete with descriptions of black performance style and the adaptation of that style to religion and work. Chroniclers frequently comment on the vitality and dynamism of the participants, although they routinely mistake survival strategy and cultural orientation for shallow merriment and contentment.[23]

The use of the body in religious expression is still highly valued by twentieth-century gospel singers. Mahalia Jackson wrote, "I want my hands . . . my feet . . . my whole body to say all that is in me. I say, 'Don't let the devil steal the beat from the Lord! The Lord doesn't like us to act dead. If you feel it, tap your feet a little—dance to the glory of the Lord.'" Thomas A. Dorsey had this to say: "Don't let the movement go out of the music. Black music calls for movement! It calls for feeling. Don't let it get away." Dorsey's attitude points to one of the most distinctive features of African American artistic expression: multidimensionality.[24]

Black people attend musical events with the expectation that the performers will appeal to their visual and aural senses. One attends a social event to hear the gutsy scream of James Brown and to witness his smooth dance moves; to see the precision stepping of black sororities and fraternities and to hear their polyrhythms, chants, and songs of allusion; to listen to the halftime music of the FAMU Marching 100 and to watch the high-stepping drum majors and musicians strut their stuff. Sidney Bechet comments on the multidimensionality of a New Orleans second-line parade: "The Marshall, he'd be a man that really could strut. . . . He'd keep time to the music, but all along he'd keep a strutting and moving so you'd never know what he was going to be doing next. Naturally, the music, it makes you strut, but it's *him* too, the way he's strutting, it gets you. It's what you want from a parade: you want to *see* it as well as hear it. And all those fancy steps he'd have—oh that was really something! . . . It would have your eyes just the same as your ears for waiting."[25]

African American musicians, dancers, and singers all testify to the spiritual dimension of their art. Many tap dancers describe tap as a "way of life." The tenor saxophonist Lester Young was totally consumed by his musical gift: "Just all music, all day and all night music. Just any kind of music you play for me, I melt with all of it."[26]

A distinctive and characteristic style is manifest in the artistic expression of black dancers, singers, and musicians. Style is an attitude, a mechanism for sizing up the world, and a mode of survival. "Behind each artist," writes Ellison, "there stands a traditional sense of style, a sense of the felt tension indicative of expressive completeness; a mode of humanizing reality and of evoking a feeling of being at home in the world." What then is the background for the strong emphasis on self-presentation among African American dancers, musicians, and singers?[27]

Because the Bakongo were constantly aware of the image they presented to others, personal appearance and other factors in self-presentation were extremely important. "The concern for elegance was dominant." The art of dressmaking and weaving was associated with royalty, and nobles of the court were always elegantly attired and richly adorned. Women of rank wore rings and heavy copper bracelets and neck bands.[28] Among the Akan of Ghana, coiffure and dress signified status. "The divine Ghana or King, according to Arab chroniclers, held court in splendid robes with gold ornaments, his horses' hooves were worked in gold, ivory and silver, and his retinue carried shields and swords embossed with gold." Yoruban art is heavily influenced by male and female hairstyles, dress, jewelry, body scarification, and painting. Some type of body art was practiced by most traditional societies; it was the Nuba's only visual art and was related to their wrestling, fighting, and dancing. The strong impulse to adorn can be identified in numerous African cultures.[29]

Slave literature shows that the importance ascribed to self-presentation and style was preserved in the Americas. Whenever possible, slaves created special attire for parties, festivals, and Sunday activities. The relationship between dress and dance is articulated in the 1789 autobiography of Gustavus Vassa, a former slave: "I laid out above eight pounds of my money for a suit of superfine clothes to dance in at my freedom, which I hoped was then at hand."[30] From the minstrel stage through traveling shows, musical theater, vaudeville, cabarets, and beyond, African American performing artists have attached great significance to personal style and dress.

The king of "strutting," George Walker, of the famous turn-of-the-century team Williams and Walker, was noted for his flashy haberdashery off and on stage.[31] Charles "Honi" Coles, who performed regularly from the thirties through the fifties, says that dancers were always very aware of the correctness and elegant arrangement of their stage clothing: "If you wore a walking outfit, it was correct down to the last detail."[32] Josephine Baker routinely required three dressing rooms, one near the stage for dressing, one for socializing, and one for housing her glamorous costumes. During a single performance she changed at least six to eight times.[33] The Cotton Club chorus line dancers were known as extremely sharp dressers: "They had about twelve dancing girls and eight show girls, and they were all beautiful chicks. They used to dress so well! On Sunday nights, when celebrities filled the joint, they would rush out of the dressing room after the show in all their finery. Every time they went by, the stars and the rich people would be saying, 'My, who is *that?*' "[34]

Many musicians developed classic styles in dress and deportment. The stride pianist Willie "the Lion" Smith elaborates: "You had to be real sharp in the way you dressed, the manner in which you approached the piano, and in the originality of your ideas. . . . Today we call it showmanship, but back then it was called 'attitude.' " "I had my own attitude and way of working at the piano. My way was to get a cigar clenched between my teeth, my derby tilted back, knees crossed, and my back arched at a sharp angle against the back of the chair. I'd cuss at the keyboard and then caress it with endearing words."[35] According to James P. Johnson, Smith's "every move was a picture." Johnson was also impressed by the attitude of the legendary Jelly Roll Morton:

> I've seen Jelly Roll Morton, who had a great attitude, approach a piano. He would take his overcoat off. It had a special lining that would catch everybody's eye. So he would turn it inside out and, instead of folding it, he would lay it lengthwise along the top of the upright piano. He would do this very slowly, very carefully and very solemnly as if the coat was worth a fortune and had to be handled very tenderly. Then he'd take a big silk handkerchief, shake it out to show it off properly, and dust off the stool. He'd sit down then, hit his special chord (every tickler had his special trade-mark chord, like a signal) and he'd be gone![36]

Louis Armstrong, Lester Young, and Duke Ellington were national style setters not just in music but also in dress, demeanor, language, and movement. The trumpeter Rex Stewart was one of many ardent Armstrong admirers: "Then Louis Armstrong hit town! I went mad with the rest of the town. I tried to walk like him, talk like him, eat like him, sleep like him. I even bought a pair of big policeman shoes like he used to wear and stood outside his apartment waiting for him to come out so I could look at him."[37]

Many classic blues singers developed reputations for their individual styles. Dance movements, gestures, and dress were no less important than their actual singing. In the midtwenties, Gertrude "Ma" Rainey's dramatic entrances shook up Thomas Dorsey:

> Ma Rainey's act came on as a last number or at the end of the show. I shall never forget the excited feeling when the orchestra in the pit struck up her opening theme, music which I had written especially for the show. The curtain rose slowly and those soft lights on the band as we picked up the introduction to Ma's first song. We looked and felt like a million. Ma was hidden in a big box-like affair built like an old Victrola of long ago. This stood on the other side of the stage. A girl would come out and put a big record on it. Then the band picked up the Moonshine Blues. Ma would sing a few bars inside the Victrola. Then she would open the door and step out into the spotlight with her glittering gown that weighed twenty pounds and wearing a necklace of five, ten and twenty dollar gold-pieces. The house went wild. It was as if the show had started all over again. Ma had the audience in the palm of her hand. Her diamonds flashed like sparks of fire falling from her fingers. . . . When Ma had sung her last number and the grand finale, we took seven [curtain] calls.[38]

The blues singer Alberta Hunter was sometimes photographed in her "King Tut" pose: "one hand on hip, the other against her forehead, her . . . nose in profile, her curvy hips hugged by a sleek long dress." During performances she typically dangled a long bright scarf that was attached to her ring: "I like to be different. . . . If I had on a black dress, I'd get a gorgeous red or yellow one, something that would be a contrast. I'd just handle it unconsciously but with flair. Jiving."[39]

Nowhere is African American style more manifest than in dance. The six definitive characteristics of African American vernacular dance are *rhythm, improvisation, control, angularity, asymmetry,* and *dynamism.*

The importance of rhythm to human existence is an ongoing theme in the writings of Katherine Dunham. She understood as early as the 1950s that the breaking of *rhythm* in an individual or society results in disintegration, malaise, and energy diffusion. It is the key to human potentials for social and personal integration. Rhythm, asserts Léopold Senghor, is "the architecture of being, the inner dynamic that gives it form, the pure expression of the life force. Rhythm is the vibratory shock, the force which, through our sense, grips us at the root of our being. It is expressed through corporeal and sensual means; through lines, surfaces, colours, and volumes in architecture, sculpture or painting; through accents in poetry and music, through movements in the dance. . . . In the degree to which rhythm is sensuously embodied, it illuminates the spirit."[40]

African American vernacular dance is characterized by propulsive rhythm. Coming from dance-beat-oriented cultures, black Americans demand a steady beat in their dance music. Although the beat can be embellished, the basic rhythm provides the dancer with dramatic exits and entrances. The jazz dancer James Berry comments: "The rhythmic motion on the beat with the music has something. You feel free to do what you want and you can't get lost, because you can always come in, you can dance with abandon but still you are encased within the beat. That is the heart of dancing."[41]

Improvisation, an additive process, is a way of experimenting with new ideas; that mind-set is Africa's most important contribution to the Western Hemisphere. One offshoot of that mind-set is the tendency toward elasticity of form in African American art. When Duke Ellington asked a candidate for his orchestra if he could read music, his reply was: "Yeah, I can read, but I don't let it interfere with my blowing!" That point of view is prevalent among jazz musicians, who thrive on improvisation. "True jazz is an art of individual assertion within and against the group. Each true jazz moment (as distinct from the uninspired commercial performance) springs from a contest in which each artist challenges all the rest; each solo flight, or improvisation, represents (like the successive canvases of a painter) a definition of his identity: as individual, as member of the collectivity and as a link in the chain of tradition."[42]

Improvisation, for the black idiomatic dancer, functions in much the same way. It is one of the key elements in the creation of vernacular dance. From the turn-of-the-century cakewalk through the Charleston of the twenties and the lindy of the thirties and forties, black dancers inserted an improvisational "break" that allowed couples to separate at various points so that they could have maximum freedom of movement. According to Thompson, "breaking the beat or breaking the pattern in Kongo is something one does to break on into the world of the ancestors, in the possession state, precisely the rationale of drum-breaks (*casée*) in Haiti." From the "breakdown" of colonial slave frolics to the break dancing of the twentieth century, the improvisational interlude has remained a cornerstone of African American dance in the United States. Indeed, throughout the Kongo-influenced communities of the African diaspora, there are many styles of " 'breaking' to the earth." For example, the "Break Out" or "Break Away" is the main section in Jamaican Jonkonnu performances, during which several dancers execute solos simultaneously.[43]

All African American social dances allow for some degree of improvisation, even in the performance of such relatively controlled line dances as the Madison and the stroll of the fifties. In this dance tradition, the idea of executing any dance exactly like someone else is usually not valued. When vocal groups perform choreographed dance movements, the audience expects each singer to bring his or her own personality to the overall movement style, thereby creating diversity within unity. Contrary to popular opinion, black idiomatic dancers always improvise with intent—they compose on the spot—with the success of the improvisations depending on the mastery of the nuances and the elements of craft called for by the idiom.

Within the context of vernacular dance performance, the "aesthetic of the cool" functions to help create an appearance of control and idiomatic effortlessness. What vernacular dance celebrates is a "unique combination of spontaneity, improvisation, and control." According to Murray, blues-idiom dance movement has nothing to do with sensual abandonment. "Being always a matter of elegance [it] is necessarily a matter of getting oneself together." Like all good dancers, practitioners of this style do not throw their bodies around; they do not cut completely loose. When the musical break comes, it is not a matter of "letting it all hang out," but a matter of proceeding in terms of "a very specific technology of stylization."[44] A loss of control and a loss of coolness places one *squarely* outside of the tradition.

Angularity is a prominent feature of African American body language, dress, and performance. Thompson has identified several Bakongo angulated gestures and body postures that show up in the sports, musical performances, religious expressions, and day-to-day conversations of African Americans. Black nonverbal communication is rife with angles. We see them in female and male stances, walking styles, and greetings. In *Jazz Masters of the 30s*, Rex Stewart contends that the "insouciant challenge" of Louis Armstrong's personal style was conveyed to the world by "his loping walk [and] the cap on his head tilted at an angle, which back home meant: 'Look out! I'm a bad cat—don't mess with me!'" Zora Neale Hurston identified this characteristic as early as the 1930s: "After adornment the next most striking manifestation of the Negro is Angularity. Everything that he touches becomes angular. In all African sculpture and doctrine of any sort we find the same thing. Anyone watching Negro dancers will be struck by the same phenomenon. Every posture is another angle. Pleasing, yes. But an effect achieved by the very means which a European strives to avoid."[45]

Hurston also identified asymmetry as a significant feature of African arts and black American literature and dance:

It is the lack of symmetry which makes Negro dancing so difficult for white dancers to learn. The abrupt and unexpected changes. The frequent change of key and time are evidences of this quality in music (Note the St. Louis Blues). The dancing of the justly famous Bo-Jangles and Snake Hips are excellent examples. The presence of rhythm and lack of symmetry are paradoxical, but there they are. Both are present to a marked degree. There is always rhythm, but it is the rhythm of segments. Each unit has a rhythm of its own, but when the whole is assembled it is lacking in symmetry. But easily workable to a Negro who is accustomed to the break in going from one part to another, so that he adjusts himself to the new tempo.[46]

The participatory nature of black performance automatically ensures a certain degree of dynamism because the demands of the audience for dynamic invention and virtuosity prevent the performer from delivering static reproductions of familiar patterns or imitations of someone else's hard-earned style.

When performers demonstrate their knowledge of the black musical aesthetic, the responses of audiences can become so audible that they momentarily drown out the performer. The verbal responses of audiences are accompanied by hand-clapping; foot-stomping; head, shoulder, hand, and arm movement; and spontaneous dance. This type of audience participation is important to performers; it encourages them to explore the full range of aesthetic possibilities, and it is the single criterion by which black artists determine whether they are meeting the aesthetic expectations of the audience.[47]

The folklorist Gerald Davis calls this phenomenon of African American performance "circularity": a dynamic system of influences and responses whose components include performers, audiences, and their traditions. Davis's model begins with an ideal form—a preacher's sermon, for example—and ends with a realized form that is shaped by all three components of the circular interchange. Davis's study concentrates on sermons but he also observes circularity in certain musical forms, selected expressions of material culture, and—quite significantly for our purposes—in some types of dance.[48]

The African American aesthetic encourages exploration and freedom in composition. Originality and individuality are not just admired, they are expected. But creativity must be balanced between the artist's conception of what is good and the audience's idea of what is good. The point is to add to the tradition and extend it without straying too far from it. The circle in black social dance is a forum for improvising and "getting down" but the good dancer does not go outside the mode established by the supporting group. "DO YOUR OWN THING," explains the playwright Paul Carter Harrison, "is an invitation to bring YOUR OWN THING into a complementary relationship with the mode, so that we all might benefit from its power." When a dancer enters the magic circle it is a way of renewing the group's most hallowed values.[49]

Among African Americans, the power generated by rhythmical movement has been apparent for centuries in forms of work, play, performance, and sacred expression. Rhythmical movement as a unifying mechanism and a profound spiritual expression is poetically voiced in an excerpt from Ellison's short story "Juneteenth." The speaker, Reverend Hickman, addresses a crowd at an Emancipation Day celebration:

> Keep to the rhythm and you'll keep to life. God's time is long; and all short-haul horses shall be like horses on a merry-go-round. Keep, keep, keep to the rhythm and you won't get weary. Keep to the rhythm and you won't get lost. . . . They had us bound but we had our kind of time, Rev. Bliss. They were on a merry-go-round that they couldn't control but we learned to beat time from the seasons. . . . They couldn't divide us now. Because anywhere they dragged us we throbbed in time together. If we got a chance to sing, we sang the same song. If we got a chance to dance, we beat back hard times and tribulations with a clap of our hands and the beat of our feet, and it was the same dance. . . . When we make the beat of our rhythm to shape our day the whole land says, Amen! . . . There's been a heap of Juneteenths before this one and I tell you there'll be a heap more before we're truly free! Yes! But keep to the rhythm, just keep to the rhythm and keep to the way.[50]

Chapter Three

Mocking and Celebrating: Freedom of Expression in Dance during Slavery

"Though outwardly yielding to the despotism of the master, the real Negro rulership was vested in that great triumvirate, instrumental music, dancing, and song."
  —Newbell Niles Puckett, *Folk Beliefs of the Southern Negro*

"For the art—the blues, the spirituals, the jazz, the dance—was what we had in place of freedom."
  —Ralph Ellison, *Shadow and Act*

It is impossible to study the evolution of African American vernacular dance in North America prior to 1950 without also studying the music of black Americans. The dancing was a visualization of the music and the musicians "danced with sound." Singers used their voices like instruments and musicians made their instruments speak. Tap dancers told stories by playing the floor with their feet and musicians told stories with their music. Dancers sang and singers danced. Both, at times, played instruments. In the same performance arenas, all three pushed the evolution of their forms along through improvisation and competition, constantly searching for freedom from rigidity and codification. They wanted to play it, sing it, dance it differently each time.

Africans who came to the Americas brought with them a rich tradition in instrumental music, song, and dance. As David Dalby, a specialist in African linguistics, observes, "A bitter aspect of the American slave trade is the fact that highly trained musicians and poets from West Africa must frequently have found themselves in the power of slave-owners less cultured and well educated than themselves." Born into cultures of "danced faiths," women and men in the Americas developed creolized versions of rituals that were centuries old.[1]

Styles of African dances, transposed in a colonial environment, made for the development of what Ralph Ellison terms America's first choreography. It was born, he asserts, of "that sense of freedom which lies within the complex unfreedom which we as a people experience in the United States." He goes on to say:

> The slaves first sensed it. They sensed it when they looked at the people in the big house dancing their American versions of European social dances. And they first mocked them—and then they decided, coming from dancing cultures, that they could do them better. And then they went on to define what surely is the beginnings of an American choreography. . . . They had the freedom of experimentation, of trying things out. . . . And in the doing, they found ways of making the human body move in stylized ways which were different.[2]

Dancing was the most popular form of recreation among the American colonists, black and white. John Playford's *The English Dancing Master*, published in 1650, greatly influenced the acceptance of dance in New England. While teaching the colonials to perform English country dances or folk dances, Playford's book also stressed the importance of dance as a mechanism for cultivating good manners and deportment: "The Art of Dancing . . . is a commendable and rare Quality fit for yong Gentlemen, if opportunely and civilly used. . . . This art has been Anciently handled . . . and much commend it to be Excellent for Recreation, after more serious studies, making the body active and strong, graceful in deportment, and a quality very much beseeming a Gentleman."[3]

Thus those colonials who did not object to dancing justified it as a teacher of manners and morals. It was acceptable, they believed, as long as it was not associated with public demonstrations, feasts, taverns, or maypole dancing. Of those ministers of New England who accepted certain kinds of dance as proper, many continued to regard mixed dancing as sinful; but they saw Playford's circle dances, performed in sets and formations, as legitimate.[4]

In New Netherlands, the Dutch danced primarily in the home, at fairs, and to celebrate Christmas and Pinkster. Further south, the ruling classes of Virginia followed the social organization of England, where dancing was essential to good breeding. Virginia planters routinely gave parties for their visitors that often lasted for several days. Having company was synonymous with having a dance; dancing was the colony's most popular amusement. All ages engaged in jigs, reels, square dances, and quadrilles, often to the music of black musicians.[5]

By the end of the seventeenth century, Virginia had an ample supply of dancing instructors who taught such court dances as the minuet and courante and probably Playford's country dances.[6] According to Eileen Southern, "the royal governor in Williamsburg gave splendid affairs at which the colonists danced country dances, minuets, and reels including their favorite *Sir Roger Coverley* or the *Virginia Reel.* . . . Colonists were also fond of a special type of lively jig called by some the 'Negro Jig.'" African American dances were performed with some regularity by whites in colonial America, although it is difficult to say how the dances looked. We are left to ponder such reports as that of a former Monticello slave who describes the brother of Thomas Jefferson as "a mighty simple man: used to come out among black people, play the fiddle and dance half the night."[7]

Engaging in the minuet required the skills of a dancing instructor to see that the dancers followed the music closely, turned out their feet and knees sufficiently, performed the steps neatly and precisely, and coordinated the gestures of the hands, arms, head, and body with the movements and steps of the feet and legs. Pierre Rameau's *The Dancing Master* (1725) outlines the importance of holding the body correctly, "the first requisite for dancing": "The head must be held erect without any suggestion of stiffness, the shoulders pressed well back, for this expands the chest and affords more grace to the body. The arms should hang at the side, the hands be neither quite open nor quite closed, the waist steady, the legs straight and the feet turned outwards."[8]

Many eighteenth-century dancing instructors were servants who provided instruction for their employer's children or were hired out by their employers to teach. After the French Revolution, French dancing instructors sought refuge in America. Working primarily in larger cities, they taught the minuet, country dances, the rigadoon, cotillions, reels, jigs, hornpipe steps, and genteel manners. During this period, young boys of the wealthier classes studied dance along with fencing, mathematics, philosophy, and languages; rich girls were taught the basic curriculum and given an ornamental education, which inevitably included dance.[9] A summary of the type of education deemed proper for young ladies appeared in an eighteenth-century book published in Philadelphia: "Merely-ornamental accomplishments will but indifferently qualify a woman to perform the *duties* of life, though it is highly proper she should possess them, in order to furnish the *amusements* of it. Yet, though the well-bred woman should learn to dance, sing, recite, and draw; the end of a good education is not that they may become singers, dancers, players, or painters; its real object is, to make them good daughters, good wives, good mistresses, good members of society and good Christians."[10]

While the planters' children were following the exacting standards of dancing instructors, those persons who could not afford lessons were dancing anyhow. At fairs, frolics, bees, marriages, and other social gatherings they danced for fun, often to the tunes of black fiddlers. In rural areas and on the frontier, formal rules of etiquette were not so important and there were few dancing instructors. Still, many gatherings ended in a dance. "The men and women of the frontier loved to dance, doing Virginia Reels, country jigs, and shakedowns."[11] In *The Cotton Kingdom*, Frederick Law Olmstead quotes a description of plank dancing in northern Mississippi: "'You stand face to face with your partner on a plank and keep a dancin'. Put the plank up on two barrel heads, so it'll kind o' spring. At some of our parties—that's among common kind o' people, you know—it's great fun. They dance as fast as they can, and the folks all stand round and holler, "*Keep it up, John!*" "*Go it, Nance!*" "*Don't give it up so!*" "*Old Virginny never tire!*" "*Heel and toe, ketch a fire!*" and such kind of observations, and clap and stamp 'em.'"[12] At the close of the eighteenth century, social dancing was popular in cities and towns—balls and dancing teachers were commonplace in American society. In the nineteenth century such round dances as the waltz, polka, mazurka, and the schottische initiated a trend toward independent couple dancing. Much of the music for these nineteenth-century European-American social dances was composed by black musicians, who sometimes had collaborative relationships with white dancing instructors.[13]

Slave trade documents prove that between 1693 and 1860, the British, French, and Dutch used dancing aboard slave ships as a means of exercising their human cargo. Many Africans continued their native music and dance once they reached solid ground. While no actual accounts of such activities have been found before the late seventeenth century, chroniclers of eighteenth- and nineteenth-century life in North America cite many instances of Africans dancing, singing, and playing music in the styles of their native countries.[14]

John Szwed and Morton Marks show that the slaves adapted their central and western African dances to a new environment, modifying the European-derived court and social dances they found in the Americas:

> It is well acknowledged that the court dances which developed in Europe from the seventeenth century onward spread to the rural areas of Europe and to the new world. What has not been properly recognized is that these dances—the quadrille, the cotillion, the contradance and the like—were taken up by Afro-Americans in North and South America and the West Indies. . . . At one extreme, they were "Africanized" for sacred purposes, at the other, they were re-formed and became the basis of a new world popular culture.[15]

The black stylization of the dances was accompanied by a stylization of the figures or dance calls. Szwed and Marks refer to these modifications as "rhymed 'raps.'" This new development in square dancing is explained by the music historian Willis James: "There were scores of Negroes throughout the South who achieved lasting reputations as 'set-callers.' In fact, their popularity rose to such heights that they were in many cases professionals, being paid a fee to bring color and entertainment to the dance. They invented an entirely new system of 'callin' sets.' As they would call the figures, frequently they would dance very original solo steps and give out their calls in a musical phrase pattern."[16]

From the slave ships to the auction blocks to the households, farms, and plantations of America, the dances of black slaves astonished European immigrants and visitors to the emerging nation. In journals, letters, diaries, newspapers, and other accounts of American life between the seventeenth and twentieth centuries, writers black and white attest to the appeal and vitality of dance performed by blacks: "Black entertainers emerged in America virtually simultaneously with the arrival of black people on the continent. In mimed song that preserved traditional African stories, in dancing and patting patterns that reflected pervasive drum and language intonations, in weeping chants that expressed the crushing burden of slavery and separation, black people . . . made a profound impression on their masters and one another."[17]

To the lively tunes of black musicians, slaves danced the cakewalk, pigeon wing, jig, buck dance, buzzard lope, juba, ring dances, quadrilles, cotillions, reels, water dances, and scores of others. In the South, on numerous occasions slaves were called upon to perform for their owners. Isaac Williams, an ex-slave, wrote: "When our masters had company staying with them, they would often collect all the slaves for a general jubilee frolic."

Robert Moton, who became president of Tuskegee Institute, recalled performing for his owners: "Sam was a favorite on the plantation . . . a remarkable acrobat . . . and could perform what were to me many very wonderful acrobatic feats, in addition to being a wonderfully good reel and jig dancer and a remarkably fine singer. . . . Under Sam's direction I practised many of his accomplishments, and with his careful tutelage became a close second. As a result, he and I were frequently called into the 'big house' to perform." The vaudevillian Tom Fletcher heard his grandfather's stories about cakewalking for his master's visitors:

> Sometimes on pleasant evenings, boards would be laid down for an impromptu stage before the verandah so the guests could have a good view of the proceedings and a real shindig would take place with singing and dancing. The *cake walk*, in that section and at that time, was known as the *chalk line walk*. There was no prancing, just a straight walk on a path made by turns and so forth, along which the dancers made their way with a pail of water on their heads. The couple that was the most erect and spilled the least water or no water at all was the winner. "Son," said my grandfather, "your grandmother and I, we won all of the prizes and were taken from plantation to plantation."[18]

Additional occasions for viewing slave performances occurred at barbecues, stores, and in the slave quarters. Church services, Saturday night dances, funerals, sports activities, and holiday frolicking also provided theater for whites. In Virginia the shucking of corn, ginning of cotton, threshing of wheat, killing of hogs, and storing away of tobacco all ended in festivities.[19] Frequently dancing contests were set up by slave owners. One ex-slave remembered an exuberantly competitive scene:

> There am dancing and singing mostest every Saturday night. He [the slave owner] had a little platform built for the jigging contests. Colored folks comes from all around, to see who could jig the best. . . . I must tell you 'bout the best contest we ever had. One nigger on our place was the jigginest fellow ever was. Everyone round tries to git somebody to best him. He could put the glass of water on his head and make his feet go like triphammers and sound like the snaredrum. He could whirl round and such, all the movement from his hips down. Now it gits noised round a fellow been found to beat Tom and a contest am 'ranged for Saturday evening. There was a big crowd and money am bet, but Master bets on Tom, of course. So they starts jigging. Tom starts easy and a little faster and faster. The other fellow doing the same. They gits faster and faster, and that crowd am a-yelling. Gosh! There am 'citement.

They just keep a-gwine. It look like Tom done found his match, but there am one thing yet he ain't done—he ain't made a whirl. Now he does it. Everybody holds he breath, and the other fellow starts to make the whirl and he makes it, but just a spoonful of water sloughs out his cup, so Tom am the winner.[20]

Roger Abrahams points out that Saturday night dances, corn shuckings, and other "permitted entertainments, provided an occasion in which the slaves not only could enjoy themselves, but were encouraged to do so in their own style. In the process, traditional features of African eloquence and improvisation in speech, song, and dance provided the basis for the development of an Afro-American aesthetic system which has been maintained to this day." Abrahams calls cornshucking ceremonies "home entertainments" or "stylized enterprises" that actively resisted acculturation by maintaining "alternative perspectives toward time, work, and status." White spectators saw the event as entertainment while the slaves used it as an opportunity for "keeping up the spirit" by celebrating shared values, experiences, and feelings. The willingness of some wealthy planters to sponsor lavish festivities was, in part, a result of a desire to dramatize the success of their slave enterprise.[21]

The attitudes of North American white slave owners toward dance ranged from forthright encouragement through indifference to suspicion and hostility.[22] But regardless of their owners' attitudes, many slaves were willing to face tremendous odds in order to "set de flo'" at a Saturday night frolic. A former Virginian slave affirmed: "Sadday nights we'd slip out de quarters an' go to de woods. Was a ole cabin 'bout five miles 'way fum de house, an' us would raise all de ruckus dere we wanted. Used to dance ole Jenny down. . . . Dat what we gals used to say. Gonna set de flo' wid Jenny tonight. Sometimes would say when Missus is roun', 'Gwine to see Jenny tonight.' An' dat mean us gonna have a dance, but Missus don't know what we talkin' 'bout. Sometimes de boys say it too—can't tell you what dey mean."[23] To make their way to these often secret dances, slaves crawled out of chimneys, faced abusive patrollers, and walked great distances.[24] Some Saturday night dances lasted through Sunday. Unwilling to end the fun, slaves stuffed old rags in the cracks of their cabin walls to block out the light. "The idea was that it would not be Sunday inside if they kept the sun out, and thus they would not desecrate the Sabbath."[25]

Although many slave owners allowed Saturday night dances, they were usually not as receptive to the idea of weekday dances. Their constant struggles to prevent impromptu partying and interplantation visiting during the week, however, were hopeless. Even "slaves who worked listlessly through the day and complained of impossible demands on their strength miraculously came to life and walked eight or ten miles to dance all night on a neighboring plantation." This determination to continue their dances is best exemplified in the words of former slave Charlie Grandy:

> Marsa ain't sayed we cain't have no dance, an' he ain't sayed we can. But sometimes feel like raisin' a ruckus—make plenty noise wid de winders wide open, shout, clap, and sing. 'Course Marsa don't take de trouble to git outen bed an' come down 'cause he know he gonna fin' ev'y slave in bed an' a-snorin'. Might whip us de nex' day, but we done had our dance. Stay as late as we want—don't care ef we is got to be in de field at sunrise. When de dance break up we go out, slam de do' ef we wants, an' shout back at de man what had de party:
>
> Eat yo' meat an' chaw yo' bone,
> Goodbye, Charlie, I'se gwine home.[26]

On the Waccamaw rice plantations in South Carolina, slaves celebrated for three days during Christmas. John Pierpont, a northern visitor, sets the scene: "On my first waking, the sound of serenading violins & drums saluted my ears, and for some time continued. . . . During almost the whole of the second and third afternoons, the portico was crowded with these dancers . . . fiddlers & drumming. . . . Some of them who were native Africans did not join the dance with the others, but, by themselves gave us a specimen of [their] sports & amusement." During the Christmas season, slave carpentry shops served as nighttime arenas for dance. For the rest of the year, weekend frolics and parties with singing, dancing, and instrumental music were most often held in the slave quarters, known among the slaves as "the street."[27]

In New Orleans, where blacks made up more than one-third of the population, African Americans gathered on Sunday afternoons and on church holy days to share the dances of their various home cultures. In *Scenes in the South and Other Miscellaneous Pieces*, J. R. Creecy reports on the sights and the sounds of black dance in early New Orleans:

> Sometimes much grace and often surprising activity and long-continued rapid motions are seen. The dancers are most fancifully dressed, with fringes, ribbons, little bells, and shells and balls, jingling and flirting about the performer's legs and arms, who sing a second or counter to the music most sweetly. . . . In all their movements, gyrations and attitudenizing exhibitions, the most perfect time is kept, making the beats with the feet, heads, or hands, or all, as correctly as a well-regulated

metronome! Young and old join in the sport and dances. . . . When a dancer or danseuse surpasses expectation, or is particularly brilliant in the execution of "flings" and "flourishings" of limb and body, shouts, huzzas, and clapping of hands follow, and numerous *picallions* are thrown in the ring to the performers by (*strange*) spectators. . . . To witness such a scene is a certain cure for ennui, blue-devils, mopes, horrors, and dyspepsia. . . . Every stranger should visit Congo Square when in its glory, once at least, and, my word for it, no one will ever regret or forget it.[28]

Along North Carolina's eastern shores, the John Canoe festival was celebrated during Christmas. Led by John Canoe, the king of the festival, participants paraded through the town to the accompaniment of cow horns, musical shouts, bells, laughter, yells, and the beating of drums, triangles, jaw bones, pots, and pans. As they danced along, the paraders sang in antiphonal chorus, responding to a leader's rhythmical songs. Gathered before the home of a prominent citizen, the blacks began their presentation. After a short play, they broke into a version of the buzzard lope, which climaxed their visit. According to Ira De A. Reid, there is a strong relationship between this festival, various prototypes in the West Indies, and an "earlier African form noted in the Yam Feasts of the Gold Coast." In Jamaica today, Jonkonnu is a street festival enacted by small groups of costumed males who perform occasionally at Christmas but are associated more often with important state events. Variations of this festival also occur in other Caribbean nations, including St. Kitts–Nevis, Belize, Bermuda, and Guyana.[29]

Holidays commemorating the passage of antislavery laws were held in some parts of the South and in cities and towns throughout the North. Characterized by parades, memorial services, and dancing to the music of brass bands, these public occasions provided nonblack observers with additional opportunities to see how blacks performed and danced. North of the Mason-Dixon line, African cultural influences were continuous and widespread during slavery. Free blacks and slaves sought out one another for cultural reinforcement. Their vitality and their determination to congregate and express themselves culturally was so strong that they often dominated northern festivals.[30] Such was the case in several New England states.

From approximately 1750 to 1850, the most significant holiday among Puritan New Englanders was Election Day. Adopted and Africanized by Yankee slaves, Negro Election Day continued an earlier practice organized by New England slaves to honor those members of the community who had come from royal families in Africa. Accounts have been found of similar practices by people of African descent in Brazil, Cuba, Jamaica, Venezuela, Mexico, New Orleans, New York, Panama, Peru, Uruguay, Colombia, Barbados, Argentina, Trinidad, and the French West Indies.[31]

In New England, slaves were given time off to elect their own kings and governors and to celebrate the holidays through song and dance. The coronation parade, the most important event of Negro Election Day, attracted people of all social classes as it wound its way through the main streets of the town. "A parade in Hartford, Connecticut, often involved as many as one hundred slaves, either mounted on horseback or marching, two by two, on foot. The procession of slaves, each dressed in his finest apparel, would advance with colors flying to the music of fifes, fiddles, 'clarionets,' and drums."[32] The tradition of the inaugural parade and the elements that gave the parade its special air of excitement and festivity— "the diversity of musical instrumentation within the parade ensemble, the polytonal texture and upbeat rhythms of the music, its percussive emphasis and the strutting and baton-twirling of the marchers"—were uniquely African and African American.[33]

During the five-day celebration cultural borrowing went both ways. Certain features of Negro Election Day represented convergences of European-American and African cultural pasts. These included "pre-election 'parmateering' (parliamenteering), the order of march during the procession, the prominence accorded military traditions, the precision drilling of troops, and the inaugural oration." William D. Piersen suggests that "the prototype for the American political parade probably owes more to these black processions in New England than to any corresponding Euro-American institution of the same era."[34]

Many African cultures have traditionally celebrated seasonal and annual festivals that bring people together to pay tribute to their ancestors and leaders and to purify their states in order to begin the new year with hope and confidence. Melvin Wade has drawn interesting parallels between the *Odwira* festival of the Ashanti and Negro Election Day rituals. Through their distorted lenses, whites saw Negro Election Day as a poor imitation of an official white holiday, but for the descendants of Africa it represented a profound linkage to their parent culture and an effective way to counter cultural and social fragmentation.[35]

In New York, however, Pinkster was the most treasured holiday among the slaves and free blacks. Initially the term was not identified with African Americans but reserved for the Dutch, who referred to the holiday as Pentecost or Whitsuntide. Between the second half of the eighteenth century and the early decades of the nineteenth century, Pinkster was adopted by African Americans, who shaped it to fit their own culture. In the process, this holiday came to represent a high-spirited time when black Americans celebrated through music, song, and dance the traditions of their African ancestors.[36]

For many years, the greatest leader of this festival in Albany was King Charley, regarded as a prince from Angola. King Charley paraded onto Pinkster Hill dressed with regal splendor in "a scarlet coat ornamented with tracings of golden lace, . . . black shoes with silver buckles, and a tri-cornered cocked hat upon his head."[37] Assembled with the master drummer and musicians, King Charley gave the cue to start the Pinkster jubilee. One nineteenth-century observer describes the setting for the dance: "In the centre of the *villa* there was a kind of Amphitheatre. . . . On the one side of which is the royal tent fronting the dancing ground, where the parties perform and around which the spectators are assembled." A special dance dedicated to the African deity Totau was one of many dances performed on Pinkster Hill during several days of vigorous and inventive movement.[38]

In a novel set in the mideighteenth century, James Fenimore Cooper's fictional character Satanstoe gives a famous account of Pinkster: "Nine-tenths of the blacks of the city, and of the whole country within thirty or forty miles, indeed, were collected in thousands in those fields, beating banjos, singing African songs. . . . The traditions and usages of their original country were so far preserved as to produce a marked difference between this festival, and one of European origin. Among other things, some were making music, by beating on skins drawn over the ends of hollow logs, while others were dancing to it."[39] Albany's Pinkster celebrations also included a carnival village where participants and spectators could purchase savory dishes and drinks or see sideshows of rope dancing, caged animals, bareback riding, and other attractions.

Although the literature on Pinkster places the most colorful festivals in Albany, the holiday was not limited to that city. All along the Hudson River Valley, in Brooklyn, and on Long Island, people of African descent organized Pinkster celebrations. Thomas Devoe's *The Market Book* contains descriptions of dancing done by slaves who visited New York City markets during Pinkster and other holidays. At Catherine Market, believed to be the first site of "public negro dancing" in New York City, slaves sold various foods for pocket change. After their goods were sold, dancing provided additional money:

> So they would be hired by some joking butcher or individual to engage in a jig or break-down . . . and those that could and would dance soon raised a collection; but some of them did more in "turning around and shying off" from the designated spot than keeping to the regular "shake-down," which caused them all to be confined to a "board," (or shingle, as they called it,) and not allowed off it; on this they must show their skill; and, being several together in parties, each had his particular "shingle" brought with him as part of his stock in trade. This board was usually about five to six feet long, of large width, with its particular spring in it, and to keep it in its place while dancing on it, it was held down by one on each end. Their music or time was usually given by one of their party, which was done by beating their hands on the sides of their legs and the noise of the heel. . . . The large amount collected in this way after a time produced some excellent "dancers;" in fact, it raised a sort of strife for the highest honors, i.e., the most cheering and the most collected in the "hat."

In time, slaves from New Jersey competed against slaves from Long Island, city slaves, and free blacks for prize money offered by spectators and market butchers. Dance and music were mutually reinforcing elements in these early displays of artistic excellence by Africans brought to North America.[40]

In Philadelphia, the last days of the semiannual fairs were reserved for slave jubilees. For many hours, blacks danced in what became Washington Square: "In that field could be seen at once more than one thousand of both sexes, divided into numerous squads, dancing and singing, each in their own tongue, after the customs of their several nations in Africa."[41]

African American dance, music, and song took on new meanings in these new settings. Recreational activities resulted in tighter communal bonds, social cohesion, and cooperation. All classes of slaves were brought together in common pursuits.[42] Slave festivities eased the pain of labor and sometimes served to disguise insurrectionary activities. A 1730 letter from Charleston, South Carolina, describes one such episode: "They soon made a great Body at the Back of the Town, and had a great Dance, and expected the Country Negroes to come & join them; and had not an overruling Providence discovered their Intrigues, we had been all in Blood." The Stono Uprising of 1739, also in South Carolina, provides a second example. A contemporary account revealed that the slaves' numbers "increased every minute by new Negroes coming to them, so that they were above Sixty, some say a hundred, on which they halted in a field and set to dancing, Singing and beating Drums to draw more Negroes to them."[43]

Music and dance gave African Americans a sense of power and control—it had a direct impact on their psychic and emotional states and allowed them to drop their masks and articulate their inner feelings. In addition, music and dance perpetuated traditions, kept values alive, and provided for individual expression. Through these art forms, slaves developed their own aesthetic standards and initiated the creation of new expressive modes.[44]

At rituals throughout the South and North, slaves and free blacks fostered the evolution of a style of dancing that was uniquely American. The bent knees and angulated bodies of their stylized adaptations were in striking contrast to the erect spines, straight legs, turned-out feet, and rounded arms of the European-American dancing instructors. Not only the shapes and movements of the black and white dances were at variance. The perspective and approach to making and learning dances were fundamentally different. The white folklorist Bessie Lomax Hawes became aware of this difference while learning ring plays from Bessie Jones, an African American of the Georgia Sea Islands:

> Suddenly the cultural gulf between us yawned very wide indeed. To me, as to all white Americans, I suspect, a person who is "with" me must do just what I am doing, must copy my movements (and my ideas and my speech and my dress and my clapping). . . . To Mrs. Jones and the Sea Islanders, to be "with" somebody means to respond to them, to complement and support their silences, to fill in their statements (musical, physical and verbal) with little showers of comment, to answer their remarks—to clap a *different* pattern.[45]

The slaves enjoyed a spontaneity, dynamism, and improvisational flair that reached back to their ancestors in central and western Africa, while the planters believed that a dance must be performed in a precise, unchanging way. Still, white Americans were entranced by the vibrancy of these slave creations and found themselves unable to resist their magnetic pull.

No wonder the influence of black dance was so widespread. It struck whites as an unthreatening black activity. Most slave owners regarded black dance as "devoid of political message, not apparently subversive, an expression that made no pretense of usurping the proper role of whites; it was technically impressive, rhythmically exciting, and possibly even sexually stimulating."[46] Furthermore it confirmed their notions that slaves were happy and contented. The process whereby black and white styles of dancing could influence one another was a painless one. Unlike other forms of communication, dance presented no language barriers. And this was a form of cultural exchange that could cross color lines without physical contact. By the early 1800s, not long after the colonies declared their independence from England, white men were carrying their versions of slave dances to the American minstrel stage.

Chapter Four

Black Dance on the Road:
Minstrelsy and Traveling Shows

I jumped around from Gonzelle White's Minstrels to the Florida Blossoms, Silas Green's Minstrels, A. G. Allen's Mighty Minstrels, Huntington's Minstrels, and back to the Florida Blossoms . . . and I saw dancers who were so good you wouldn't believe it.
— Pigmeat Markham, *Jazz Dance: The Story of American Vernacular Dance*

From the 1840s through the 1890s, minstrel shows—wherein white men in blackface portrayed caricatures of black Americans and of African American song and dance styles—were the most widespread form of American entertainment. Although the exploitation of African American performance styles for American theatrical entertainment gained tremendous momentum in the early 1800s, it actually had started decades earlier on both English and American stages.

The earliest specific reference to a black dance appeared in the *New York Journal*, which described "Mr. Tea, a 'Negro Dance, in Character,' in a stage entertainment on 14 April 1767."[1] The theatrical portrayal of blacks in the nineteenth century shifted from tragic or pitiful to comic, and they were ridiculed primarily through two caricatured impersonations: the plantation slave (Jim Crow) and the city dandy (Zip Coon). Many blackface minstrels helped start and promote this shift in emphasis, but the presentations of Thomas Dartmouth Rice had the greatest initial impact in America.

After copying the dancing and singing of a black deformed stable hand, Rice appropriated the song and dance intact, clothes and all, and put it on the stage. According to Marshall Stearns and Jean Stearns, "the dance, not the melody, made Jump Jim Crow a national craze. The first of many Afro-American dances to become a worldwide success, Jump Jim Crow's appeal was universal—the fascination of rhythmic tensions set up and neatly resolved." Rice immediately proceeded to accumulate a fortune performing his "Jim Crow" song to enthusiastic audiences in the United States and Europe. Others followed suit, and in 1843 four white men, Dan Emmett, Frank Bower, William Whitlock, and Dick Pelham, formed the first full-fledged white minstrel company, the Virginia Minstrels.[2]

Soon hundreds of blackface minstrel performers were appropriating African American art forms and successfully crisscrossing the Atlantic to showcase their stolen goods. While early minstrelsy did involve some blendings of white and black dances, the arena in which early minstrelsy showed the strongest debt to African Americans was dance. "The normal direction of the adaption," reports Robert Toll, "was from blacks to blackface, and the 'borrowers' were white men who consciously learned from blacks."[3]

As a young man, E. P. Christy, leader of the well-known Christy Minstrels, was greatly influenced by blacks in the South. His supervision of a ropewalk staffed by slaves in New Orleans in 1827 provided significant exposure to African American songs. During that period he also visited Congo Square on a regular basis. By the late 1830s, Christy had settled in Buffalo, New York, where he performed in blackface and continued to appropriate black material. One-legged Harrison, a black church singer, was one of his primary sources. Dan Emmett of the Virginia Minstrels also had extensive exposure to black material. Emmett served as a fifer in Kentucky and on Mississippi riverboats. He also played with Thomas Dartmouth Rice and traveled through the West with a circus company, which usually included at least one black dancer.[4]

Two very early New Orleans sources of minstrel material for white impersonators were Old Corn Meal, a singing street vendor who first appeared on the stage of the St. Charles Theater in 1837, and John "Picayune" Butler, a black banjoist. Thomas Dartmouth Rice went to New Orleans in 1835, 1836, and 1838; during his second season, Rice's act included a skit called "Corn Meal." Butler, a native of the West Indies, emigrated to New Orleans in the 1820s and is celebrated in an 1850 minstrel song, "Picayune Butler's Come to Town." The white minstrel performer and clown George Nichols got ideas and songs for his act from both of these black men.[5]

By the middle of the nineteenth century, minstrelsy's basic structure was in place and dancing was prominently featured in each section. The first part began with the entire company seated in a semicircle, an interlocutor in the middle, and two comedians, Mr. Tambo and Mr. Bones, on the ends. Between songs and dances, the interlocutor engaged in banter with the tambourine and bones players. A group song-and-dance routine closed the act. The second part, called the olio, consisted also of song-and-dance acts along with acrobats, a stump speaker, and various other novelties. Part three showcased a one-act skit that included individual dances and songs and ended in a lively group rendition of a song and dance.[6]

Hans Nathan, author of *Dan Emmett and the Rise of Early Negro Minstrelsy,* describes the "vigorous leg and footwork," "expressive arms and hands," and "sliding steps" of the blackface minstrels: "The body of the dancer was always bent and twisted and his legs were wide apart. In the early fifties we find a variant of this gesture: with the pelvis drawn in and the torso leaning forward precariously, the dancer added to the eccentricity of his act by stiffening his right leg and extending his left arm with a beckoning gesture of his hand which corresponded to the naughty one of his partner." Important steps included cutting the "long J bow," "walking jawbone," "double shuffle," "Grape Vine twist," "Grand Congo Dance," "Five Miles out of Town," "Louisiana toe-and-heel," "Virginny Breakdown," and "Long Island Juba."[7]

For the most part, white men dominated the stage during this period of classical minstrelsy. The most important exception to this rule was William Henry Lane, born free in about 1825. Marian Hannah Winter describes Lane as the "most influential single performer of nineteenth-century American dance" and "a prodigy of our entire theater history." Lane, known as Master Juba, honed his skills as a champion jig dancer in the "academy of the vernacular." His mentor, "Uncle" Jim Lowe, was an exceptional black jig and reel dancer who was well known in dance halls, saloons, and other venues outside the conventional theater. As a teenager, Lane engaged in contests against the top minstrel dancers of the day and by 1845 was acclaimed "beyond question the very greatest of all dancers." Charles Dickens claimed to have witnessed a performance by Juba in a dance hall of New York's Five Points district: "Single shuffle, double shuffle, cut and cross-cut; snapping his fingers, rolling his eyes, turning in his knees, presenting the backs of his legs in front, spinning about on his toes and heels like nothing but the man's fingers on the tambourine; dancing with two left legs, two right legs, two wooden legs, two wire legs, two spring legs,—all sorts of legs and no legs—what is this to him?"[8]

When Master Juba toured New England with the Georgia Champion Minstrels, his billing read: "The Wonder of the World Juba, Acknowledged to be the Greatest Dancer in the World. . . . No conception can be formed of the variety of beautiful and intricate steps exhibited by him with ease. You must see to believe." Similar accolades, expressed not by promoters but by critics, awaited him in England when he arrived there in 1848 to appear with Pell's Ethiopian Serenaders. One London critic marveled that there had never been displayed such "mobility of muscles, such flexibility of joints, such boundings, such slidings, such gyrations, such toes and heelings, such backwardings and forwardings, such posturings, such firmness of foot, such elasticity of tendon, such mutation of movement, such vigor, such variety, such natural grace, such powers of endurance, such potency of pastern." An anonymous clipping commented on Master Juba's rhythmical skills: "The manner in which he beats time with his feet, and the extraordinary command he possesses over them, can only be believed by those who have been present at his exhibition."[9]

Lane ingeniously combined the Irish jig and reel with African-derived movements and rhythms to lay the foundation for what we know as American tap dance. Every tap dancer after Juba is in some sense a student of the William Henry Lane School. The ability of twentieth-century rhythm tap dancers to play the floor with their feet reaches back to Lane's ability to use his body as a musical instrument. Referring to tap dance, Winter tells us that Master Juba was "an initiator and determinant of the form itself."[10]

No permanent African American minstrel companies were established until after the Civil War. But black minstrel troupes were touring as early as 1855, and by the 1870s, black minstrelsy had established a place on the American stage. Advertising themselves as "real," "genuine," or "bonafide Negroes," hundreds of freed slaves saw minstrelsy as a possible escape from poverty as well as an opportunity to cultivate and nurture their artistic talents. "Father of the Blues" W. C. Handy, vaudevillian Tom Fletcher, musical comedy and ragtime composer Ernest Hogan, Gertrude "Ma" Rainey, Bert Williams, and Bessie Smith—along with many, many others—began their careers as minstrel performers. During the 1880s and 1890s, the three largest black owned and managed companies were the Hicks and Sawyer Minstrels, the McCabe and Young Minstrels, and the Richards and Pringle Minstrels. The unrelenting efforts of such black company owners as Charles Hicks and Lew Johnson helped to construct models of African American entrepreneurship in the theatrical world.[11]

Although the format for American minstrelsy already was set when African Americans themselves went on stage as minstrels, they brought with them a new vivacity, cleaner and more genuine humor, and expertise on numerous musical instruments. James Weldon Johnson comments on modifications made by black minstrel performers: "These performers could not help bringing to professional minstrelsy something fresh and original. They brought a great deal that was new in dancing, by exhibiting in their perfection the jig, the buck and wing, and the tantalizing stop-time dances."[12] In her discussion of black minstrel performers, Winter cites additional characteristics of black performance style on the minstrel stage: "rhythmic treatment of this material," "the intangibles of performance," and "a phenomenal virtuosity in 'trick' dances."[13]

Billy Kersands, black minstrelsy's most famous comedian and an excellent dancer, was noted for his perfect execution of the Virginia essence. This was minstrelsy's most famous dance and probably the first popular professional dance drawn from the African American vernacular. The ragtime composer Arthur Marshall offers a description: "If a guy could really do it, he sometimes looked as if he was being towed around on ice skates. . . . The performer moves forward without appearing to move his feet at all, by manipulating his toes and heels rapidly, so that his body is propelled without changing the position of his legs." Eventually the essence became the soft shoe. When taps were added, the result was referred to as "picture dancing."[14]

The Bohee Brothers, James and George, were excellent soft-shoe dancers and the first polished public performers on the banjo. They were among the first singing and dancing musicians. Their specialty was playing the banjo while singing and performing a soft shoe in the calcium light. "William Allen's *Pedestal Clog* was danced on a surface fifteen inches square and four feet high; [in minstrel shows] stunt dancing on a peck measure or a square of glass one inch thick was commonplace." The cakewalk became an important part of minstrelsy and was initially performed by men before women appeared on the minstrel stage. Dressed in wigs, makeup, and dresses, men played the women's roles for their male walking partners. Winter reports that the cakewalk was made a part of the walkaround in minstrelsy's final days, adding "an authentic American note at a period when imported operetta and extravaganza were eclipsing most of our indigenous theatrical forms."[15]

Black minstrelsy included numerous song-and-dance artists. Tom Fletcher offers an explanation for the existence of so many versatile performers: "Back in those days you were not hired or even considered in show business unless you could sing, dance, talk, tumble, or play some instrument in a brass band." Among the two hundred performers at a Cincinnati minstrel festival in 1883 were twenty banjo players, sixteen vocalists, and twenty song-and-dance artists. Black minstrels composed songs or had special ones written for them. The songs "belonged" to the minstrels who introduced them publicly; likewise, specialty dances were associated with the individual performers who created or introduced them.[16]

Black minstrel performers carried their dances, songs, and jokes to Ireland, Canada, Scotland, Germany, Java, Australia, New Zealand, England, Asia, and to towns and cities throughout the United States. Billy Kersands taught dancing in royal circles, and the Bohee Brothers gave banjo lessons to the Duke of Windsor, the Prince of Wales, and King George V of England. Black minstrels gave numerous command performances for European royalty.[17]

An 1894 advertisement offering jobs to forty black minstrels brought two thousand interested performers to a New York office. Minstrelsy provided essential stage training for African American men and women who had virtually no other access to theatrical experience. In spite of minstrelsy's cruelly stereotyped caricatures, African American artists made America aware of the diverse talents of black people. In so doing these performers subtly modified the standard plantation images of blacks as inept, without culture, and "happy." Indeed, through the use of direct protest material in their songs, they provided an undercurrent of independence and anger. The theater historian Thomas Riis sheds some light on this phenomenon: "Afro-American tricksters, used to wearing the mask for white slave owners, could show the white minstrel audiences what they wanted them to see. . . . The roles played and the masks worn in minstrelsy were shared superficially by both black and white entertainers, but they were used for quite different purposes." Riis notes that "the professional and plastic transformation by black performers" and the attraction of orally based stage performance help explain the success of black troupes with African American audiences. No doubt part of the appeal, too, lay in this use of the minstrel mask as a cover for the expression of dissatisfaction and anger.[18] Furthermore, black minstrelsy opened new opportunities to black performers and provided a new set of cultural heroes to the black populace in general. Everybody knew, for example, that songwriter James Bland, comedians Billy Kersands and Tom McIntosh, and banjoists Horace Weston, James Bohee, and George Bohee were internationally famous.[19]

Black minstrel performers, male and female, retained much authenticity in their presentations of black religious music; they also included in their programs such genuine black vernacular elements as symbolic animal characters. Furthermore, thanks to the tremendous impact of William Henry Lane, "the minstrel-show dance retained more integrity as a Negro art form than any other theatrical derivative of Negro culture."[20] And African American minstrel women and men of the nineteenth and twentieth centuries not only helped "retain" aspects of black American dance; they actually added to the rich bedrock of black vernacular dance from which they had drawn to give power to their stage shows. In the circling patterns of American cultural influences, black social dance of the twentieth century drew heavily on the dances of black minstrelsy, which in their turn drew freely from the social dances that the slaves had done with rags in the cabin cracks to keep out the sun.

By the 1890s, the popularity of American minstrelsy was beginning to decline and the genre eventually splintered into revues, operettas, vaudeville, burlesques, and farces. The minstrel roots of these forms had a great impact on their evolution. Around the turn of the century, artists readily switched back and forth between various performance venues. Minstrels traveled with musical comedy companies and road shows while actors and singers toured with minstrel companies. Black minstrel shows continued to be a significant performance arena for African American artists, but as other avenues opened, the largest companies dwindled. Nonetheless, small nondescript shows continued as late as the 1940s.[21] Twentieth-century black minstrel shows were greatly influenced by the nineteenth-century formats; but minstrelsy was not a static institution, and African Americans increasingly brought their flavor to these stage presentations.

Traveling Shows

The nineteenth century in America was an age of touring performers. Variety, or the "performance of brief entertainment acts," had been present in American theater from its inception. Through the 1840s, a typical evening at the theater could last three hours and feature a conglomeration of theatrical fare, including Shakespearean plays, magic acts, minstrelsy, acrobatics, dancing, music, and singing. "Popular" culture was eclectic and played simultaneously to all classes. According to Lawrence Levine, nineteenth-century Americans "shared a public culture less hierarchically organized, less fragmented into relatively rigid adjectival boxes than their descendents were to experience a century later."[22]

During the decades when minstrel shows were touring the United States, other important performance vehicles were becoming institutionalized, including the circus, freak shows, burlesque, vaudeville, Wild West shows, and carnivals. Although some of these forms did not originate in the United States, they took on a uniquely American character as they evolved in the towns and cities across this nation.[23]

The numerous traveling shows of the late nineteenth century became training grounds for the cultivation of black artistic talent. Dancers, singers, and musicians shared the spotlight, maintaining the close relationship between instrumental music, song, and dance that was at the core of African American culture. Road shows, tent shows, minstrel shows, circuses, medicine shows, carnivals, and gillies featured a wide cross-section of black performance styles and provided arenas in which dancers, comedians, blues singers, acrobats, instrumentalists, and many others could rub elbows. These theatrical venues were extraordinarily conducive to creative freedom and experimentation. Emerging and established performers could try out new ideas and advance the evolution of their particular art forms. Many of these "academies" lasted through the first half of the twentieth century and allowed for the widespread dissemination of classic American indigenous dances.

James Weldon Johnson reports that African Americans made significant progress on the theatrical stage between 1875 and 1900. Although black artists were limited by the trappings of blackface minstrelsy, "many black or black-derived stage shows of the nineteenth century featured dance—especially vigorous and inventive dance." The performance settings for these presentations served as springboards for the many exciting stage versions of black vernacular dance that dazzled audiences in the United States and abroad during the twenties, thirties, and forties.[24]

In the late 1800s, black concert companies actively toured the country and offered an alternative to the images of the minstrel stage. Among these groups was the Hyers Sisters Concert Company. Anna Madah Hyers and Emma Louise Hyers first performed in 1867 at the Metropolitan Theater in Sacramento, California. In 1869 a Boston reviewer wrote: "We were invited with some fifty other persons this forenoon to hear the singing of two colored young ladies, named Anna and Emma Hyers. . . . They are aged respectively sixteen and fourteen years, and, after a casual inspection, may be called musical prodigies. They are, without doubt, destined to occupy a high position in the musical world." By 1871, they were successfully touring western and northern states under the management of their

father, Sam Hyers. The Hyers troupe changed its format in 1876, establishing the first black repertory company. Their themes grew out of black
American life and their original dramas featured plantation songs, operatic presentations, ballads, comedy, and authentic African American dances. It is very important to note that these shows were the forerunners of
the black musicals that surfaced in the 1890s.[25]

During the last quarter of the nineteenth century, white road shows
generally did not open their stages to black actors and actresses, but some
did feature black dancers and choral groups. Nine months after the publication of Harriet Beecher Stowe's novel *Uncle Tom's Cabin* in March
1852, several dramatic versions of the novel were being performed in the
United States and Europe; but not until the 1870s did theatrical companies begin hiring African Americans for reenactments of the book's plantation scenes. Once that venue was available to black performers, it became an increasingly important one, offering employment and early
training to such stars as Ernest Hogan, who helped lay the foundation for
the groundbreaking black musicals of the twenties.[26]

As the vaudevillian Tom Fletcher observed, "*Uncle Tom's Cabin* show
companies all carried lots of dancers with them. The Buck-and-Wing, the
Virginia Essence, and the Knockabout Song and Dance were the big routines then." By the 1890s, some of the largest *Uncle Tom's Cabin* companies featured singers, dancers, and several instrumental groups along with
show wagons, floats, military drill demonstrations, and animal acts. Eventually, *Uncle Tom's Cabin* shows—demonstrating virtually no interest at
all in the antislavery message of Stowe's novel (except perhaps the will to
counterstate it)—presented the public with virtually the same point of view
and images as those of the minstrel shows of the nineteenth century.[27]

One of the first black road shows to appear in major music halls and to
eliminate blackface makeup was *The Creole Show*, developed in 1890 by
Sam Lucas, a black actor, and Sam T. Jack, a white manager. This show
was structured according to the standard minstrel format, but women replaced men in the front semicircle and Florence Hines, a male imperson-
ator, served as the interlocutor (the orchestra and endmen were males).
The show's use of a sixteen-woman chorus was another innovation for a
minstrel troupe. As in all large black shows of the late 1800s, cakewalks
were featured. The tremendously influential cakewalkers Dora Dean and
Charles Johnson met while performing with *The Creole Show*.[28]

In Old Kentucky premiered in St. Paul, Minnesota, in 1892 and from
its inception had black dancers and singers in its cast. The importance of

this show to African Americans was its regular Friday night dance contest, open to anyone courageous enough to accept the challenge. Willie Covan, at age sixteen, was practicing vigorously in Chicago and eagerly anticipating his chance at stardom when *In Old Kentucky* arrived there in 1915: "I came jumping out with a Wing, a Grab Off, and a Roll and managed to get in a lot of new stuff before my time ran out." With his prize in hand, Covan was carried out on the shoulders of his fans and on the way to becoming a legend in American tap dance. Bill "Bojangles" Robinson also won a Brooklyn dance contest sponsored by this show.[29]

South before the War (1893) played in burlesque houses for several seasons. This predominantly black show featured plantation, levee, and camp-meeting scenes and a huge cakewalk. "Players often used the production as a showcase for introducing new songs and dances to the public, as in 1895, for example, when Billy Williams introduced the 'possum-ma-la dance.'" *South before the War* featured several great dancers. Among them was Katie Carter, dubbed "queen of the female *buck and wing* dancers." Her performances helped establish buck and wing dancing as a major attraction in black shows.[30]

According to Tom Fletcher, the original idea for *South before the War* was conceived by Billy McClain, a minstrel performer born free around 1866 and referred to by one reporter as the Frederick Douglass of the theatrical world. McClain toured with minstrel troupes and the Sells Brothers and Forepaugh's Circus in the 1880s and was instrumental in creating jobs for thousands of African American artists. He succeeded in securing financial backing for *Black America*, a summer outdoors extravaganza that employed more than five hundred performers when it premiered in 1895. Among them were Charles Johnson of the famous cakewalking team Johnson and Dean, musician May Bohee, comedian Billy Farrell, dancer Katie Carter, sixty-three vocal quartets, and a drill team of men who had served with the United States Ninth Cavalry. A *New York Times* reviewer proclaimed the dances "peculiar in their attractiveness. The efforts that the white man has made to reproduce them will be seen to be but a faint imitation of what they really are. The naturalness and spontaneity of action on the part of the negroes will be at once recognized and appreciated. Their dances beggar description, and must be seen to be appreciated." The actual performance was presented in a large amphitheater and consisted of three parts: dance and song recreations of African episodes, American dances and songs in the African American and European traditions, and a grand cakewalk contest for the finale. With this show, black Americans made white managers aware of the vast numbers of talented black performers seeking work in the theater.[31]

Following the example set by Sam T. Jack in 1890, another white manager, John W. Isham, also realized that substantial money could be made sponsoring African American casts. In 1895, he produced *The Octoroons*, a musical farce. Dances were prominently displayed in Isham's new format, which also included a playlet, songs, and specialty acts. *The Octoroons* ended with "a cakewalk jubilee, a military drill, and a 'chorus-march-finale.'" Another Isham production, *Oriental America* (1896), was the first black show to play on Broadway and presented some of the best formally trained black singers available, including J. Rosamond Johnson, then a music student in New York City. Songs, dances, and specialty acts linked the main storyline that preceded the finale. One innovation was the replacement of the typical military drill–cakewalk ending with operatic selections.[32]

The star of Black Patti's Troubadours, an all-black touring company, was Matilda Sissieretta Joyner Jones, one of the most accomplished concert artists of the nineteenth century. While touring as a solo singer, a newspaper critic called her "Black Patti," an allusion to the Italian soprano Adelina Patti. Her distinguished career included an engagement with Patrick Gilmore's Band at the Pittsburgh Exposition of 1893, an extensive European tour, and an appearance at the White House. When Jones returned to America in 1896, she began touring with Black Patti's Troubadours, managed by the white producers Rudolf Voelckel and James Nolan. A typical Troubadours show had three parts: a buck dancing contest ended part one, a cakewalk ended part two, and the final section presented songs and operatic selections by Black Patti and the chorus. Ida Forsyne recalls her days with the company: "We had a cakewalking contest every performance, and my partner and I won it seven nights straight in a row. We added legomania and tumbling in the breaks."[33] This legendary all-black show lasted approximately twenty years and at varying points featured such stellar artists as Bob Cole, who also wrote some of the shows, comedian Tom McIntosh, buck dancer King Rastus Brown, and singer and dancer Stella Wiley.[34]

Although several all-black traveling shows formed after 1900 and became significant incubators for vernacular dance, the greatest developer of dancing talent by any stretch of the imagination was the Whitman Sisters Troupe (1900–1943). Hundreds of dancers got their first break with this company. The Whitman Sisters "featured dancers *as dancers*—a hint of what was to come on Broadway—and sold the show to the public largely on the strength of this dancing."[35]

Essie, Mabel, Alberta, and Alice Whitman were the daughters of a Methodist bishop who taught them the double shuffle when they were young girls. Their early apprenticeship in church socials and benefits led to the formation of a singing act comprised of the two eldest sisters, Essie and Mabel. By 1911, the four sisters headed an established road show with Alberta performing flash dancing and her little sister Alice "billed as 'The Queen of Taps.'" Tap dancer Jeni LeGon describes the dancing skills of Alice Whitman: "She was the best there was. She was tops. She was better than Ann Miller and Eleanor Powell and me and anybody else you wanted to put her to. Oh, she was just an excellent dancer. I mean she did it all. She could do all the ballet-style stuff like Eleanor. And then she could hoof! But she never went out on her own, you know, she stayed with the sisters."[36] Alice Whitman's son, Pops Whitman, "developed into one of the first great acrobatic tap dancers, a master of cartwheels, spins, flips, and splits—swinging with the rhythm." The internationally famous Pops Whitman toured with several big bands of the thirties. Count Basie first saw Catherine Morgan, the woman who would become his second wife and a dancer with the Three Snakehips Queens, while playing for the Whitman Sisters. Basie thought "that was really the big time. The Whitman Sisters had a show that was second to none in show business. They had a top company for years. . . . Alice was the baby sister, and she was one of the greatest tap dancers around."[37]

The Whitman Sisters' shows typically featured dancing comedians, a chorus line, female singers, a few excellent dancers, and a small jazz band. The comedian Pigmeat Markham felt the impact and popularity of this group: "They was like the Bible to Negro audiences—people saved up their money for a whole year to hear them when their show came to town.[38]

In 1902 the Smart Set was organized by Billy McClain, Ernest Hogan, and Gus Hill, a white producer. Built on successive scenes, its show was structured like a musical comedy rather than a variety show and featured the singer Marian Smart. But the star was always a dancer-comedian. Tom McIntosh, Sherman H. Dudley, and Ernest Hogan were among the most famous of these Smart Set comedians who danced.

Wednesday night buck and wing contests were held from New Jersey to Georgia and points further south, where the company traveled during winter months. In this context it is quite notable that the only black Mardi Gras marching club in New Orleans, the Zulu Social Aid and Pleasure

Club, was developed after a Smart Set appearance there in 1909: "Early in 1909, a group of laborers, who had organized a club named 'The Tramps,' went to the Pythian Temple Theater to see a musical comedy performed by [the] Smart Set. The comedy included, 'There Never Was and Never Will Be A King Like Me,' a skit about the Zulu Tribe. . . . As soon as the Tramps saw the skit, they put their heads together in a wood-shed on Perdido Street and emerged as the Zulus."[39]

That same year J. Homer Tutt and Salem Tutt Whitney organized the Smarter Set, also known as the Southern Smart Set. Soon this company merged with the original Smart Set, forming a collaboration that lasted until 1923. Tutt and Whitney were talented songwriters and successful performers who wrote many musicals for the company. Other writers included James Reese Europe, Luckey Roberts, James Vaughn, Will Vodery, and Henry Creamer.[40]

The Rabbit Foot Minstrels (1900–1950s), popularly known as "the Foots," was organized by Pat Chappelle, a former minstrel performer, and toured primarily in the South. The company employed comedians, blues singers, novelty acts, jugglers, and vaudeville teams. When Ma Rainey and her band toured with "the Foots," she performed, in addition to the blues, dancing, comedy, novelty, topical songs, and popular songs.[41]

Silas Green from New Orleans (1907–58) toured exclusively in the South and was owned, managed, and controlled by African Americans. Its founder, Professor Eph Williams, was reputedly the only black American circus owner during the 1890s. The comic story of Silas Green was interspersed with blues singers, several chorus line numbers, and specialty acts that presented a broad range of versatile talents. "The band played ragtime, jazz, and swing tunes composed by southern and northern blacks, heralding and disseminating the music of its people throughout the South." Some of America's most outstanding artists performed with this company, including Ma Rainey, Bessie Smith, Butterbeans and Susie (Jody Edwards and Susie Edwards), and Nipsey Russell.[42]

Such tent show companies as the Rabbit Foot Minstrels and Silas Green from New Orleans took vaudeville to the South. While road shows appeared in northern and southern theaters, tent show performers worked under canvas mainly in the Midwest and the South. Small-town and rural audiences crowded into tents to see dramatic performances interspersed with popular singers, dancers, black blues singers, novelty bands, and a range of specialty acts. "Almost 400 tent-show companies traveled the nation in 1925 . . . visiting 16,000 communities and entertaining 76,800,000 people."[43]

Many African American performers of the early twentieth century had to engage in a kind of leapfrogging from show to show in order to stay employed, increase their salaries, and move up the theatrical ladder. The experiences of Pigmeat Markham in the twenties is typical of the kind of mobility that allowed for a tremendous amount of cross-fertilization and sharing of artistic ideas: "I jumped around from Gonzelle White's Minstrels to the Florida Blossoms, Silas Green's Minstrels, A. G. Allen's Mighty Minstrels, Huntington's Minstrels, and back to the Florida Blossoms . . . and I saw dancers who were so good you wouldn't believe it."[44]

In addition to road shows and minstrels, African American dancers gained experience in circuses, medicine shows, carnivals, and gillies. These touring enterprises "provided the seeds on a grass-roots level for the growth of a professional style of dancing."[45]

Circuses first appeared in America during the late 1700s. Primarily city shows, they were initially more accessible to northerners, though some shows traveled to the South as well. By the 1890s, the arrival of the circus was a major event in southern towns. During those years, approximately forty groups toured annually between April and December. Loyal followers came into towns early to enjoy the parades and the opening ceremonies; major cities hosted thousands of visitors arriving on excursion trains. North and South, the appeal was universal.

From 1870 to 1920 was the golden age of American circuses. The country's leading circus entrepreneurs, the Ringling Brothers, P. T. Barnum, W. C. Coup, and George F. Bailey, added multiple rings, making shows much more elaborate. According to the cultural historian Robert Bogdan, the freak show was already an integral component of the circus when tent size and sideshow attractions increased around 1890. "Bands with black musicians, blackface minstrel bands, and troupes of dancers dressed as Hawaiians were used to attract crowds and provide a festive atmosphere inside the freak show tent."[46]

Black vaudeville acts were introduced as side shows in 1899, when Perry G. Lowery presented his group with the Sells Brothers and Forepaugh's Circus at Madison Square Garden in New York City. Prior to that time, circuses had hired blacks primarily as musicians.[47] Tom Fletcher saw Wilbur Sweatman—who later became an important jazz clarinetist—as he performed with a circus band in the early 1900s:

> I met Wilbur Sweatman when he came to New York in the early 1900s to join the Sells Brothers and Forepaugh's Circus as a member of Pro-

fessor P.G. Lowery's Band. P.G. was one of the great colored cornet soloists and band leaders. . . . In the summer seasons, his band and orchestra played for the different acts and freaks in the side show, plus the colored minstrel and cakewalk company. In those days, when the circuses played at old *Madison Square Garden* there would be a street parade the night before the opening, with bands, animals, actors, clowns, everything except the freaks. The colored band made the parade in New York and the season Sweatman was with the bands the crowds that lined the sidewalks started following the band just to hear Sweatman playing his clarinet. Everybody was saying they had never heard anybody play the instrument like that before. Sweatman was the sensation of the parade.[48]

The clarinetist Garvin Bushell, who also later became a jazzman, played for dancers in a circus band during the summer of 1916:

This was a three-ring circus, but our band only performed in the sideshow. . . . Each attraction had its own platform. . . . The last attraction was the black band—it was minstrel entertainment, more or less. We had two or three girl dancers, a male dancer, and a blackface comedian. . . . The emcee would announce, "Straight from New Orleans, the Cotton Town Minstrels," and the chorus girls would come out and do gags, dance, and sing. We had about twenty or twenty-five minutes for our act. We'd go on four times a day. The parade was usually around ten in the morning, then we'd do an afternoon show at two that lasted 'til about 4:30. In the evening we'd play in the sideshow before and after the big top performance.[49]

According to the jazz clarinetist Buster Bailey, "fellows that played the circus were the top musicians of the day and, during the off season, a lot of them would play in the local bands like those led by Handy, George Bynum, Stewart, et cetera."[50]

Nettie Compton worked for the Ponsell Brothers Circus as a singer and dancer in 1902. Dressed in "fancy frocks," the women danced the cakewalk with their male partners, who wore top hats and carried canes: "I can still see it—the girls kind of flirted, and the boys strutted and pranced. You used a lot of strut in the Cakewalk—lots of fellows walked like that just for notoriety—and they could really show off. The girl would stop and applaud her partner, while he made up four steps of his own, sometimes regular tap steps, and then he'd end it, maybe with a somersault. We had some nice dancers and a good band."[51]

Medicine shows toured the United States and Canada from approximately 1870 to 1930 and provided jobs for large numbers of black dancers, singers, and musicians. The companies usually ranged in size from two to forty performers and revolved around the sale of cheap, ineffective patent medicines. Small operations consisted of a "pitchman," or "Doctor," and one or two assistants whose performances were designed to attract large crowds so that the pitchman could hawk the goods. Although some of the largest medicine shows traveled by rail, most journeyed by wagon before 1900, when trucks came into use. The operator of a large medicine show was in some sense a theatrical producer who put together packages that were interrupted periodically for sales pitches. A third of the show was reserved for demonstrations, lectures, and sales.

The New Orleans black song and dance team called Pork Chops and Kidney Stew traveled with one of the larger troupes promoting a miracle tonic called Hadacol. They appeared in the first part of the show, which also included an acrobatic act, a harmonica player, a comic act, Sharkey Bonano's Dixieland Band playing "The Hadacol Boogie," a female tumbler, and a danced version of the "Darktown Strutters' Ball" featuring backbends and other exuberant movements to show what was possible after a dose of Hadacol.[52]

Many famous performers got their start with medicine shows. When George Walker of the legendary Williams and Walker Company decided to start an act of his own, he found work with quack doctors who discovered that Walker's ability to dance and sing, rattle bones, and beat the tambourine drew large crowds of eager customers for the patent medicine. Ulysses "Slow Kid" Thompson began performing as a dancer with a small medicine show at the age of fourteen or fifteen: "We had a canvas tent in back where we dressed and a small platform out front where we danced— any step was okay—clapping our hands for accompaniment. Then the doctor went into his sales talk." Stearns and Stearns describe medicine show dancing as "a crazy-quilt blend of [movements] such as shuffles, struts, hops, twists, and grinds, with a touch of the flat-footed Buck. . . . The emphasis was on eccentric dancing, that is, highly individual and inventive movements following no set pattern, but rather exploring new ways of capturing attention."[53]

Musicians in training were equally well served by their experiences with medicine shows. Eubie Blake performed briefly in 1901 as a buck dancer, musician, and singer on the portable wagon stage of Dr. Frazier's Medicine Show. The careers of bluesmen Sonny Terry, Blind Willie McTell, and T-Bone Walker included performances with medicine shows.

Walker gained valuable experience in this arena: "Dr. Breeding . . . hired me and another boy, Josephus Cook, to ballyhoo for him. . . . I'd play and feed jokes to Seph, and he'd start in to dance. I'd pick up from there, and we built on our breaks. Then we'd stack up the bottles and Doc would come on."[54] Walter Fuller, born in 1910, was a featured trumpeter with the Earl Hines Band during the thirties. But before then his summers with a medicine show band proved invaluable to his early development: "Every year after school, I would travel with Dr. Stoll's Medicine Show through the states up as far as the coal region in Pennsylvania. I was twelve when that started, and a fellow from my hometown, a tuba player named Benny Stratton, was like my guardian and tutor. They had a very, very fine band, and they would carry me out to what they called the 'woodshed' and teach me, and make me study an hour each day. That went on all through the summer for three years." Buster Smith, who played with the Blue Devils and later with the bands of Bennie Moten and Count Basie, explains the pre-jazz influence of medicine show musicians in Texas:

> I'll tell you, a lot of it started around here on these medicine shows. We used to have them all over town here. . . . A medicine show used to have four or five pieces: trombone, clarinet, trumpet, and a drummer, every man blowing for himself as loud as he could blow to attract a crowd for the "doctor." Then there would be a couple of comedians clowning a little bit, then the doc would have the boys blow again to attract another crowd after he'd sold the first crowd. He'd sell them this patent medicine—good for anything—at a dollar or a dollar-fifty a bottle and the comedians would go through the crowd selling it. Then the boys would get up and blow again to attract another bunch of suckers. That's how that jazz started down in these parts.[55]

Around the 1890s and the first decade of the twentieth century, while medicine shows were flourishing, the American carnival provided even more forms of entertainment. The beginnings of the carnival date back to the 1893 World's Columbian Exposition, a Chicago-based exhibition that included fun houses, outdoor rides, and games of chance. Between World Wars I and II, carnivals thrived in the United States. Large elaborate shows traveled to cities while smaller places hosted limited operations that featured shooting arcades, porn shows, fortune tellers, mechanized rides such as roller coasters and Ferris wheels, freak shows, and a midway, which offered cotton candy, popcorn, and other food.[56]

Miniature carnivals were called gillies, the name given to specially equipped trucks that were used for traveling from town to town. A gilly normally consisted of two or three rides, a few tent attractions, and several games of chance. For dancers, movement from a medicine show to a gilly or a carnival allowed for more range, scope, and opportunities to portray characters and choreograph roles. It also meant more stability, better salaries, and a chance to perform and build a reputation before consistently large audiences in the "Jig Top," the tent where African American shows were held. Gilly shows usually included a chorus line of three or four women, a musician, a straight man, and the featured dancer, who was also a comedian. Carnivals had much larger Jig Top casts. By the 1930s some presentations resembled cabaret shows or revues. One such show, *Harlem in Havana*, was operated by the black producer Leon Claxton as part of the Royal American Shows. It lasted over thirty years.[57]

Throughout the country, many famous jazz musicians served apprenticeships in the sideshows of carnivals. Lester Young played in his father's carnival band. Sidney Bechet "paid dues" on the clarinet in carnival bands, and Jo Jones not only drummed but also danced, played the piano, and sang in carnivals:

> At that time, when musicians were advertised for they had to do more than just play. You might have to be a dancer or a straight man. . . . Many jazzmen came up from or through the carnivals. There were good musicians too in the Ringling Brothers band. P.G. Lowery was the band leader and a lot of good musicians would join his band to make the season. In the carnivals you had some great drummers. There was Snag Jones, for example, out of Chicago. The carnival drummers were flashy but they also could play. Then a lot of men came up through the minstrel shows like the Riverboat Minstrels, and a lot also came up through traveling rodeo shows like The One-O-One Ranch.[58]

The impact of touring shows on the evolution of American dance in the twentieth century has been extraordinary. Pigmeat Markham explained the significance of these shows to the training of black dancers:

> In the old days, show business for a colored dancer was like going through school. You started in a medicine show—that was kindergarten—where they could use a few steps if you could cut them, but almost anything would do. Then you went on up to the gilly show, which was like grade school—they wanted dancers. If you had something on the ball, you graduated to a carnival—that was high school—and you sure had to be able to dance. College level was a colored minstrel show, and as they faded out, a vaudeville circuit or even a Broadway show.[59]

Such stellar dancers as Peg Leg Bates, Leonard Reed, and Willie Covan moved through these venues to vaudeville circuits and beyond. In these settings, black dancers, many of them great or on their way to greatness, learned and perfected their craft. Using the tricks of improvisation and propulsive rhythm, these sideshow dancers worked their magic to create new blendings of shuffles, grinds, twists, spins, and struts and found new ways of making the body move. These early stylists would become the shining standard bearers for amateur and professional dancing in the twenties and thirties—as, increasingly, American choreography came into its own.[60]

Chapter Five

Dancing Singers and Singing Dancers: Black Vernacular Dance on Stage, 1890–1940

> Motion pictures of African choruses accompanying their soloists show
> that even handclapping can become a dance, while in the New World
> this tendency to "dance the song," whether it is religious or secular, is
> a commonplace.
> —Melville J. Herskovits, *The Myth of the Negro Past*

Many touring shows began and ended in New York around 1900. With more theaters than any other American city and a solid theatrical tradition for black artists, it was a logical place to plant the seeds for the development of black musical theater.[1]

In 1897, Bob Cole and Billy Johnson left Black Patti's Troubadours to begin working on the production of *A Trip to Coontown*, "the first full-length black musical comedy actually written, performed, and managed" by African Americans. James Weldon Johnson described Cole as "the most versatile theatrical man the Negro has yet produced: a good singer and an excellent dancer, and able to play several instruments. He could write a dramatic or a musical play—dialogue, lyrics and music—stage the play and act a part. . . . He was educated and a serious student of the whole history of the theater and the drama." *A Trip to Coontown* featured several specialty acts, including the Freeman Sisters (Pauline and Clara), who were contortional dancers. The first act of the show closed with an "elaborate ballet" that included impersonations of Japanese, Arab, Spanish, Egyptian, and Chinese dancers. According to one critic, the dancing was "pretty and vivacious in a manner not specially recalling the usual ragtime steps."[2]

Three months after *A Trip to Coontown* opened, Will Marion Cook

premiered *Clorindy—The Origin of the Cakewalk* featuring veteran minstrel performer Ernest Hogan in the starring role supported by twenty-six
singers and dancers. Cook had studied violin at the Oberlin Conservatory and in Berlin. Later he returned to New York and attended the National
Conservatory of Music, where he studied composition with Antonín
Dvořák and harmony and counterpoint with John White.[3]

Clorindy set a new standard on Broadway. Never before had New York
audiences seen such power and energy on the musical stage. Pandemo-
nium followed the closing number. Cook describes the show: "The Darktown finale was of complicated rhythm and bold harmonies, and very tax-
ing on the voice. My chorus sang like Russians, dancing meanwhile like
Negroes, and cakewalking like angels, black angels! When the last note
was sounded, the audience stood and cheered for at least ten minutes."
The exuberant dancing and the introduction of "Negro syncopated music" created a model that was adapted for the white stage by George Lederer, who produced *Clorindy* at the Casino Roof Garden. James Weldon
Johnson explained that Lederer

> judged correctly that the practice of the Negro chorus, to dance stren-
> uously and sing at the same time, if adapted to the white stage would
> be a profitable novelty; so he departed considerably from the model of
> the easy, leisurely movements of the English light opera chorus. He also
> judged that some injection of Negro syncopated music would produce
> a like result. . . . Ironically, these adaptations from the Negro stage, first
> made many years ago, give many present-day critics reason for condemn-
> ing Negro musical comedy on the ground that it is too slavish an imita-
> tion of the white product.[4]

Bert Williams and George Walker formed a vaudeville act in the early
1890s. By late 1896 they were cakewalking in a forty-week run at Koster
and Bial's, Broadway's top variety theater. In addition to Williams, Walker, and their cakewalking partners, the cast included seven couples and a
blackface host who was led on stage by a baton-flourishing drum major.
After the host introduced the competing couples, Williams and Walker
strutted on stage with their partners and "everything was set up for them
to win the cake with their ludicrous burlesque of the others' eccentric
steps."[5]

At the end of the nineteenth century, the cakewalk became the rage of
Manhattan, with Williams and Walker the "dancing masters" for white
New York society. The cakewalk had a tremendous impact on American

dance in its time. Its popularity equalled that of the Charleston in the twenties and the lindy in the thirties. Cakewalk contests were held throughout the country, and Madison Square Garden became the home of the national championships. Tom Fletcher described a typical contest in *One Hundred Years of the Negro in Show Business:*

> The Madison Square Garden competition was always a sell-out. Before the contest there would be a big plantation scene with the cast of about 150 singers and dancers and some great vocal soloist of the period. After this show was over, the judges, including many of New York's prominent brokers, sportsmen and athletes, especially prize fighters, would take their places on the stage. Walter F. Craig and his orchestra of fifty pieces would be seated on the stage to provide the music.
>
> The inside of Madison Square Garden on such occasions was arranged like a race track. . . . When the contest music started, first would appear a drum major who would go through a routine with his baton then return to his place as leader. Then the curtain would part and 50 or 60 couples would come from behind the stage on to the floor, prancing and dancing to the tempo of the music. It was very reminiscent of the grand entry at a circus. The girls' dresses were of all colors. The men wore full dress, clown clothes or comedy costumes with the big checks. When all the walkers were on the floor, then the 50 or 60 couples could all be seen doing different prances and dance steps ranging from buck-and-wing to toe dancing and, in fact, practically everything known to the terpsichorean art.[6]

Cakewalking couples were judged by style, time, and execution. The winners often stayed together as vaudeville acts. According to Fletcher, participating couples were all good dancers and singers who knew the value of individual inventiveness. The cakewalk offered seemingly unlimited possibilities for dance and sometimes encompassed tap or even Russian dances; but cakewalk couples always finished with an exaggerated high-stepping strut. A strong influence on many twentieth-century steps, the cakewalk set the stage for the evolution of American social and theatrical dances that would upstage and then replace the nineteenth-century cotillions, schottisches, and waltzes. The Williams and Walker vehicle *In Dahomey* lifted the cakewalk to the status of an international dance craze after the show's smashing London run of 1903. After a month there, the cast was invited to perform at Buckingham Palace.[7]

Obviously, dance played a tremendous role in the success and appeal of the Williams and Walker Company. Both of the company leaders were excellent dancers. Bert Williams, an eccentric dancer, performed very much like southern tent-show comedians. His movement consisted of a lazy grind with rotary hip-slinging that was coupled with a shuffle or hop. George Walker was also a comedy dancer whose reputation as a strutter remains unsurpassed. Walker's wife, Ada Overton, was an accomplished artist in her own right; she was a singer and dancer who created much of the company's choreography. Fletcher saw her perform with the company: "As a dancer she could do almost anything, and no matter whether it was buck-and-wing, cakewalk, or even some form of grotesque dancing, she lent the performance a neat gracefulness of movement which was unsurpassed by anyone. Those of us who can actually remember her, are pretty well agreed that she was a Florence Mills and Josephine Baker rolled into one."[8]

The Williams and Walker Company worked with some of the best musicians and lyricists of that period. Will Marion Cook was its musical director and composer. His assistants included Alex Rogers, James Vaughn, and J. Leubrie Hill, the songwriter who later produced *Darktown Follies.* Williams and Walker starred in two more shows, *Abyssinia* (1906) and *Bandana Land* (1907). But by 1910 a severe illness had forced Walker into early retirement and Williams was performing with the Ziegfeld Follies.

At the same time that the Williams and Walker Company was presenting musicals, Bob Cole and his new partners, the brothers J. Rosamond and James Weldon Johnson, were collaborating on white musicals and writing two operettas of their own, *The Shoo-Fly Regiment* (1906) and *The Red Moon* (1908). Ernest Hogan also produced *Rufus Rastus* (1905) and *The Oyster Man* (1907). Although Hogan's dance skills were obscured by his reputation as a comedian, he was truly a magnificent dancer. He had introduced the pasmala in the early 1890s when he toured with a minstrel company, the Georgia Graduates. Eubie Blake, Flournoy Miller, and pianist Luckey Roberts all testify that Ernest Hogan was the best dancing comedian and the greatest black performer of his day. By 1912, Hogan, Bob Cole, and George Walker had died, leaving a tremendous gap in New York's black theatrical leadership.[9]

Between 1910 and 1920, black theater developed away from Broadway, allowing African American musical theater to grow without the constraints of white critics. Beginning in 1913, Harlem's Lafayette Theater offered the best opportunities for composers and playwrights to stage new musicals, and the actor J. Leubrie Hill was one of the first to do so. Assisted by the composer Will Vodery and the songwriter Alex Rogers, Hill produced *My*

Friend from Kentucky (1913), better known by the name of its company, the Darktown Follies. This was by far the most important musical of the teens. And it was a show that exploded with dances—ballin' the jack, the Texas tommy, the cakewalk, and the tango. Riis explains the importance of dance in this production: "Hill realized . . . that the novel impact of black performers lay in the special ways they could use their bodies and their voices, making the trappings of the nineteenth-century extravaganza or European operettas seem irrelevant."[10]

The show's dances and songs were performed by an outstanding cast that included the tap dancers Eddie Rector and Toots Davis, the ballroom dancers Ethel Williams and Johnny Peters, and the pianist Luckey Roberts, who sang and danced with five other men of the chorus. Tumbling was Roberts's specialty. Davis performed "over the top" and "through the trenches," two tap air steps that would catch on with tap dancers of the thirties and forties.

Ethel Williams and Johnny Peters were already partners when they were hired for the show. In 1912 they worked as a duet at a downtown cabaret, where they performed the maxixe, waltz, one-step, tango, and Texas tommy. Williams spent glorious years with the *Darktown Follies*: "We had some wonderful dancers, a featured dance called the Texas Tommy, and a fine cakewalk for the finale, but the most fun was a circle dance at the end of the second act. Everybody did a sort of sliding walk in rhythm with their hands on the hips of the person in front of them and I'd be doing anything but that—I'd 'Ball the Jack' on the end of the line every way you could think of—and when the curtain came down, I'd put my hand out from behind the curtain and 'Ball the Jack' with my fingers."[11]

Several critics agreed with the *New York World's* claim that the dancing surpassed anything Broadway had ever seen. Astounded by the energy, vitality, and dynamic dancing of the cast, these critics eventually lured downtown visitors to Harlem. Florenz Ziegfeld, one such visitor, bought the rights to "At the Ball," the *Darktown Follies's* finale. James Weldon Johnson described this finale as "one of those miracles of originality which occasionally come to pass in the world of musical comedy. . . . The whole company formed an endless chain that passed before the footlights and behind the scenes, round and round, singing and executing a movement from a dance called 'ballin' the jack,' one of those Negro dances which periodically come along and sweep the country." When Ziegfeld put this finale in his *Follies of 1914*, it was "one of the greatest hits the Ziegfeld Follies ever had." Ethel Williams, considered by many to be the reigning

American female dancer of that era, was brought in to coach Ziegfeld's cast, but neither she nor anyone else from the original show was hired to perform downtown. Nor did the name of J. Leubrie Hill, the original show's producer, ever appear on the program.[12]

Nevertheless, the longstanding and ubiquitous presence of African American comedy, music, song, and dance—as performed not just by imitators but by black performers themselves—was too much a part of the American theatrical scene to be uprooted. Despite Ziegfeld's attempts to simplify the routines and the dances, his cast could not ball the jack convincingly. Certainly, they could not do it the way he had seen it done at the Lafayette. Carl Van Vechten's review mirrored that of several other critics: "The tunes remained pretty; the *Follies* girls undoubtedly were pretty, but the rhythm was gone, the thrill was lacking, the boom was inaudible, the Congo had disappeared."[13]

The rise of black theaters in American cities during the teens allowed African American performers to play before black audiences, free of the taboos imposed by American racism. Harlem's theaters developed stock companies that served both as performance outlets for those who had worked in the companies of Williams and Walker and Cole and Johnson and as training grounds for newcomers whose day would come in the twenties. For a while, dramatic plays dominated the productions at the Lafayette and Lincoln Theaters, but eventually musicals resurfaced and were kept alive through the work of Sherman H. Dudley, Salem Tutt Whitney, J. Homer Tutt, Irving C. Miller, and J. Leubrie Hill.[14] Black theatrical experimentation in Harlem and on the road led straight to those black musicals of the twenties that left an indelible imprint on American musical theater.

In the late teens the enterprising and talented Eubie Blake and Noble Sissle spent their days "hustling up and down Broadway" trying to sell their songs.[15] Eubie Blake was a pianist, composer, and conductor from Baltimore; Noble Sissle was a singer and lyricist who had served in World War I as a member of the famous 369th Regiment band led by James Reese Europe. Around the same time, the actor-comedians Flournoy Miller and Aubrey Lyles, graduates of Fisk University and vaudeville stars, were trying to find songwriters for a new show based on *The Mayor of Dixie*, a 1907 production that Miller and Lyles had staged at the Pekin Theater in Chicago. The four artists joined forces and created the most important musical comedy of the twenties, *Shuffle Along*.

After a difficult start, *Shuffle Along* opened on 23 May 1921 and became a soaring success. James Weldon Johnson recalled how "all New York flocked to the Sixty-third Street Theater to hear the most joyous singing and see the most exhilarating dancing to be found on any stage in the city. *Shuffle Along* was a record-breaking, epoch-making musical comedy. . . . Its dances furnished new material for hundreds of dancing performers. . . . Within a few weeks *Shuffle Along* made . . . it necessary for the Traffic Department to declare Sixty-third Street a one-way thoroughfare."[16] The dancing in *Shuffle Along* included buck and wing, slow-motion acrobatics, tap air steps, eccentric steps, legomania, the soft shoe, and much prancing and high kicking. Of the show's dancers, one critic said with enthusiasm that "every sinew in their bodies danced; every tendon in their frames responded to their extreme energy." Perhaps *Shuffle Along*'s greatest contribution and innovation was the dancing of its sixteen-woman chorus line. Because of that electrifying line of dazzling dancers, Stearns and Stearns observe, "musical comedy took on a new and rhythmic life, and [white] chorus girls began learning to dance to jazz."[17]

Several members of the cast later became international stars: Paul Robeson, Josephine Baker, Florence Mills, and Caterina Jarboro. With an extraordinary pit orchestra that included William Grant Still and Hall Johnson, Sissle, Blake, Miller, and Lyles created a model of success that inspired other black writers and composers to produce musicals.[18]

Shuffle Along was followed by a wave of African American cast shows that continued to feature exciting dance. Among these were *Put and Take* (1921) and *Strut Miss Lizzie* (1922). Such dancers as Maxie McCree, an innovator of tap styles from straight tap to acrobatic dancing, and Grace Rector astounded critics, who praised the dance but had no cultural context for understanding what was being stylized and absolutely no vocabulary for describing it. Dressed in top hats and tails and sporting canes and monocles, the acknowledged predecessors of the "class acts," Rufus Greenlee and Thaddeus Drayton danced the Virginia essence and sang in *Liza* (1922). *The Plantation Revue* (1922) was the first in a long series of black musical revues backed by the white producer Lew Leslie, who routinely raided black vaudeville to find artists for his shows. Florence Mills was lured away from *Shuffle Along* when Leslie offered to triple her salary.[19]

According to Allen Woll, Leslie's "success in the 1920s was [based on] his ability to discover and exploit new black talent." His revue format "capitalized on the most popular elements of the black musical show" and "blurred the line between nightclub and theater for the audience." Focused on talent rather than scenery and costumes, these shows were less expensive to produce. *The Plantation Revue* was comprised of the best acts from revues at Leslie's restaurant, the Plantation Club. In the show, U.S. Thompson and Lou Keane presented their tap and acrobatic specialties to the music of Will Vodery's pit band including the dancing cornetist Johnny Dunn. The featured dancers in such revues, unhampered by flimsy plots or storylines, could refine their skills and tighten their acts by concentrating totally on dancing.[20]

The international dance craze of the twenties went into full swing when the choreographer Elida Webb introduced the Charleston in *Runnin' Wild* (1923). The Dancing Redcaps (including Sammy Dyer, Derby Wilson, Pete Nugent, and Chink Collins) stopped that show with stomping, clapping, and stepping to James P. Johnson's raggy tune called "The Charleston." James Weldon Johnson saw *Runnin' Wild* in the early twenties: "When Miller and Lyles introduced the dance in their show, they did not depend wholly upon their extraordinarily good jazz band for the accompaniment; they went straight back to [early] Negro music and had the major part of the chorus supplement the band by beating out the time with hand-clapping and foot patting. The effect was electrical. Such a demonstration of beating out complex rhythms had never before been seen on a stage in New York." *Runnin' Wild* also featured tappers Mae Barnes, Lavinia Mack, and Tommy Woods and George Stamper, who performed a slow-motion dance with splits. Noble Sissle reported to Jean Stearns and Marshall Stearns that Woods did everything in tempo: "He'd start with a Time Step and go into a flip, landing right on the beat."[21]

How Come, an earlier musical of 1923, featured the tapper Johnny Nit as well as the legendary clarinetist Sidney Bechet, who played the role of a police chief. *Dinah* (1924), produced by Irving C. Miller at the Lafayette Theater in Harlem, introduced the black bottom, a dance sensation of the twenties that was slightly less popular than the Charleston. *Chocolate Dandies* (1924) featured Josephine Baker, who had performed in the chorus line of *Shuffle Along;* the dancer and choreographer Charlie Davis; and the dancers Bob Williams and Johnny Hudgins. The female chorus line presented swinging and complex ensemble tap sequences, Davis's latest creation.[22]

The 1924 opening of Lew Leslie's *Dixie to Broadway* helped stabilize a trend that stifled the evolution of black musicals for years to come: all the performers were black, but all the producers and off-stage creative talents were white. Black lyricists, directors, stage managers, composers, and conductors were virtually boycotted as black shows became white commodities.

Fortunately, the dancers were almost always responsible for their own choreography—though white dance directors often got the credit.[23]

The undisputed star of *Dixie to Broadway* was Florence Mills, dancer, singer, actress extraordinaire. Critics were stunned by her dancing ability. When asked to comment on her dancing, she explained: "It all depends on the audience. . . . I make up the dances to the songs beforehand, but then something happens, like one of the orchestra talking to me, and I answer back and watch the audience without appearing to do so. It's great fun. Something different at each performance. It keeps me fresh. . . . I'm the despair of stage managers who want a player to act in a groove. No grooves for me. The stage isn't large enough for me at times."[24] Other fine dancers in this show were Willie Covan, U. S. Thompson, and Johnny Nit.

By the midtwenties, black shows were losing ground with the critics and "becoming more white oriented," but the dancing remained exciting. The stiff competition from Harlem cabaret revues probably helped spark the quality of musicals that opened in the latter part of the decade.[25]

The first important musical of the late twenties was *Rang Tang* (1927), with a plot by Miller and Lyles, music by Ford Dabney, and featured dancers Mae Barnes, Byron Jones, and Lavinia Mack. *Blackbirds of 1928*, with Bill Robinson and Snake Hips Tucker, ran for 518 performances. *Harlem*, a play produced in 1929, introduced the slow drag as part of a rent party scene. Bessie Smith performed "sundry dance steps at intervals" in *Pansy*, but the hit of that year was *Hot Chocolates*, which began as a revue at Connie's Inn in Harlem.[26]

For *Hot Chocolates*, Fats Waller, Andy Razaf, and Harry Brooks provided the music and lyrics; Leroy Smith's band swung the show from the orchestra pit; and, for part of the show's run, Louis Armstrong played his trumpet during intermission. But even with all this musical talent on hand, it was dance that prevailed in the reviews. Jazzlips Richardson, a former carnival comedian, performed his eccentric dance. The Six Crackerjacks, the acknowledged kings of acrobatic dancing, were a late addition to the show.[27] Archie Ware, one of the six dancers, described their style: "We had an acrobatic *variety* act—we tumbled in different costumes, we tapped, we sang, we danced, we featured lots of comedy—and our act was the fastest and *the first to do it in swinging rhythm*."[28] Roland Holder, sporting top hat and tails, danced the soft-shoe routine he had learned from Buddy Bradley, one of a long list of black choreographers who put together steps for black and white dancers.

The tap dancer Derby Wilson appeared in the short-lived *Bomboola*

(1929) and the dancing of Mae Barnes and Eddie Rector carried *Hot Rhythm* (1930). Working as a team rather than as solo specialties, the Four Flash Devils performed tap and acrobatic feats in *Change Your Luck* (1930). The tightly rehearsed ensemble dazzled audiences with their dramatic splits, flips, and slides. Bill Robinson continued to amaze the critics in *Brown Buddies* (1930).

Blackbirds of 1930, starring Ethel Waters, lasted through sixty-two performances, much to the credit of the tap team Buck and Bubbles, Jazzlips Richardson, and the Berry Brothers, who combined strutting with routines calling for precise acrobatics. But the ability of dancers to keep a Broadway show going was beginning to wane. By the early thirties, American vernacular dance was slowly disappearing from Broadway shows. Such spectacular dance teams as the Nicholas Brothers did appear in Hollywood films of the thirties and forties, but for the most part American theater turned its back on black indigenous dance.[29]

Vaudeville and TOBA

The black theater of the early twentieth century was more than a place to see recent vaudeville acts and musical comedies. It was "a secular temple for black communities," a place to see dramatic troupes and to hear orchestral groups, choral organizations, concert companies, and instrumental and vocal recitalists.[30] Chicago was the site of America's first black-owned theater, the Pekin, founded by Robert Motts in 1905, and it served as a model for the establishment of such black theaters in other major American cities, as the Howard Theater in Washington, D.C., the Lafayette and Lincoln Theaters in New York City, the New Standard and Dunbar Theaters in Philadelphia, and the Booker T. Washington Theater in St. Louis.

In New York, the Lafayette, known for its female orchestras, was a refuge from the discriminatory policies of Broadway. Washington's Howard Theater (and concert hall), established in 1910, exchanged shows with the Lafayette on a regular basis. Black theaters brought actors, instrumentalists, singers, comedians, dancers, composers, and playwrights before black audiences.

Thousands of African Americans were involved in show business by 1910. The U.S. census of that year reported 5,606 black musicians and 1,279 black actors and actresses. Their performances were by no means limited to the United States. The successes abroad of nineteenth-century black artists opened the way for large numbers to travel between 1910 and 1914. Dan Washington and Minnie Washington appeared in several European countries before touring Syria, Czechoslovakia, Turkey, and Russia. The *New York Age* mentioned, in 1913, "the successful engagement of Hen Wise and Katie Milton at the Apollo Theater, Shanghai, China," and "a new vaudeville route for black acts between Honolulu and [Asia]."[31]

By the second decade of the twentieth century, many blacks began to turn away from so-called book shows (ones with storylines and fully plotted scripts) in favor of the more loosely organized variety shows. They joined those African Americans who had already switched to vaudeville just after the turn of the century. Prejudice, a decline in financial sponsorship, and a decrease in black entrepreneurial leadership all caused the swing to vaudeville. The overall decrease in the viability of American touring companies likewise made the situation for white companies very problematic. Both black and white performers were affected by the increasingly high costs of transportation nationwide and by the growing popularity of talking picture films. Black touring shows found themselves relegated to second-class theaters.[32]

Outraged at the prevailing situation, Sherman H. Dudley, a musician-actor who had traveled with carnivals and minstrel shows, left the Smart Set Company in 1913 to begin working on his plans for a consolidated black theater circuit. He contacted theater owners around the country, offering them a part in his scheme. By the beginning of 1915, his weekly black newspaper column, "What's What on the Dudley Circuit," listed twenty-three cooperating black owned or operated theaters. African American companies could finally book their shows for the entire season through one professional agency.[33]

Dudley's efforts led to the founding of a black vaudeville circuit in 1920, the Theater Owners' Booking Association (TOBA). He joined forces with Milton Starr, a white theater owner, and by 1921, there were 300 theaters nationwide that presented black acts; 94 were owned and managed by African Americans. Of the 107 theaters devoted to black road shows and variety acts, TOBA controlled 80 and provided performance outlets for over 50 companies and 179 vaudeville acts.[34]

Dancing acts abounded on the TOBA. Black dance teams had been rising in popularity since 1900, and many original and inventive combinations of comic, tap, and acrobatic routines thrilled audiences and inspired emerging artists throughout the country. The legendary trainers of black dancers, the Whitman Sisters, were headliners on the TOBA circuit for many years. The hoofer Pete Nugent told Marshall Stearns and Jean Stearns, "You found out if you could dance on T.O.B.A. and if you couldn't you were fired on the spot."[35]

The actor Clarence Muse described TOBA shows as "tabloid editions of musical comedies." Each night three forty-five-minute revues were presented by a group of about thirty-five persons. Ernest "Baby" Seals, a dancer-producer, carried his own show on the circuit. He featured a dancing comedian and a blues and ballad singer in an eight-part, seventy-five-minute show made up of chorus numbers, solo specialties, comedy skits, and, as always, lots of dancing performed to the swinging rhythms of a small jazz band. On the road, new talent was discovered continuously. Things changed on a moment's notice, depending on the talent and inspiration. According to Seals, "I made up some material, we'd see things on the road, other guys had ideas—we'd try anything."[36] This flexible approach to show making helped cultivate an atmosphere that encouraged improvisation on a wide scale and allowed for the emergence of new choreographers. Free of the constraints imposed on aspiring artists in schools and studios, black artists in this setting could experiment and push the evolution of vernacular dance along at an incredible speed.

Jack Wiggins, Bill Robinson, Eddie Rector, the Berry Brothers, and a host of other star dancers served their apprenticeships on TOBA. For many dancers, the TOBA circuit was not their first brush with vaudeville. The practice of using children, especially young African Americans who could sing and dance sensationally, had been widespread in white vaudeville for years. Numerous white female stars, including Sophie Tucker, Nora Bayes, Eva Tanguay, Grace LaRue, and Emma Kraus toured alongside "picks," short for pickaninnies. The head of one vaudeville circuit reputedly said, "If the bill is weak, add a Negro act, and if that don't do it, hire some Negro kids."[37]

Mayme Remington's act served as an early training ground for some of America's most talented artists: Luckey Roberts, Bill Robinson, Coot Grant, Toots Davis, Dewey Weinglass, Eddie Rector, Lou Keane, and Archie Ware. Tiny Ray, a dancer, described his stage work with Gussie Francis, a white actress: "We played all kinds of circuits and wore opera hats, tuxedo jackets, short pants, and black silk stockings. . . . We worked out all our own routines, too." Ray and his cohorts performed a soft shoe, then sat on stage and sang "Won't You Come Down, Rainbow Queen" while their employer rocked back and forth in a swing. Henry "Rubberlegs" Williams worked with Naomi Thomas's Brazilian Nuts: "She had a boy named Rastus who was sensational. He jumped down from a high drum into a split and came up dancing the Charleston." Another act led by Nora Bayes appeared in the same show: "She'd sing 'Mississippi Mud' and when she came to the line 'the darkies beat their feet' her six picks would do the Pasmala around her." The Whitman Sisters and other black performers also employed black children, but this was by and large a practice exercised by white adults, who reaped the profits, while black children tolerated injustices in order to gain stage experience.[38]

Vaudeville featured a wide array of acts. In the early 1900s black acts included such novelties as jugglers, acrobats, ventriloquists, magicians, and animal trainers. Fletcher recalled "the Kratons, hoop-rollers and jugglers, who made the hoops do everything but talk," the Spiller's Musical Bumpers, the Wangdoodle Comedy Four, and the Golden Gate Quartet. Eph Thompson presented trained elephants and the Sunny South Company included a singing and dancing male quartet. Impersonation and body contortion were also popular. TOBA and other African American circuits featured "jubilee," or spirituals, singers; the yodeler Charles Anderson; Harrison Blackburn, "the one-man circus"; and Bronco Billy Verne, who performed his "weight-lifting, balancing, and lariat-throwing demonstration."[39]

Thomas Riis observed, "On the circuit, one learned the art of improvising in the dance and comedy traditions of earlier black shows, as well as the art of survival. Days were long, travel difficult, audiences demanding and pay low." Nevertheless it was a training ground for many of America's artistic standard bearers and style setters. Some of the best known were Ethel Waters, Butterbeans and Susie, the Whitman Sisters, Ma Rainey, and Bessie Smith.[40]

Scores of pre-jazz and jazz musicians played in vaudeville. W. C. Handy and James Reese Europe toured with their bands on vaudeville circuits. One of America's greatest ragtime composers, James Scott, spent ten years in vaudeville theaters, accompanying silent films, slide shows, a variety of acts, and audience sing-alongs that filled the time between acts. Playing for silent films encouraged unconventional instrumental sounds because it required artists to imitate trains, planes, snores, screams, laughter, steam whistles, and animal noises. Pianists played an indispensable role in vaudeville theaters. Usually theaters opened at noon and offered two shows per day that were accompanied by one pianist. At 6:00 P.M. an orchestra was on hand to play for the evening shows, which usually ended around midnight. Jazz giants Fats Waller, Ben Webster, Count Basie, and many other black musicians took a turn playing for silent movies.[41]

The growing appeal of films gave a crushing blow to vaudeville. As early as 1910, short films were included as specialty acts on theater bills. By the end of the twenties, many vaudeville houses had become movie theaters. Weakened by the Great Depression and the increasing dominance of the sound film industry, the Theater Owners' Booking Association slowly disintegrated in the early thirties.[42]

Cabarets and Nightclubs

While TOBA and black musicals were enjoying their golden years, Harlem was fast establishing itself as one of the entertainment meccas of the world. By 1925, the country's main center of jazz development had shifted from Chicago to New York. African American artists from all over the country congregated there to participate in one of the most exciting artistic flowerings of the twentieth century later termed the Harlem Renaissance. In Harlem cabarets and nightclubs, dancers, musicians, and singers participated jointly in revues that rivaled Broadway shows. Willie "the Lion" Smith had this to say about Harlem in the twenties: "Instead of fights on the street corners after the cabarets closed, there would be people dancing the Charleston."[43]

American nightclubs evolved from the late nineteenth- and early twentieth-century cabarets that replaced standard restaurants in many major American cities. By 1914, New York had at least twenty first-class cabarets, where some of its wealthiest citizens dined and listened to music. The subsequent addition of floor shows and dancing helped provide an intimate atmosphere in which women and men could enjoy themselves in close proximity to each other and to the stars who entertained them. Since cabarets could offer long-term employment, they shared major dance headliners with vaudeville and theater shows.[44]

The forerunners of cabarets in New York were the city's saloons and rathskellers of the nineteenth century. Music, dancing, and entertainment were standard fare in many of these early drinking establishments, owned by blacks as well as whites. In 1880, one of the most famous spots was managed by Ike Hines, a black former banjo player who had traveled with Hicks and Sawyer. The blues pioneer Perry Bradford described Hines's club:

> Ike's new style of entertainment was started in the basement of an old Greenwich Village house that was located on Thompson Street near

Minetta Lane, at Third and McDougal. He opened it as a get together place for all the folks in the neighborhood. The natives would congregate every evening to drink large schooners of beer, and sing, dance and play their old favorite pieces of long time remembrance. It was an informal style of entertainment. If you could dance, sing or play an instrument, you were always welcome. The Germans named Ike's place a rathskeller, because it was located downstairs in a basement and had orthodox entertainment. The girls would dance from table to table, shaking like jelly on a plate while the men did some comical steps. Some smart promoters copped Ike's style of shows and introduced it at Chicago's World's Fair in 1893. Ike's show has gone down the corridor of time to be attempted today as the Shake Dance, but it ain't nothing but what the oldtimers used to call the "Hootchie Kootchie," which Ike had started 'way back in 1880.[45]

As black residents were pushed out of lower Manhattan by new immigrant groups, they relocated further uptown west of Sixth Avenue in the lower thirties and upper twenties. By 1900, there was another shift northward to the fifties and sixties. Ike's Professional Club moved to this area, where black honky tonks, gambling clubs, and professional clubs thrived. James Weldon Johnson's description of a club like Hines's first appeared in his novel *The Autobiography of an Ex-Coloured Man:*

In the back room there was a piano, and tables were placed round the wall. The floor was bare and the centre was left vacant for singers, dancers, and others who entertained the patrons. . . . In this back room the tables were sometimes pushed aside, and the floor given over to general dancing. The front room on the next floor was a sort of private party room; a back room on the same floor contained no furniture and was devoted to the use of new and ambitious performers. In this room song and dance teams practised their steps, acrobatic teams practiced their tumbles, and many other kinds of "acts" rehearsed their "turns."[46]

The professional clubs served as meeting places for working dancers, singers, musicians, composers, actors, writers, actresses, and athletes. Frequented by blacks and a few whites, Ike's Professional Club, the Douglass Club, Barron Wilkins's Little Savoy, Joe Stewart's Criterion, the Anderson Club, the Waldorf, and others provided opportunities for African American artists to get together and share their ideas and talents.

Honky-tonks, on the other hand, were "places with paid and volunteer entertainers where both sexes met to drink, dance, and have a good time; they were the prototype of the modern night-club." Some of these establishments moved to Harlem when blacks began migrating there after 1900.[47]

Leroy's Restaurant (1910–1923) was the first Harlem cabaret opened for black patronage. Willie "the Lion" Smith, James P. Johnson, and Fats Waller were some of the musicians Leroy Wilkins hired for his restaurant. According to Smith, at Leroy's the pianist was the person "in charge. . . . He had to be an all-round showman and it helped if he could both dance and sing. . . . The show actually consisted of the pianist, occasionally accompanied by several instrumentalists, six or seven sopranos, and a bunch of dancing waiters who also sang." On any given night the audience might include Florence Mills, Bert Williams, Bill Robinson, Flournoy Miller, Aubrey Lyles, Rufus Greenlee, Thaddeus Drayton, the comedian Mantan Moreland, or Clarence "Dancin'" Dotson. Ethel Waters, a regular at Edmond's Cellar, might drop in and rock the house with her "Shim-Me-Sha-Wabble" number. Or members of the chorus from the Smart Set shows might stop by and take over the floor with their spectacular dancing.[48]

The dance called the Texas tommy was still in full swing when the Lion played at Leroy's in the teens: "The sharp dancin' cats . . . would hop-skip three times and then throw a doll over their shoulders. Then they would hop-skip three more times and squat on their knees as they skated right on down the floor." Leroy's was a favorite hangout for Russell Brown, a dancer who often performed for tips on street corners and in saloons and cabarets. Brown was best known for a "Geechie dance" that was later called the Charleston. At first referring to himself in the third person, Willie "the Lion" Smith described Russell Brown:

> He took a special liking to the way the Lion played the piano for him so I let him get in the show and share our tips. Brown . . . was given a nickname by the people in Harlem. When they met him on the street they would holler at him. "Hey, Charleston — do your Geechie dance!" Some folks say that is how the dance known as the Charleston got its name. I'm a tough man for facts and I say the Geechie dance had been around New York for many years before Brown showed up. The kids from the Jenkins Orphanage Band of Charleston used to do Geechie steps when they were in New York on their yearly tour.[49]

Garvin Bushell played jazz at Leroy's in the early twenties with several alumni of the Jenkins Orphanage Band. He recalled that "there was a small dance floor in front of the bandstand. The dancers were our inspiration."

It was at Leroy's that Bushell first witnessed three- and four-hour-long piano battles that involved such stalwart "gladiators" as James P. Johnson,
Fats Waller, and Willie "the Lion" Smith. According to Bushell, "one man
would play two or three choruses, and the next would slide in. Jimmy was
on top most of the time. . . . You got credit for how many patterns you
could create within the tunes you knew, and in how many different keys
you could play. You had to know how to play in every key, because all those
players had been baptized in cabarets. You never knew what kind of key
the entertainer wanted."[50]

Another early Harlem cabaret was J. W. Connor's Cafe (1913–30).
Connor's was one of the first locations hosting afternoon teas during which
customers gathered to socialize and listen to music. At the Astoria Cafe,
Barron Wilkins expanded the concept by offering tango teas, which gave
patrons the added advantage of dancing with professionals who had been
hired to demonstrate and teach the new dance called the tango. This practice spread to similar businesses, thereby providing jobs for many emerging artists. Goldie Cisco, who later danced in the chorus line of *Shuffle
Along*, was among those who taught the tango at Wilkins's cabaret. The
Astoria Cafe went through other names before emerging as the Barron
Wilkins' Exclusive Club, one of Harlem's top four night clubs during the
early twenties. In 1923, Duke Ellington played there with the Washing-
tonians, led by banjoist Elmer Snowden.[51]

By the middle twenties, Harlem nightclubs and cabarets were in the vanguard of New York night life. Business was booming in these places that
employed hundreds of singers, dancers, and instrumentalists, along with
waiters, doormen, cooks, and coatroom checkers. On the scene when these
night spots flourished, James Weldon Johnson noted: "The larger clubs
maintain permanent companies of performers; and such clubs as Connie's
Inn, the Cotton Club, and Smalls' Paradise put on revues that are often
better than what may be seen in the theaters downtown. The night-clubs
have been the training ground for a good part of the talent that has been
drawn upon by musical comedy and revues in the professional theater."[52]

The exclusive black-owned Smalls' Paradise was known for its colorful
floor shows, its big-band jam sessions, and its singing, roller skating, and
dancing waiters who did the Charleston "while balancing full trays on their
fingertips." At the original Smalls' basement spot, whose full name was
Smalls' Sugar Cane Club (1917-25), strutting, tapping, shuffling waiters
"slid up to a table with a cutaway step (a heel pivot and a dip). They also
sang in quartets, trios, and solos during the floor shows."[53]

Connie's Inn opened in 1923 with Wilbur Sweatman's Rhythm Kings on the bandstand. During the second half of the twenties, it was one of Harlem's top clubs and the home of the hit musical *Hot Chocolates*, produced first as a floor show by the choreographer Leonard Harper.[54]

The corner of 142d and Lenox was the location of Harlem's most well-known nightclub, the Cotton Club (1923–40), made famous by the transcontinental broadcasts of the Duke Ellington band. Albert Murray attested to the impact of Ellington's band: "Those radio waves and those phonograph records penetrated the entire culture to its very core, making for a much bigger statement than anyone imagined at the time. . . . Ellington wove his music into contrived 'primitive' show segments that satisfied the needs of performers, choreographers, and patrons, while the technology of the time sent his work across the country and around the world on its own terms."[55]

The revues featured singers, comedians, dancers, and a band; opening nights there featured all the pomp and circumstance of Broadway premieres and were fully reviewed by downtown critics and reporters. Cab Calloway offered his first impression of the Cotton Club:

> I had seen some elaborate shows in Chicago, but nothing to compare with a Cotton Club revue. A large part of it was the club itself. It was a huge room. The bandstand was a replica of a southern mansion, with large white columns and a backdrop painted with weeping willows and slave quarters. The band played on the veranda of the mansion, and in front of the veranda, down a few steps, was the dance floor, which was also used for the shows. The waiters were dressed in red tuxedos, like butlers in a southern mansion, and the tables were covered with red-and-white-checked gingham tablecloths. . . . I suppose the idea was to make whites who came to the club feel like they were being catered to and entertained by black slaves. The sets and costumes were stunning and elaborate, like operatic settings almost. The chorus girls changed costumes for every number, and the soloists, dancers, and singers were always dressed to the hilt—the women in long flowing gowns, if that was appropriate, or in the briefest of brief dance costumes.[56]

Performers were required to do three shows per night—at 8:30, 11:30, and 2:00. In addition, on special evenings a Cotton Club revue might be taken en bloc to a theater downtown. Or, for no extra pay, performers were also required to play impromptu smokers and conventions for local politicians, gangsters, or other big shots.[57] Underpaid and overworked, such African American artists as Ethel Waters and Avon Long used this venue as a steppingstone for their careers, despite the club's blatant practice of exploiting black stereotypes in order to satisfy the psychological needs of white downtowners who flocked there nightly in search of what they considered exotic.

Although cultural historians have long recognized the Cotton Club as a vital springboard for jazz music as a national (and then international) phenomenon, few scholars have acknowledged the club's significance to the history of American dance. Cotton Club revues were usually built around such popular dance fads as truckin', the Susie Q, the Charleston, peckin', the shorty George, and the skrontch. When Lena Horne joined the club's chorus line in the fall of 1933, she performed the fan dance, made famous by Sally Rand at the Chicago World's Fair. Horne recalled that she and the other members of the chorus line "weren't quite as naked as Miss Rand, but we were pretty close — my costume consisted of approximately three feathers. We did a semi-tap-semi-jazz kind of step, choreographed by our captain, Elida Webb."[58]

The eccentric dancers Earl "Snake Hips" Tucker and Bessie Dudley dazzled all-white audiences with their inimitable and classic quivers, grinds, and hip rolls. Many of America's most exciting dance acts appear on the roll call of Cotton Club dancers: the Berry Brothers, the Nicholas Brothers, Anise and Aland, Dynamite Hooker, Mildred and Henri, Bill Robinson, Peg Leg Bates, Tip Tap and Toe, the Four Step Brothers, the Three Chocolateers, Son and Sonny, Buck and Bubbles, Henry "Rubberlegs" Williams, and Whitey's Lindy Hoppers. The choreographers Elida Webb and Clarence Robinson maintained extraordinarily high standards for the chorus line dancers, who were backed by the top-notch bands of Duke Ellington, Andy Preer, Cab Calloway, Jimmy Lunceford, Claude Hopkins, Andy Kirk, or Lucky Millinder. Cab Calloway pointed out the hard work that spelled excellence in the Cotton Club shows: "The club was alive with music and dancing at night, but it was also alive all day long. If the chorus line wasn't rehearsing, then the band was. If the band wasn't rehearsing, then one of the acts was." "We knew we had a standard of performance to match every night. We knew we couldn't miss a lick. And we rarely did."[59]

At 3:30 or 4:00 A.M., when the last show was over, many performers and patrons from the Cotton Club went next door to Happy Rhone's Orchestra Club (1920–25), one of the first Harlem clubs to present floor shows. In this plush setting, Noble Sissle often served as master of ceremonies until the club changed hands in the midtwenties and reopened as the

Lenox Club, an important early morning meeting place for musicians and the originator of the city's breakfast dance fad.[60]

According to Willie "the Lion" Smith, this area was the jumpinest spot in town: "Talk about Fifty-second Street—that wasn't the first swing alley. 133rd Street was IT. Things were swinging to beat all hell on 133rd between Lenox and Seventh avenues in the mid-twenties. They called it 'jungle alley' back in those days and it was only two blocks from the place where late in the afternoon you could find all the big-time musicians gathered around the Tree of Hope. As soon as it was dark, the cellar joints started to open up for a long night which sometimes extended to noon of the following day." Jungle Alley was the home of the Clam House, Tillie's Chicken Shack, Mexico's, the Nest Club, and Pod's and Jerry's, a basement speakeasy that always featured a talented singer, dancer, or musician.[61]

At the Nest Club, the floor shows were less elaborate than those at the larger clubs and the emphasis was on music. The Nest Club opened in 1923 with a Leonard Harper revue and Sam Wooding's band. Dressed in bird costumes, the performers did a show based on the theme "Where do the birds go every night? To the Nest! To the Nest!" Garvin Bushell played there in the twenties: "We'd start playing about 9:00, and the revue would go on about 11:00 or 11:30. The second show would begin about 3:00 a.m. We'd be finished by 4:30 or 5:00 a.m. Then we'd often go some place for breakfast." In the early thirties Dickie Wells of the dance team Wells, Mordecai, and Taylor became the host at the new Nest Club, renamed the Dickie Wells's Shim Sham Club.[62]

Mexico's, a favorite late night spot of the Ellington band, was also located on 133d. Sonny Greer believed that "the most authentic jam sessions were at Mexico's. He specialized in that. Monday would be trumpet night, Tuesday saxophone night, Wednesday trombone night, Thursday clarinet night, Friday piano night, and so on."[63] But the number one hangout for jazz musicians in New York City was the Rhythm Club, where they could jam free of the limits imposed by floor shows. Young musicians would go there to be heard and to learn from the experts.

Eventually dancers and other performers joined the action. When the Rhythm Club moved further uptown in 1932, the original site, renamed the Hoofer's Club, became the headquarters and stomping grounds of America's most innovative tap dancers. Dancers and musicians found a common ground for exchange and mutual enrichment at the Hoofer's Club. Jazz musician Dicky Wells sets the scene: "While you're blowing, cats are dancing. Or if you're singing, cats are dancing, you know. And I

mean, really dancing. . . . It would invigorate you because you'd be playing better while people were dancing. That's the reason the concert is kind
of stiff, cold."[64]

During its golden years between 1920 and 1940, Harlem was "known
for abundant and inspiring stylizations of life in music, dance, speech,
walks, and dress."[65] In the Harlem cabarets and nightclubs of the twenties and thirties, vernacular dance took a giant leap forward. Uptown clubs
were hotbeds of artistic developments that had a profound influence on
the American theater that ultimately affected cultures throughout the
world.

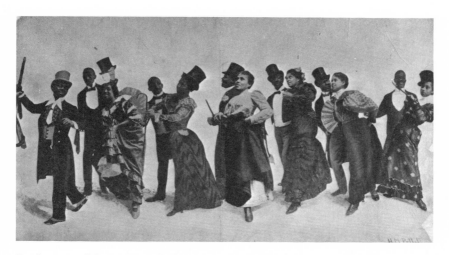

By the turn of the century, fancy steps, elegant clothes, and mock aristocratic attitudes made the cakewalk an international dance craze (circa 1900). (Courtesy of the Photographs and Prints Division, Schomburg Center for Research in Black Culture, the New York Public Library, Astor, Lenox, and Tilden Foundations)

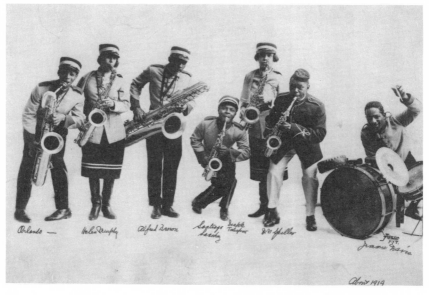

The Musical Spillers, a popular vaudeville touring act (1919). (Courtesy of the Photographs and Prints Division, Schomburg Center for Research in Black Culture, the New York Public Library, Astor, Lenox, and Tilden Foundations)

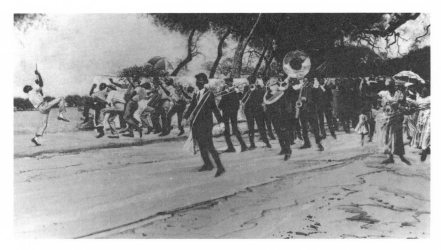

Second line dancers (*left*) strut and high step during a New Orleans street parade. Painting by Morton Roberts (1958). (Courtesy of Morton Roberts, N.A.)

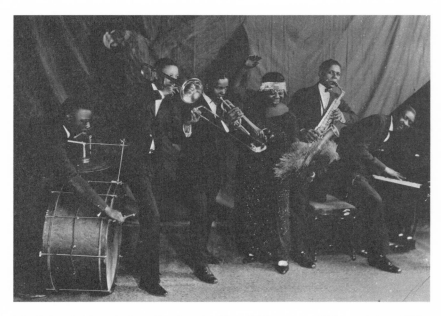

Ma Rainey's Georgia Jazz Band at the Grand Theater in Chicago (circa 1923–24). *From left*: Gabriel Washington, Albert Wynn, Dave Nelson, Ma Rainey, Eddie Pollack, and Thomas Dorsey. (From the Frank Driggs Collection, courtesy of Frank Driggs)

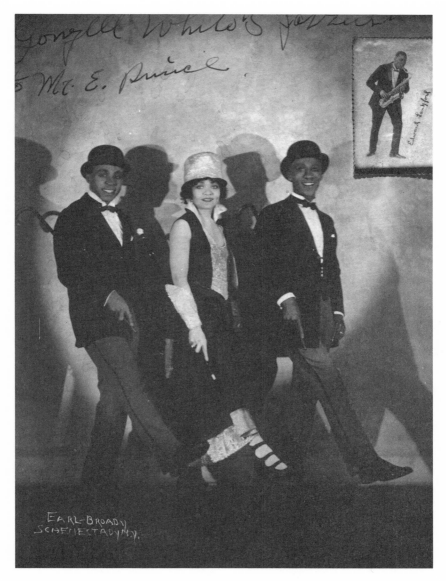

Gonzelle White (*center*) and her husband Edward Langford (*insert*) led an act that featured young musicians like the young Count Basie as well as comedians and dancers. White, the show's star, sang, danced, and blew alto saxophone (1920s). (Courtesy of the Photographs and Prints Division, Schomburg Center for Research in Black Culture, the New York Public Library, Astor, Lenox, and Tilden Foundations)

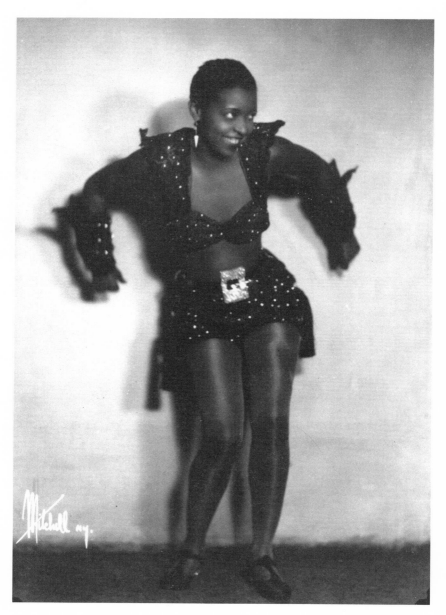

Ethel Waters, "Sweet Mama Stringbean," started her career as a dancing singer. Her classic version of the shimmy broke up the house every night (1920s). (Courtesy of the Yale Collection of American Literature, Beinecke Rare Book and Manuscript Library, Yale University)

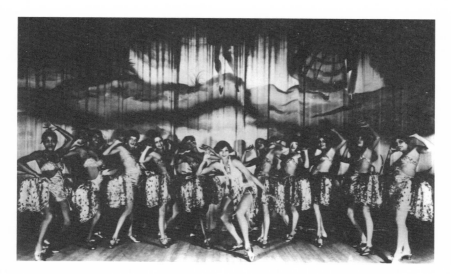

Maude Russell and Her Ebony Steppers appear in *Just a Minute*, a 1929 Cotton Club show. (Courtesy of the Photographs and Prints Division, Schomburg Center for Research in Black Culture, the New York Public Library, Astor, Lenox, and Tilden Foundations)

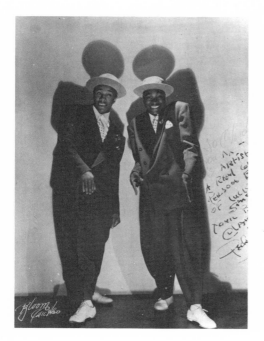

Peck and Peck, a jazz dance duo, performed during the big band era, but their vernacular body English has survived through the 1980s and 1990s and has traveled all over the world (late 1930s). (Courtesy of the Photographs and Prints Division, Schomburg Center for Research in Black Culture, the New York Public Library, Astor, Lenox, and Tilden Foundations)

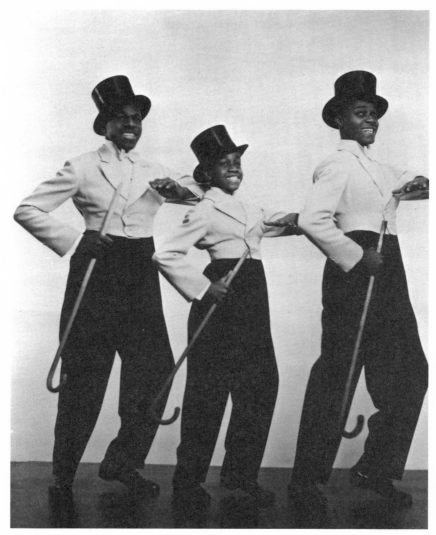

The Berry Brothers, known for their strut and cane act, dazzled audiences with breathtaking acrobatics performed precisely on the beat. *From left:* James Berry, Warren Berry, and Ananias Berry (circa 1936). (Courtesy of the Dance Collection, the New York Public Library for the Performing Arts, Astor, Lenox, and Tilden Foundations)

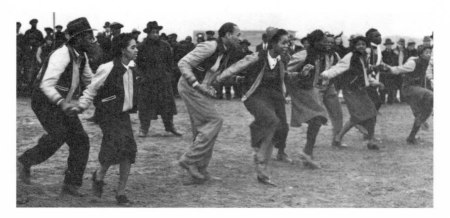

Whitey's Lindy Hoppers at the New York World's Fair (1938). *From left:* Thomas Lee, Wilda Crawford, Herbert White (watching his group), William Downes, Mickey Jones, Mae Miller, Russell Williams (partially hidden), Connie Hill, and two unidentified dancers. (Courtesy of Monica B. Smith and the Morgan and Marvin Smith Collection, Photographs and Prints Division, Schomburg Center for Research in Black Culture, the New York Public Library, Astor, Lenox, and Tilden Foundations)

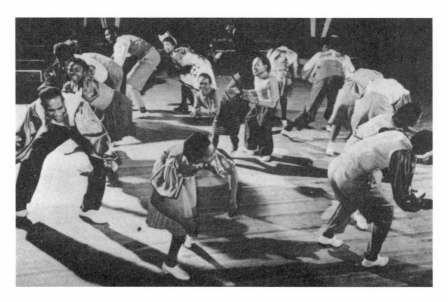

Doing the Big Apple at Harlem's Savoy Ballroom (circa 1938). (Courtesy of the Photographs and Prints Division, Schomburg Center for Research in Black Culture, the New York Public Library, Astor, Lenox, and Tilden Foundations)

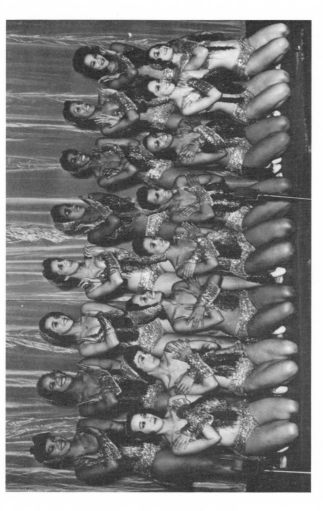

The Apollo's number one line reputedly featured the best chorus line dancers in New York City. Front row (*left to right*): Doris Dawson, Mimi Lynn, Henrietta Campbell, Olive Prince, Vernice Crawford, Aline Crawford, Marion Coles, and Margret Hart. Back row (*left to right*): Helen Holland, Claudia Heyward, Frenchie Bascomb, Ristina Banks (the group's leader), Dorothy Preston, Carolyn McLaughlin, Bobby Vincent, and Elaine Dash (1940). (Courtesy of the Monica B. Smith Morgan and Marvin Smith Collection, Photographs and Prints Division, Schomburg Center for Research in Black Culture, the New York Public Library, Astor, Lenox, and Tilden Foundations)

Chapter Six

Jazz Music in Motion: Dancers and Big Bands

> Dancing is very important to people who play music with a beat. I think that people who don't dance, or who never did dance, don't really understand the beat. . . . I know musicians who don't and never did dance, and they have difficulty communicating.
> —Duke Ellington, *The World of Duke Ellington*

The infancy of jazz coincided with extensive artistic and commercial efforts to get black musical theater established on Broadway. As a result, jazz musicians had a recognized connection with professional dance acts prior to the thirties. From the orchestra pit, musicians backed professional dancers and singers in theaters across the country. Throughout the twenties, jazz musicians, singers, and dancers worked together in night clubs and cabarets; and they performed jointly in revues that toured the United States and abroad. As early as 1921, when Garvin Bushell toured with Mamie Smith and Company, his co-performers included a comedian, a dance team, a magician, and some singers. Many of America's jazz giants gained experience playing for these small revues. Bushell recalled hiring a pickup musician while appearing in Kansas City: "When we got there for the first rehearsal we met this youngster on saxophone who played all his parts and didn't miss a note. When we told him to take a solo, he took a tremendous one. We said, 'What's your name?' 'Coleman.' 'Coleman who?' 'Coleman Hawkins.' . . . We had to read our parts when we played in the pit, and Hawk never hit a bad note."[1]

Garvin Bushell was a member of Sam Wooding's orchestra when it toured Europe in 1925 with a revue called *Chocolate Kiddies* that included over thirty dancers, comedians, and chorus line members. The hit of the show was "Jig Walk," created by the choreographer Charlie Davis. According to Bushell, "That's where we got to do the Charleston." That same year the Claude Hopkins band toured Europe with the Josephine Baker Revue. These were just a few of many shows that afforded opportunities for professional dancers and jazz musicians to inspire one another.[2]

As jazz bands became increasingly popular, they moved up from the pit to take center stage. Earl Hines helped pioneer the move from the pit to the stage at the Apollo Theater:

> We had to play the show from the pit and then go up onstage for our specialty. I had written three weeks before we got there that we wanted to wear the white suits and be onstage all the time, and they had agreed. "I'm not going in the pit," I said, getting salty. The producer called the manager, and he came and said, "You *are* going in the pit!" I told all the boys to pack up then, and we left the show standing there. Next morning I went to the theater and said, "Well, what about it?" The stage manager said, "We've got you set up on the stage."[3]

Vaudeville declined rapidly around the early thirties and a new performance format called presentation evolved. By this time, radio broadcasts had helped create a demand for jazz bands throughout the country at hotels, supper clubs, theaters, colleges, night clubs, high schools, affluent prep schools, and at such dance halls as the Savoy and Roseland in New York City. Big city movie houses also featured bands on vaudeville-like bills that were presented between motion pictures.[4] According to Cholly Atkins, a tap dancer, choreographer, and director, the most popular venues of the thirties were dance halls, hotels, and theaters. Dance halls were scattered across the United States, and any town with more than 150,000 people had at least one hotel with a reasonably sized dance floor. And though they were often presented as part of a musical package, bands were the headliners in these performance arenas. During the era of presentation, these packages were called "revues" or "units" and included dancers, solo singers, comedians, a chorus line, and, of course, a big-name band.

Many bands had two or three dancing acts that they secured through booking agencies. For example, if Cab Calloway saw an act he liked, he would have his band manager find out which agency was handling the dancers and see if they were available for a future engagement. A booking agency allowed the tap duo of Honi Coles and Cholly Atkins to take their class act on the road with numerous bands. Typically they might hook up with the Basie band for a cross-country tour on a northern route from

New York to California and come back with the Billy Eckstine Band on a southern route through Oklahoma City, St. Louis, Atlanta, and then up to Washington, D.C., as a final stop. But most dance acts didn't do extended tours with big bands; rather, they were hired for "spot bookings." During the thirties, Jimmy Lunceford carried his own revue, called *The Harlem Express*.

In the thirties, the most well-known African American theater circuit was called 'Round the World. Its tour comprised such independent theaters as the Howard in Washington, D.C.; the Lafayette in Harlem; the Royal in Baltimore; the Lincoln, Standard, and Pearl in Philadelphia; and the Regal in Chicago. Ninety-nine percent of the artists featured in this big city loop were black. Revues generally opened with a couple of numbers by the band followed by a singer, a comedy dance act, more pieces by the band, a straight dancing act, another band appearance, and a closing number that featured a popular singer.[5]

Honi Coles counted as many as fifty top-flight dance acts "in the late 20s and early 30s." Coles explained the importance of these acts: "Back a while, when show business was show business, and there were all sorts of variety presentations, the dancing act was the nucleus of every show. Dancing acts were always surefire crowd pleasers. . . . Generally speaking, [they] were used to strengthen the show." Coles insisted that at one point tap dancers were more important than any other act on most bills because they could not only open and close the show but they could also fill the trouble spots. They were "the best dressed, the best conditioned, the most conscientious performer[s] on any bill, and in spite of being the least paid, [they were] the act[s] to 'stop the show.'"[6]

The diversity of dancing acts during the thirties and forties was astonishing: ballroom, adagio, eccentric, comedy, flash, acrobatics, and tap—the most prevailing style. Harold Norton and Margot Webb, who had studied ballet and performed a repertory of rumba, waltz, tango, and bolero numbers, made up one of the most famous African American ballroom teams from 1933 to 1947. Webb's solo work included a jazz toe dance (en pointe). During the thirties, this team enjoyed extended bookings with the Earl Hines Band at Chicago's Grand Terrace; toured England and France with Teddy Hill's band as part of the *Cotton Club Revue*; and performed as a single act on variety stages in Italy, France, and Germany. Before meeting Norton, Webb appeared in revues choreographed by leading black "dance directors," including Clarence Robinson and Leonard Harper.[7]

"Adagio" dancers performed a style that consisted of ballroom dance with various balletic and acrobatic lifts, spins, and poses. Honi Coles referred to Anise Boyer and Aland Dixon as the "fastest . . . adagio act." They traveled extensively with the Cab Calloway Band, sharing the dance spotlight with stand-up tap single Coles and with the Chocolateers, who introduced a dance called peckin'.[8]

Eccentric dance, a favorite with many jazz band leaders, "may include elements of contortionist, legomania, and shake dancing, although these styles frequently overlap with others, and a dancer can combine something of all of them. A few involve tap, for tappers are generally regarded as the dancing elite and imitated whenever possible. . . . 'Eccentric' is a catchall for dancers who have their own non-standard movements and sell themselves on their individual styles." One of the most famous of these dancers was Dynamite Hooker, who toured during the thirties with the bands of Cab Calloway, Duke Ellington, and Jimmy Lunceford.[9]

The big band era coincided with the most fruitful years for comedy-dancing acts. As a result, bands provided steady employment for such two-man teams as Chuck and Chuckles, Stump and Stumpy, Moke and Poke, and Cook and Brown, who combined superb dancing with acrobatics and tumbling. Straight acrobatic teams were also featured in traveling units. They combined gymnastic material with music and performed it precisely on the beat. Most of the black acrobatic acts used jazz music.[10]

By the midthirties, many dancers in search of new and exciting ideas had developed what became known as flash dancing—a compression of acrobatics and jazz dancing. The flash acts "spice their routines with *ad lib* acrobatics. Without any warning or apparent preparation, they insert a variety of floor and air steps—a spin or flip or knee-drop or split—in the midst of a regular routine, and then, without a moment's hesitation, go back to the routine."[11]

The connection between big bands and tap dancers is one that has resurfaced in the last decades of the twentieth century. As jazz music has commanded a broader and broader audience, jazz lovers have discovered again one of the most sophisticated representations of jazz music by dancers, rhythm tap, created by African American tap innovators of the twentieth century. King Rastus Brown's flatfooted hoofing preceded the legendary Bill Robinson's "up on the toes" approach. Eddie Rector added elegance and body motion, and John Bubbles's crowning achievement—dropping the heels—added extraordinary rhythmical complexity.

Baby Laurence, tap dancer extraordinaire, explained that "tap dancing is very much like jazz music. The dancer improvises his own solo and expresses himself." Rhythm tappers are jazz percussionists who value improvisation and self-expression. Jazz musicians tell stories with their instruments and rhythm tappers tell stories with their feet. In a 1973 obituary for Baby Laurence, Whitney Balliett wrote, "A great drummer dances sitting down. A great tap-dancer drums standing up."[12]

Rhythm tap's close relationship to jazz music is evident in the large number of top caliber jazz drummers who could tap: Philly Joe Jones, Buddy Rich, Jo Jones, Big Sid Catlett, Eddie Locke, and Cozy Cole, who once had a dance act along with tapper Derby Wilson. Louis Bellson, who played drums with Duke Ellington in the fifties, commented on the relationship between drumming and tapping: "You get a guy like Jo Jones, all those guys can do a time step and the shim-sham-shimmy because that's what you did in the theater. . . . We base all of our rhythms on dancing. When I play a drum solo, I'm tapping. My brother-in-law Bill Bailey, oh, what a tap dancer. I mean that's one of the greatest drum solos I've heard in my life, Bill Bailey did it on stage. All he had was a rhythm section and he danced up and down that stage. I've got films on him. I look at them every once in a while. I study those films." According to Bellson, Duke Ellington always referred to the drummers as dancers. "I remember Ellington telling me that the great thing about Africa is that the drummers and dancers are like one." He would introduce the drummer by saying, "And now Dave Black is going to perform a little dancing for you." Bellson added, "And I know every time I get ready to play the brushes, I say 'I'm going to tap dance for you now, and these are Jo Jones' licks that he taught me.'"[13]

At the start of their careers, the drummers Max Roach, Kenny Clarke, and Art Blakey were greatly influenced by rhythm tappers. Roach accompanied Groundhog and Baby Laurence and learned steps from them. He recalled performing with Laurence: "We usually did our act as an encore. I would play brushes on the snare and he would just dance and we'd exchange things, call and response. I would imitate him and then I would play time over it." In 1961, while playing with the Charlie Mingus band, Dannie Richmond enhanced his drumming technique by studying Laurence's feet every night:

> The band would play the head on the theme and Baby Laurence played the breaks. Little by little we worked it where at first I was just doing stop-time, fours, so much that I'd memorized every lick of his. I learned that it wasn't just single strokes involved in the drums. My concept was that if you had the single strokes down, you could play anything. It's not

true. It's almost true, but not totally. And the way Laurence would mix paradiddles along with single strokes. He could do all of that with his feet. It got to where we're doing fours together. He'd dance four, then we played threes, twos, one bar apiece, but I was copying him. I'd more or less play what he danced. I was trying to keep it in the context of melody dance and, mind you, to me that was the same as a saxophone player trying to play like Charlie Parker. He was the only one who could dance to Charlie Parker tunes. . . . It was a gas for me to duplicate what Laurence danced. When he switched up on me and changed the time, there was no way I could play that.

According to Philly Joe Jones, "the drummer who has been a dancer can play better than someone who has never danced. See, the drummer catches the dancer, especially when a dancer's doing wings. And the cymbals move at the same time to catch the dancer."[14]

In the thirties and forties, rhythm tap's greatest exponents functioned in closely knit circles that included singers, comedians, jazz musicians, and chorus line dancers. The various types of performers shared rehearsal and performance spaces, jam sessions, and living quarters; they attended sports events and parties; they belonged to the same fraternal clubs. Billy Strayhorn, Duke Ellington's co-composer, was the last official president of the Copasetics, a club organized by tap dancers but with musicians such as Dizzy Gillespie and Lionel Hampton among its membership.

The impact of the jam session, or "cutting contest," on rhythm tap's evolution parallels much of what Ellison has to say about the relationship of the jam session to the development of jazz instrumentalists. Ralph Ellison called the jam session the "jazzman's true academy":

It is here that he learns tradition, group techniques and style. For although since the twenties many jazzmen have had conservatory training and were well grounded in formal theory and instrumental technique, when we approach jazz we are entering quite a different sphere of training. Here it is more meaningful to speak, not of courses of study, of grades and degrees, but of apprenticeship, ordeals, initiation ceremonies, of rebirth. For after the jazzman has learned the fundamentals of his instrument and the traditional techniques of jazz—the intonations, the mute work, manipulation of timbre, the body of traditional styles— he must then "find himself," must be reborn, must find, as it were, his soul. All this through achieving that subtle identification between his instrument and his deepest drives which will allow him to express his own unique ideas and his own unique voice. He must achieve, in short, his self-determined identity. In this his instructors are his fellow musicians, especially the acknowledged masters, and his recognition of manhood depends upon their acceptance of his ability as having reached a standard which is all the more difficult for not having been codified. This does not depend upon his ability to simply hold a job but upon his power to express an individuality in tone.[15]

In nightclubs and on street corners tap dancers participated in jam sessions — exchanging ideas, inspiring one another, and battling for a place in the rhythm tappers' hierarchy of artistic excellence. Jimmy Crawford jammed with many rhythm tap artists: "Dancers influenced the music a whole lot in those days. Sometimes we'd have jam sessions with just tap dancers, buck dancers and drums. Big Sid Catlett was one of the greatest show drummers who ever lived. He could accompany, add on, improvise, so well. And believe me, those rhythm dancers really used to inspire you."[16] No jam sessions were as exciting as those held at the legendary Hoofer's Club, where the reigning tap kings of the early thirties included Raymond Winfield, Honi Coles, Harold Mablin, and Roland Holder.

In 1932, when Baby Laurence went to New York as a singer with the Don Redman Band, he headed straight to the Hoofer's Club: "Don discouraged my dancing, but when we hit town my first stop was the Hoofer's Club — it was the biggest thrill of my life." The cardinal rule there was "Thou Shalt Not Copy Another's Steps — Exactly." Those foolish enough to break that rule in public had to suffer the consequences. Dancers lined up to get front row theater seats when tap acts performed at local theaters. According to Laurence, "they watched you like hawks and if you used any of their pet steps, they just stood right up in the theater and told everybody about it at the top of their voices."[17] Leonard Reed's first stop in New York was also the Hoofer's Club:

> You could hear dancing the minute you got in the building. There was always dancin' going on, known dancers and unknown dancers. Bubbles would come occasionally. Bill Robinson came in occasionally. . . . All the dancers would hang out, and they would trade ideas. That was affectionately called "stealin' steps." Everybody did it. That's how you learned. You would do something, and you'd say to the other dancers, "You tryin' to steal it? Alright, do it!" "Let me see you do this!" And they'd try it. Of course, when they did it, it was slightly different. But that's how it was. Everybody was always showin' steps and trying to steal steps. It was an amazing time.[18]

The very best dancers in this tradition have unique styles that are immediately recognizable aurally and visually, although the emphasis, of course, is on sound. This drive toward individual expressiveness grows right out of an African American aesthetic sense that puts supreme value on what the African Americanist John Vlach calls "freewheeling improvisation and innovation, . . . distinctive dynamism, . . . and delight in the surprise value of new, not completely anticipated discovery." What these dancers value most is not the exactness of frozen choreography and set routines developed by others, but the joy that is inherent in improvisational flights of freedom. Perhaps Baby Laurence said it best: "From my point of view, having a choreographer tell me what to do would ruin everything. I wouldn't be able to improvise or interpret the music, and I couldn't express myself."[19]

During the early sixties, Stanley Dance conducted a "Spontaneous Opinion" poll in *Metronome* of twenty-eight jazz musicians. One of the questions asked was "Who is the greatest dancer you ever saw?" Twenty-six named tap dancers and over half of the votes went to Baby Laurence— a tap artist with a jazz musician's sense of his craft.[20]

Jazz musicians and rhythm tap dancers were obviously in pursuit of identical artistic goals. Their partnership in the thirties and forties mirrored much more than a convenient musical package. Their mutual admiration grew out of a special kinship based on similar aesthetic points of view and what Albert Murray calls a shared "idiomatic orientation."

Numerous rhythm tappers performed with jazz bands during the thirties and forties. Honi Coles worked as a single with Count Basie, Claude Hopkins, Jimmy Lunceford, Fats Waller, Duke Ellington, Lucky Millinder, Louis Armstrong, and Cab Calloway. Coles felt "it was such a kick to work with the great bands, especially with guys like Fats Waller—the looser of the band leaders. . . . People like Fats Waller and Louie Armstrong were people who enjoyed and loved life and showed it every instant of the day."[21] Buster Brown toured with Count Basie, Jimmy Lunceford, and Dizzy Gillespie; Bunny Briggs with Duke Ellington, Earl Hines, Count Basie, and Charlie Barnet; Jeni LeGon with Fats Waller and Count Basie; Baby Laurence with Count Basie, Duke Ellington, and Woody Herman; the Miller Brothers and Lois with Jimmy Lunceford and Cab Calloway; Coles and Atkins with Billy Eckstine, Count Basie, and Charlie Barnet; and Peg Leg Bates with Erskine Hawkins, Claude Hopkins, Duke Ellington, Louis Armstrong, and many others.[22]

Although dancers appeared with big bands in theaters throughout the country, the premiere stage and number one testing ground in America was Harlem's Apollo Theater. Beginning in 1934, stage shows were built around such well-known jazz bands as those led by Duke Ellington, Count

Basie, Don Redman, Chick Webb, Lucky Millinder, and Fletcher Henderson.[23] The Apollo opened around 10:00 A.M. and offered four to five shows per day starting with a short film, a newsreel, and a featured film, followed by a revue. Presented in the spring of 1934, *The Golliwog Revue* was a typical show that consisted of seven acts including Don Redman's band, the headliner; chorus line dancers; the Jack Storm Company, an acrobatic act; Leroy and Edith, the Apollo lindy hop contest winners; Myra Johnson, a singer; the Four Bobs, tap dancers; and Jazzlips Richardson, an eccentric dancer. Throughout the show Johnny Lee Long and Pigmeat Markham, comedians, joked with Ralph Cooper, the host.

In addition to their own presentations, the featured bands played for the chorus lines and for all the dance acts. Andy Kirk backed Bill Robinson at the Apollo: "Playing the Apollo was different from playing a dance hall, because in a dance hall the dancers had to dance to your music. At the Apollo, with a star like Bojangles, we had to play music for *him* to dance to. . . . We always had regard for the artist, whatever he was doing, and our music was background. We wanted to play it right—the way he wanted it." The Apollo had a good floor for dancers. And the place was known for unusually demanding and discriminating audiences. "When big name dancers played the Apollo, there was nothing in the audience but dancers with their shoes," said Sandman Sims. "Up in the balcony, dancers, and the first six rows, you saw nothing but tap dancers, wanta-be tap dancers, gonna-be tap dancers, tried-to-be tap dancers. That's the reason a guy would want to dance at the Apollo."[24]

Under the direction of black producer-choreographers (who maintained their own chorus lines), the Apollo revues changed each week. Charlie Davis, Leonard Harper, Addison Carey, Teddie Blackman, and Clarence Robinson also took their chorus lines on the independent theater circuit 'Round the World. The Apollo chorus line was the best in New York. Honi Coles "was astounded at the dancing ability that most of these young ladies had. A dancing act could come into the Apollo with all original material and when they left at the end of the week, the chorus lines would have stolen many of the outstanding things that they did. . . . The production numbers that these girls did were often as effective as anything the stars or any of the acts would do."[25]

The role of chorus line dancers in the development of jazz has been consistently overlooked by jazz and dance historians. According to Dicky Wells, many jazz musicians felt a kinship with chorus line dancers: "They used to be the biggest lift to musicians, because we thought alike." "They were more important than people realize. You might say we composed while they danced—a whole lot of swinging rhythm. That's when we invented new things and recorded them [the] next day."[26]

The Apollo's dance contests featured some of the most dedicated big band followers in the country. Their intricate steps devised to the swinging rhythms of America's jumpingest jazz bands could only be matched in enthusiasm by the contests held further uptown at Harlem's legendary dance hall the Savoy Ballroom, known among the initiated as "the track." The artist Romare Bearden went there three nights a week during the early thirties: "The best dancing in the world was there, and the best music. . . . You'd want to be either in Harlem then or in Paris. These were the two places where things were happening."[27]

When the Savoy opened its doors on 12 March 1926, over five thousand people rocked the city block–long building to the rhythms of Fess Williams and His Royal Flush Orchestra and the Charleston Bearcats. "Few first-nighters will ever forget the dynamic Fess, whose eye-catching trade mark was a shimmering, glittering diamond studded suit and whose showmanship and musicianship eventually catapulted him to national fame from the newly-born Savoy's No.1 bandstand."[28]

That first night, Fletcher Henderson's Roseland Orchestra made a guest appearance at the Savoy as did the legendary tap dancer Eddie Rector. Leaders of Harlem's benevolent, social, cultural, civic, educational, and welfare groups were present along with Hollywood and Broadway stars, social leaders, church dignitaries, sports and newspaper personalities, and federal, state, and city government officials. The Savoy offered quite a showcase for this grand event: "Architecturally, the Savoy dazzled with a spacious lobby framing a huge, cut-glass chandelier and marble staircase, an orange and blue dance hall with soda fountain, tables, and heavy carpeting covering half its area, the remainder a burnished dance floor 250 feet by 50 feet with two bandstands and a disappearing stage at the end."[29]

This institution of international fame surpassed all of America's top dance halls in grandeur and impact on American music and dance. The Savoy's twenty-fifth anniversary booklet was justified in boasting: "From [the] Savoy's mammoth mahogany floor, there was launched a long succession of dance fads, styles, and crazes that 'caught fire' almost overnight, capturing the imagination of dancers in every nook and corner of this country and sweeping far to the four winds and the seven seas for universal popularity." Dances that started or were made popular at the Savoy include the lindy hop, the flying Charleston, the big apple, the stomp, the jitterbug jive, the snakehips, the rhumboogie, variations of the shimmy and the peabody, and new interpretations of the bunny hug and the turkey trot.[30]

Charles Buchanan, the Savoy's manager, paid such dancers as Shorty Snowden to come in and "perform" for his clientele. Couples went there to practice during the day, and the most skillful "rug cutters" were constantly vying for first place honors in the northeast corner of the dance floor, known as "the Corner." There an invisible rope surrounded a dancing area that met the requirements of ritual, recreation, and performance. The "Saturday night function" that is associated with affirmation, celebration, and freedom was played out in this setting, where individual expression and inventiveness were as prized as technical virtuosity and the ability to execute carefully rehearsed maneuvers. As at the Apollo, no one could copy another dancer's steps. Shorty Snowden, the self-styled introducer of the lindy, was king for many years. Although his expertise was limited to the floor lindy (as opposed to the lindy, which had aerial steps), his dancing skills still far exceeded the capabilities of the average dancer.[31]

The lindy revolutionized American dance. Its fundamental approach can still be seen in social dancing. The breakaway, its most important element, allows for improvisation that might incorporate old steps or create new ones. An influential predecessor of the lindy was the Charleston swing. Barbara Engelbrecht explains that "this 'swing' infused the Lindy Hop's basic step—the syncopated two step, with the accent on the off-beat—with a relaxed and ebullient quality. And this relaxed and ebullient style of execution gives the impression, like the music, of the beat moving 'inexorably ahead.' The dancers' feet appear to 'fly' in syncopated rhythms, while the body appears to 'hold' the fine line of balance in calm contrast to the headlong rush of the feet." According to Stearns and Stearns, the lindy flowed more smoothly and horizontally than the earlier two-step, had more rhythmic continuity, and was more complicated.[32]

At the Savoy, black musicians and dancers, armed with the musical innovations of Louis Armstrong, helped develop the formula for what was eventually call "swing music," which swept the country during the Great Depression and ricocheted far beyond the Western Hemisphere. The relationship between dance halls and jazz is eloquently explained by Ralph Ellison:

> Jazz, for all the insistence of the legends, has been far more closely associated with cabarets and dance halls than with brothels, and it was these which provided both the employment for the musicians and an

audience initiated and aware of the overtones of the music; which knew the language of riffs, the unstated meanings of the blues idiom, and the dance steps developed from, and complementary to, its rhythms. And in the beginning it was in the Negro dance hall and night club that jazz was most completely a part of a total cultural expression; and in which it was freest and most satisfying, both for the musicians and for those in whose lives it played a major role.

"The Savoy Ballroom was the ultimate conferrer of postgraduate degrees in big bandsmanship," asserts Nat Hentoff. Only the best bands were allowed to return and Charles Buchanan, the Savoy's manager, called the best bands the ones that kept the floor filled. Night after night, the dancers and musicians at the Savoy spurred one another on to greater heights and earthier depths—always with an attitude of elegance.[33]

During the forties, Dicky Wells played trombone at the Savoy for six months with Jimmy Rushing's band: "There was plenty of competition on the next stand then, with all the different bands coming and going. And the Lindy Hoppers there made you watch your P's and Q's. The dancers would come and tell you if you didn't play. They made the guys play, and they'd stand in front patting their hands until you got the right tempo."[34]

Countless jazz musicians have commented on the importance of dance to their music:

William "Cat" Anderson: "I enjoy having a floor full of dancers. It seems to me that everybody enjoys the music more, even those who are not dancing but just standing there watching the dancers. We play more swinging things then than we would at a concert, because people like to get up and move about in rhythm."[35]

Duke Ellington: "They used to have great dancers up at the Ritz, Bridgeport. Every now and then you go into a ballroom like that where they have great dancers. It's a kick to play for people who really jump and swing. On two occasions up there we were using a substitute drummer, but we didn't have to worry about him because the dancers were carrying the band and the drummer. You start playing, the dancers start dancing, and they have such a great beat you just hang on![36]

Pops Foster: "In about 1935 or 1936 we started playing for audiences that just sat there. I never liked this, I always liked to play for an audience that dances."[37]

Lester Young: "I wish jazz were played more for dancing. I have a lot of fun playing for dances because I like to dance, too. The rhythm of the dancers comes back to you when you're playing. When you're playing for dancing, it all adds up to playing the right tempo. After three or four tempos, you find the tempos they like. What they like changes from dance date to dance date."[38]

Baby Dodds: "When I first went to New York it seemed very strange to have people sitting around and listening rather than dancing. In a way it was similar to theater work. But it was peculiar for me because I always felt as though I was doing something for the people if they danced to the music. It never seemed the same when they just sat around and listened. We played for dancing and quite naturally we expected people to dance."[39]

Jimmy Crawford: "In ballrooms, where there's dancing like I was raised on, when everybody is giving to the beat, and just moving, and the house is bouncing—that inspires you to play. It's different when you go to those places where it's 'cool' and the people just sit listening. I don't care too much for the 'cool,' harsh pulsation. I don't like music where it's simply a matter of 'Listen to my changes, man!', and there's no emotion or swing. I think Louis Armstrong has done more to promote good feeling among earthy people than anyone. He can't speak all those foreign languages, but he lets a certain feeling speak for him. You can play too many notes, but if you make it simple, make it an ass-shaker, then the music speaks to the people."[40]

Frankie Manning, Norma Miller, and many other lindy hop experts attest to the ability of the Savoy big bands to "speak to the people." Constantly driven toward excellence and technical perfection, the Savoy Lindy Hoppers perfected the lindy in direct response to the dynamics of the musicians. According to Stearns and Stearns, the stage was set for movement innovations with the appearance of a group of Kansas City musicians in 1932. The power and drive of the Bennie Moten Band "generated a more flowing, lifting momentum. The effect on the dancers was to increase the energy and speed of execution."[41]

During the midthirties, a monumental change in the lindy took place when Frankie Manning and his partner Freida Washington introduced the first aerial or air step (called "over the back") in a Savoy dance contest against Shorty Snowden's Lindy Hoppers. What followed was the development and perfection of numerous air steps by Savoy dancers. Manning and Washington were members of Whitey's Lindy Hoppers, a group of excellent dancers organized by Herbert White, the Savoy's floor manager. In 1936, Manning developed the first ensemble routines, which made it possible to easily adapt the lindy hop to stage presentations.[42]

As the dance became airborne, its popularity spread the length and breadth of America. By the fall of 1936, White managed three teams, each comprised of three couples. Frankie Manning became the main choreographer for the first-string team; during his years with Whitey's Lindy Hoppers, they became internationally known. The Savoy dancers traveled with many great jazz bands, including those of Duke Ellington, Count Basie, Chick Webb, and Cab Calloway. Manning was a member of the teams that traveled to Europe, Australia, New Zealand, and South America. The Savoy dancers appeared in a production of *The Hot Mikado* with Bill Robinson at the 1939 World's Fair, at the Cotton Club and Radio City Music Hall in New York City, at the Moulin Rouge in Paris, and in a musical short, *Hot Chocolate* (1941), with Duke Ellington. In addition to *Hot Chocolate*, White's teams appeared in the films *A Day at the Races* (1937), *Radio City Revels* (1938), and *Hellzapoppin'* (1941). With the exception of *A Day at the Races*, Frankie Manning was the choreographer for all of the film appearances.

Between 1935 and 1950, Savoy lindy hop teams won fourteen championships at the annual Harvest Moon Ball, a competitive dance spectacle held at Madison Square Garden in New York. During the thirties and the forties a significant number of Savoy regulars made the transition from amateur to professional. Whitey's Lindy Hoppers disbanded after Manning and most of the group's other men were drafted during World War II.[43]

The Savoy's success owes as much to the famous "battles of the bands" staged there as it does to the music and the dancers who created visualizations of the music. For most of the thirties, the all-time favorite at the Savoy was the hard-driving band of Chick Webb. When a band battle was scheduled, Webb's musicians trained like prize fighters and had special section rehearsals to prepare for the "kill." "The brass used to be downstairs, the saxophones upstairs, and the rhythm would get together somewhere else. We had the reputation of running any band out that came to the Savoy. But just forget about Duke!" Another tough opponent was the Count Basie Band. Dicky Wells called Basie's rhythm section "nothing less than a Cadillac with the force of a Mack truck." The alto saxophonist Earle Warren recalled one occasion when the Count reigned supreme.

> *Swingin' the Blues* was built to be a house breaker. . . . "We began working on it when we were on the road and getting things together for a battle of jazz with Chick Webb at the Savoy. The battle of jazz was something to be reckoned with and we had to have something fresh and new to bring to the Savoy or we would falter at the finish line. So we proceeded to rehearse diligently. . . . By the time we got it together we were

cookin'. At the Savoy we saved it until about halfway down in the program. Chick did his thing, *God Bless*, and then we reached into our bag and pulled out this powerhouse. When we unloaded our cannons, that was the end. It was one of those nights—I'll never forget it." Nor will anyone else who heard it, for that was one of the few nights at the Savoy when Chick Webb lost a battle of jazz.[44]

One of the most famous battles at the Savoy was the night the Benny Goodman Band faced Chick Webb and His Little Chicks. The Savoy was packed and many more people waited outside. For blocks, traffic was backed up in every direction—with approximately twenty-five thousand people trying to attend. Goodman pulled out all of his guns, but could not win the crowd. When Webb ended the session with a drum solo, the dancers exploded in a thunderous ovation. "Goodman and his drummer, Gene Krupa, just stood there shaking their heads."[45]

The Savoy was Webb's "musical home," and he played on and off there for ten years until his death in 1939. His phenomenal success is explained by Duke Ellington:

> Some musicians are dancers, and Chick Webb was. You can dance with a lot of things besides your feet. Billy Strayhorn was another dancer—in his mind. He was a dance-writer. Chick Webb was a dance-drummer who painted pictures of dances with his drums. . . . The reason why Chick Webb had such control, such command of his audiences at the Savoy ballroom, was because he was always in communication with the dancers and felt it the way they did. And that is probably the biggest reason why he could cut all the other bands that went in there.[46]

Ralph Ellison has written that after the church and the school, the third most vital institution in the lives of African Americans has been the public jazz dance. There the artistry of dancers, musicians, and singers converged to create a union that personifies what jazz is all about. Ellison spent time in Oklahoma watching Jimmy Rushing on the bandstand: "It was when Jimmy's voice began to soar with the spirit of the blues that the dancers—and the musicians—achieved that feeling of communion which was the true meaning of the public jazz dance. The blues, the singer, the band and the dancers formed the vital whole of jazz as an institutional form, and even today neither part is quite complete without the rest." Wynton Marsalis's conception of an ideal forum for jazz is an intimate communal setting in which members can choose to participate by dancing or by engaging in "call and response" with the musicians: "We love to have the people get into the music even if we're in a concert hall. . . . People should be able to come in and out of the hall, it's like a community event. We're community musicians."[47]

In the late fifties, the Savoy Ballroom closed and later the building was demolished. Ralph Ellison had this to say about the Savoy's importance as a cultural institution of the thirties.

> In those days, for instance, the Savoy Ballroom was one of our great cultural institutions. In the effort to build much needed public housing, it has been destroyed. But then it was thriving and people were coming to Harlem from all over the world. The great European and American composers were coming there to listen to jazz — Stravinsky, Poulenc. The great jazz bands were coming there. Great dancers were being created there. People from Downtown were always there because the Savoy was one of the great centers of culture in the United States, even though it was then thought of as simply a place of entertainment.[48]

The musicians, dancers, and singers that walked through the doors of the Savoy infused American culture with elegance and brilliance in music and movement and an unmistakable style that has been embraced by cultures worldwide. Albert Murray observed, "No institutions had more to do with the development or the sophistication, the variety, the richness and the precision of jazz than institutions like the Savoy ballroom. But dance has always been central and I always want to see jazz connected with dance. What we should try to reach in a concert hall is the same kind of ambience that one reaches in a dance hall."[49]

Vernacular Dance on Stage: An Overview

The dances that began on the farms, plantations, levees, and urban streets of colonial America evolved through minstrelsy and moved onto the "stages" of traveling shows, vaudeville, musical theater, cabarets, and night clubs. The development and growth of this country's preeminent vernacular dance paralleled the evolution of African American music and took a giant leap forward in the twenties, thirties, and forties, when the connections between black singers, dance acts, and jazz musicians revolutionized American culture.

Throughout his life, Duke Ellington, arguably America's greatest twentieth-century composer, never severed the tie between his music and dance. Even the sacred concerts, late in his career, featured such dancers as Geoffrey Holder, Baby Laurence, Bunny Briggs, and Buster Brown. Ellington always preferred having musicians in his band who could dance: "I used to be a pretty good dancer at one time. I think it's very important that a musician should dance. . . . Dancing is very important to people who play music with a beat. I think that people who don't dance, or who never did dance, don't really understand the beat. What they get in their minds is a mechanical thing not totally unacademic. I know musicians who don't and never did dance, and they have difficulty communicating." According to Albert Murray, one of the first Ellington musicians that played and danced in front of the band was Freddy Jenkins, known as "Little Posey," but the all-time king of the dancer-musicians in this band was Ray Nance, nicknamed "Floorshow." During his years with Ellington, he was featured on trumpet and violin and as a dancer and singer.[50]

As Wynton Marsalis perceptively remarked, "Duke Ellington understood the importance of romance in body movement, the romantic aspect of body movement to jazz music." When Ellington reached his sixties, he danced in front of the band much more than he had in previous years. Still, movement was important to him all along. According to Albert Murray, earlier in his career "there was that subtle thing, the way he would walk and as [Count] Basie and those guys would say, 'It was all such a picture.'" Many jazz musicians knew how to move with style: "Ellington had that big wide-legged stride and Earl [Hines] had that flashy patent leather tip and Nat King Cole put it like his shoes were velvet, like they were socks and Basie would come out there like he didn't know what was happening. He was doing the hell out of that stuff. They all had that — Hamp [Lionel Hampton] always danced, Cab [Calloway] could sing and dance."[51]

Louis Armstrong, America's quintessential twentieth-century musician/singer/dancer, was "considered the finest dancer among the [jazz] musicians" of the twenties. During the midtwenties, at Chicago's Sunset Cafe, Armstrong played in a show that included Buck and Bubbles, Edith Spencer, Rector and Cooper, and Mae Alix. On Friday nights Charleston contests were held. The show's producer staged the finale of the main show as a dancing act for four musicians in the band: Armstrong, Earl Hines, Tubby Hall, and Joe Walker. Armstrong remembered: "We would stretch out across that floor doing the Charleston as fast as the music would play it. Boy, oh boy, you talking about four cats picking them up and laying them down — that was us."[52]

Another sparkling partnership on the dance floor consisted of the jazz singer Sarah Vaughan and Dizzy Gillespie. Vaughan recalled that during the early forties when she and Gillespie toured with Earl Hines, "we'd get to swinging so much, Dizzy would come down and grab me and start jitterbugging all over the place." Ella Fitzgerald had similar memories: "We used to take the floor over. Yeah, do the Lindy Hop because we could do it. Yeah, we danced like mad together. . . . We'd go with the old Savoy steps." Gillespie, noted for a "snake hips" dance specialty at the start of his career, always created dances to his music: "A feeling for dancing was always a part of my music; to play it right, you've got to move. If a guy doesn't move properly when he's playing my music, he ain't got the feeling. Thelonious Monk, Illinois Jacquet, and all those instrumentalists who move a lot, are playing just what they're doing with their bodies."[53]

Thelonious Monk, like Ellington, never severed the connection between jazz music and dance. According to the pianist Randy Weston, "not only is Monk such a master pianist and composer, but when you watch him play, he does a complete ballet. He doesn't just play the piano, but he puts his whole body into the piano. . . . It's a whole dance." Monk would often rise from the piano and break into bodily visualizations of his music. "When his music was happening," according to Ben Riley, a jazz drummer, "then he'd get up and do his little dance because he was feeling good and he knew you knew where you were and the music was swinging and that's what he wanted. So, he'd say, 'I don't have to play now, you're making it happen.'"[54]

Early in his career, Count Basie played with Gonzelle White and Her Jazz Band, a stand-up act that featured dancing musicians who performed all kinds of tricks with their instruments. Basie would play behind his back, stand on one foot, play with his leg on the piano, or perform fancy tricks with his hands and arms. Gonzelle White's trumpet player, Harry Smith, was featured as a dancer who tapped, did splits, buck and wing, kicks, and the soft shoe. Basie was knocked out by the group's drummer: "Freddy Crump was a top-notch drummer, and he did all of the fancy things that show-band drummers used to, like throwing his sticks in the air and catching them like a juggler without losing a beat. He was a whole little act by himself, especially when it came to taking bows. He used to come dancing back in from the wings and hit the drum as he slid into a split. He used to grab the curtain and ride up with it, bowing and waving at the audience applauding."[55]

But the all-time experts of show-band novelties were the dancing-singing musicians that played with Jimmy Lunceford. Eddie Durham, an arranger, believed that Lunceford's band had the slickest, most precise stage presentation in the business: "There was nobody could play like that band! They would come out and play a dance routine. The Shim Sham Shimmy was popular then and six of the guys would come down and dance to it—like a tap dance, crossing their feet and sliding."[56] What followed were impersonations of other bands and glee club–like song presentations. Nat Pierce, a jazz pianist, saw Lunceford's band perform in Boston: "His four trumpet players were throwing their horns up to the ceiling. It was a big, high hall, and they'd throw them up twenty or thirty feet, pick them out of the air, and hit the next chord. I was just amazed by the whole thing."[57]

Commenting on the relationship between jazz and dance, Murray observes that

> whatever else it was used for, it was always mostly dance music. Even when it was being performed as an act in a variety show on a vaudeville stage, the most immediate and customary response consisted of such foot tapping, hand clapping, body rocking, and hip rolling as came as close to total dance movement as the facilities and the occasion would allow. Nor was the response likely to be anything except more of the same when the most compelling lyrics were being delivered by Ma Rainey or Bessie Smith, whose every stage gesture, by the way, was also as much dance movement as anything else.[58]

From Billy Kersands's captivating Virginia essence to the dynamic glides, spins, and splits of James Brown, African American dancing singers have captured the imaginations of people throughout the world. The long-standing tradition of dancing singers in African American culture reaches back to central and western Africa, where song was always coupled with bodily movement. Many of America's most outstanding twentieth-century singers began as dancers or included dancing in their performances.

Just after World War II, the relationship that dancers, musicians, and singers had enjoyed for so many years was fractured by federal, state, and city governments. In 1944, a 30 percent federal excise tax was levied against "dancing" night clubs. Later it was reduced to 20 percent. "No Dancing Allowed" signs went up all over the country.[59] Max Roach argues that the new tax signaled the end of variety entertainment as it had been known: "It was levied on all places where they had entertainment. It was levied in case they had public dancing, singing, storytelling, humor, or jokes on stage. This tax is the real story behind why dancing, not just tap dancing, but public dancing per se and also singing, quartets, comedy, all these kinds of things, were just out. Club owners, promoters, couldn't afford to pay the city tax, state tax, government tax."[60]

Dancers, singers, and comedians suffered. Only jazz instrumentalists were able to thrive under these conditions. According to Roach, "if somebody got up to dance, there would be 20 per cent more tax on the dollar. If someone got up there and sang a song, it would be 20 per cent more. If someone danced on the stage it was 20 per cent more." As a result jazz gradually lost its dancing audience. People began sitting down in clubs, and as agents began pushing small combos, only a few big bands were able to survive.[61]

Social dancing suffered, but as usual African Americans found other avenues for public dancing. Professional dancers, on the other hand, were faced with a serious dilemma. Many tap dancers turned away from dance to other careers. The eccentric dancer Bessie Dudley eventually found a job in a Long Island factory. By the early fifties, promoters were pushing vocal groups instead of dancers.[62] With the help of Cholly Atkins, these groups became the new disseminators of vernacular dance on stage. They comprised a new generation of dancing singers.

The extremely rich cross-fertilization of African American vernacular dance, jazz, and singing in the twenties, thirties, and forties brought character and style to American culture. The dance that evolved during that period in America's history is "classic jazz dance." Duke Ellington had this to say about a renewal of the association between jazz music and jazz dance: "With the new music that already is, and what is coming, there's no predicting what effect the disassociation from dancing will have in the future, but my own idea is that it is going to make a big fat curve and come right back to where it was, except that it will be on a slightly higher musical plane."[63]

Chapter Seven

"Let the Punishment Fit the Crime": The Vocal Choreography of Cholly Atkins

> He's the wellspring from whence we flow. And the groups that want to be viable go back to Cholly. . . . What he uses is more of a scientific approach than a fad approach. Cholly understands the way that the human body moves, he understands the grace of dance.
> —Interview with Melvin Franklin

From the twenties through most of the forties, American tap dance in the jazz/rhythm tradition experienced its heyday. Suddenly in the late forties, the bottom dropped out for many rhythm tap dancers who had established successful careers in vaudeville, in musicals, and with big bands. By the sixties, even the great champion and chronicler of American vernacular dance, Marshall Stearns, wondered if classic jazz dance was vanishing forever. Although we know now that black vernacular dance evolves in a cyclical pattern, no one could have predicted in the sixties that dance movements from the twenties, thirties, and forties would live on through the nineties and beyond in many of the performance traditions that span African American culture.

The lively existence of such black dancing vocal groups as those in the *Motor Town Revue* helped preserve and recycle much of the vocabulary of classic jazz dance, including some tap. The man largely responsible for this particular cultural transference was Cholly Atkins, a jazz dance artist who worked as a choreographer for Motown Records from 1965 to 1971.

On 30 September 1913, Charles Atkinson was born to Sylvan and Christine Atkinson in Birmingham, Alabama. Four years later, the couple broke up, and Charles and his brother relocated with their mother to

Buffalo, New York. Christine Atkinson was a fine social dancer who, like many black parents, danced around the house with her children to tunes played on an old victrola. When he was ten years old, Charles won a Charleston contest at a local theater, and by the time he was in high school he was alternating basketball practice with rehearsals for musicals. The school's physical education teacher, a Russian who was an excellent dancer, directed these shows and taught many of the students to soft-shoe. When the Chocolate Steppers appeared at a local theater with Cab Calloway, Atkins copied their steps, practiced to Teddy Wilson records at home, and became solidly convinced that he was going to become a dancer. By the early thirties, he had earned enough of a reputation for his dancing skills that he was occasionally choreographing chorus line routines at small black midwestern clubs.[1]

In 1933, Atkinson worked as a singing waiter at a club near Buffalo, where he met William Porter, a dancing waiter who taught him rhythm tap. Their friendship led to the formation of the Rhythm Pals, a vaudeville-style song-and-dance duet. Three years later, with his name changed to Cholly Atkins, he and his partner sang and danced their way along the California coast, working at nightclubs, performing in black musical shorts, and appearing as extras in Hollywood films. Atkins also did tap sound tracks for white chorus line dancers who backed such stars as Eleanor Powell. Although the Hollywood appearances were all typecast roles—he was cast as a Mongolian in *The Charge of the Light Brigade*—this period in his life was to have an extremely important influence on his future endeavors: "I used to take my food in a cardboard box—a sandwich, a bottle of milk, and an apple—and visit other sets during lunch hour. Nobody ever chased me away, and I saw a lot of choreographers at work."[2] At one such session, he witnessed the Nicholas Brothers rehearsing their "Chattanooga Choo Choo" routine with dance director Nick Castle. While choreographing and staging routines for female chorus line dancers in small black nightclubs, Atkins never missed an opportunity to learn from other artists. "My friends called me a rehearsal freak because I used to watch everybody else's rehearsals. That's how I learned to produce, direct and choreograph."[3]

By 1939, the Rhythm Pals sought work in New York, where the partnership soon dissolved. But Atkins's newly acquired choreographic skills landed him a job dancing and helping to choreograph acts for the renowned Cotton Club Boys, who were appearing with Bill Robinson in *The Hot Mikado* at the World's Fair in New York. At the time, Atkins happened to be living in the same building with Honi Coles. "Everyday we'd go to

Mt. Morris Park to play ball, and that's how we got to be real close friends."[4] Coles, with his professional reputation already established in New York, took him under his wing, introducing him to dancers and producers. When one of the Cotton Club Boys became ill, Coles suggested Atkins as a replacement: "That's the best thing that ever happened to the Cotton Club Boys because they were just six dancing boys who did what the producer told them. . . . Cholly made an act out of them."[5]

Honi Coles had the fastest feet in the business: "He could do all of [John] Bubbles' steps but faster." In the twenties and thirties, Philadelphia was a tap dance heaven—even paper boys would put down their bags and join the street-corner competition. In 1931, Coles had left Philadelphia to serve a short stint with the Miller Brothers, who performed one of his routines on narrow planks suspended five feet over the stage. Later he worked with the Lucky Seven Trio, also called the Three Giants of Rhythm. Coles had toured with the Cab Calloway Band since 1940, and in 1942, he suggested that Cholly Atkins and his second partner, the singer and dancer Dottie Saulters, join Cab's revue. In April 1943, Coles was inducted into the army, and Atkins was drafted the following September.[6]

Three years later they were living at 2040 Seventh Avenue in Harlem with the Mills Brothers, Billy Eckstine, and several other black performers. Their formation of a class act team, Coles and Atkins, led to a series of tours from 1946 to 1949, including a very successful European tour in 1948. They appeared primarily with big bands, including those of Count Basie, Cab Calloway, Johnny Otis (featuring the Ink Spots), Charlie Barnet, Louis Armstrong, Lionel Hampton, and Billy Eckstine. In the film *Over the Top to Bebop*, Marshall Stearns explains that the class act "started with the soft-shoe, the sand and the shuffle; and it grew up and became a dance in which you showed elegance and dignity and precision. And every class act in the Thirties and Forties had their own soft shoe." Coles and Atkins's particular soft shoe was inspired by Ethel Waters, who was present at many of their early rehearsals and hummed "Taking a Chance on Love" as they pieced together bits of tap and authentic jazz dance to develop a routine that is now a tap classic.[7]

By 1949, with no lines and one song, Coles and Atkins were stopping the show every night in the Broadway musical *Gentlemen Prefer Blondes*. Finally they had landed a steady job for three years, but it proved to be merely a temporary godsend: "I think one of the most discouraging times in my life was when Cholly Atkins and myself had just finished 3 years with *Gentlemen Prefer Blondes*. We did 2 years on Broadway and one year

on the road. We laid off for six months after that. We couldn't find a job."
Unwilling to give up dancing completely, Atkins accepted a job as head
of the tap department at the Katherine Dunham School of Arts and Research, and Coles opened a studio with Pete Nugent. During this same
period, Atkins also taught at the International School of Dance at Carnegie Hall and choreographed for the June Taylor Dancers. Although jobs
were scarce, the duo did manage to squeeze out a few club dates. They
were back in full force again in 1955, working with Tony Martin's Las
Vegas act and later with Pearl Bailey for about a year and a half. But tap
was fast becoming a thing of the past. By 1960, in order to make ends meet,
Atkins was coaching again, while Coles replaced Leonard Reed as production manager at Harlem's Apollo Theater.[8]

When asked what caused the demise of tap, many of the living experts
point to rock and roll or Agnes de Mille. But a close look at the political
and socioeconomic events from the late forties through the fifties reveals
a series of factors that hurt American vernacular dance in general and the
rhythm tap tradition in particular: the sudden shift in taste on the Broadway stage; the false depiction of and eventually the absence of tap in
movies; the advent of bebop, with its emphasis away from big bands and
toward small jazz combos; the 1944 tax levied against "dancing" night
clubs;[9] the gradual disappearance of variety shows; and, finally, the infat-
uation of America's youth culture with the sounds of rhythm and blues,
newly renamed rock and roll.

Although Broadway never encouraged "plain hoofers," tap reigned supreme on the Broadway stage from the early twenties until the late thirties. In white musicals and revues, the tradition of making the dancing
secondary to the acting had been established early with performers such
as George White and George M. Cohan, who were primarily dancers
rather than actors. Black dancers had the added disadvantage of facing
owner-producer-directors who wanted them to Europeanize (whiten) their
styles and critics who had difficulty not only in understanding this art's
subtleties but in appreciating them as well. Although *Shuffle Along* and
other black musicals of the twenties had a tremendous impact on the
musicals that followed them, these strongholds of American vernacular
dance did not survive on the Broadway stage. Aesthetic and economic
factors caused the death of tap on white Broadway. Tap was overexposed
and carelessly presented.[10]

Chorus lines performed clichéd and preformulated routines behind
specialty acts who executed dangerous, flashy steps. Tap's rhythm got lost,

and in the process, tap lost its heartbeat. The depression shut down theaters on Broadway; and with the takeover of the entertainment scene by the motion picture industry, many of the vaudeville houses that were not closed outright were converted into movie theaters. Finally, the 1936 musical *On Your Toes*, choreographed by George Balanchine, helped shift Broadway's emphasis toward ballet. Then came *Oklahoma* (1943), about which the choreographer Buddy Bradley succinctly declared: "Agnes de Mille did a fine job of making the dance advance in the plot in *Oklahoma*, but she turned her back on real American dance and everybody followed her example."[11]

A study of tap's representation in film discloses that the Jim Crow persona was reinvented over and over: black dancers were depicted as excelling in creative energy but mindless.[12] This association still prevailed in the fifties, when the stage was being set for the black awareness movement of the sixties and the subsequent African American identification with Africa. By the midsixties, the Hollywood image of Bill Robinson and Shirley Temple merely represented for many black Americans another version, still offensive, of Little Eva and Uncle Tom. For the black community's younger generation, coming of age in the black-and-proud sixties but knowing nothing about the famous black tap teams of the past, this art form was hopelessly linked to the minstrel stage and to stereotyped film roles, to "Tomming."

In an article entitled "Hearing Dance, Watching Film," the dance historian and critic Sally Sommer points out that high-budget, widely disseminated movies of the thirties and forties presented tap as a flimsy, unserious art whose greatest practitioners were white stars like Fred Astaire and Eleanor Powell. Not only did this practice exclude tap's true originators and innovators but it also convinced the American public that tap was not worthy of the respect given to more "serious" dance forms like ballet and modern dance.[13]

In these films, tap was usually presented within arenas of light-hearted play, such as bowling alleys or living rooms, rather than on a stage. Consequently, this promoted the idea that tap was entertainment, not art. In addition, Hollywood's tap dance sequences were usually staged in a way that made this difficult art form appear to be nothing more than spontaneous outbursts erupting from one's nature instead of one's culture:

> Tap dancing is often presented as an explosion of joyous energy that seems to strike from nowhere, as opposed to the rehearsed artifice of

ballet. Gene Kelly in the famous "Singin' in the Rain" sequence, [is] walking down the street in the rain jumping into all the puddles that he can possibly find, spinning round with his umbrella, leaping on and off the kerb. He is confronted by a policeman clad in sensible rainwear who frowns [at] Kelly's frivolous activities, upon which he is forced back into his everyday existence—hunching his shoulders as he walks away in the rain. The sequence is represented as . . . an effortless and seemingly unchoreographed dance which expresses the man in love as delightfully playful.[14]

On the music scene, the swinging rhythms of big band music shifted in the midforties to the more angular tempos of such modern virtuosos as Dizzy Gillespie and Charlie Parker. The catchword was bebop. These men, building on the creations of Charlie Christian, Lester Young, and Louis Armstrong, routinely met at Minton's, a nightclub on West 118th Street in Harlem. Bored with commercial jazz and feeling that the primary function of jazz players was to communicate as soloists directly with their listeners, many leading "boppers" started experimenting in small groups, most often in quintets. Ralph Ellison has eloquently described the scene at Minton's:

> It has been a long time now, and not many remember how it was in the old days; not really. Not even those who were there to see and hear as it happened, who were pressed in the crowds beneath the dim rosy lights of the bar in the smoke-veiled room, and who shared, night after night, the mysterious spell created by the talk, the laughter, grease, paint, powder, perfume, sweat, alcohol and food—all blended and simmering, like a stew on the restaurant range, and brought to a sustained moment of elusive meaning by the timbres and accents of musical instruments locked in passionate recitative.[15]

Eileen Southern has defined bebop as a music "characterized by complex polyrhythms; steady but light and subtle beats; exciting dissonant harmonies; new tone colors; and irregular phrases." Honi Coles pointed out that to a great extent it was tap dancers who gave birth to bebop—through the work of John Bubbles: "If you listen to any band before the thirties, the drummer was used just to keep time, then drummers started listening to Bubbles." Ironically enough, these same Bubbles-inspired drummers helped cut tappers out of jazz shows. In bop's tighter arrangements, the spaces formerly reserved for tappers was gone, and all the percussion was now being done by the drummers. Coles vividly remembered the change from tap's heyday in the thirties: "We had arrangements written for the taps to be the syncopation in the band—for the taps to be the percussion. We were our own percussion." But by the forties, the bebop drummers "dropped bombs in unexpected places." The tap dancer of the thirties seemed in the way. According to Buster Brown, a bebop tap dancer, only those tap dancers who could adjust to the new music continued to exchange creative ideas with jazz drummers: "Honi always said tap dancers taught drummers, but I thought we taught one another. But we did give them the idea of using a lot of things they weren't using before, like triplets. . . . The proudest moment of your life, as a dancer, was when a musician said, 'Hey man, I dig what you're doing.' That was a compliment. We were respecting one another."[16]

Bebop posed a problem for the average listener. Jazz had been closely associated with dance halls and cabarets, and the development of dance steps had paralleled the development of the music. In these settings pre-bebop jazz had satisfied the musicians and the audience while helping to create a total cultural experience, which included music and dance. The average listener, accustomed to the clear driving pulse of earlier jazz styles, could not easily anticipate the elusive and fragmented rhythms of bop. Finally, bebop lost its dance audience. Not surprisingly, many of the older musicians resented this new form, which was jarring to swing-tuned ears and difficult to master. Then once the federal tax was levied on dance floors, jazz was relegated to small clubs, where there was no room for chorus lines or even dancing duos with their sometimes elaborately choreographed teamwork. To an extent white America did stop dancing. African Americans, however, filled that public dance void of the forties by continuing to dance at rent parties, family gatherings, and any other occasion that offered even the slightest opportunity to "get down." Bop or no bop, blacks found there to be sufficient bands around that continued to lay down a steady, danceable beat.[17]

During the early forties the standard format at the Apollo was the variety show, and major dance acts played there on a regular basis. In addition, the big bands who headlined usually featured one or more dance acts. Frank Schiffman, the owner of the Apollo, hired Coles and Atkins before they had even performed together on the professional stage because of their obvious talent:

> The orchestra is playing "Taking A Chance on Love" as if it will never reach the second note of the melody. The dancers walk, wheel, and tap with leisurely elegance, as the tune gradually emerges. Their dancing

holds it together and at the same time makes it flow. The audience at Harlem's Apollo Theater is transfixed. One graceless motion could shatter the poise and hover, but it never occurs. Relaxed and smiling, Coles and Atkins toss off gliding turns, leaning pull-ups, casual slides, and crystal clear taps. The suspense is continuous, the execution flawless.[18]

Throughout the fifties, Billy Eckstine used Coles and Atkins to reopen the Apollo after summer renovations. The variety show format was gradually on its way out and rock and roll dominated the charts. Coles and Atkins found themselves on bills with vocal groups like the Clovers. This group and similar ones had the support of a new American social class — teenagers, both black and white. Having more money and more leisure time than ever before, white teenagers became bored with singers like Perry Como and Doris Day and began listening to stations that played black rhythm and blues. The Chicago disc jockey Alan Freed was a major voice in this revolution, and although he played all kinds of rhythm and blues, he was definitely partial to black vocal harmony groups.[19]

By the late forties and fifties, as Bobby Schiffman began to play a more influential role in his father's business, vocal groups displaced the long-standing variety acts. Many of these young performers knew absolutely nothing about show business and turned up at rehearsals not only looking unpolished but lacking even sheet music. To rehearse, Reuben Phillips, manager of the house band, was forced at times to go across the street to the local record shop, buy the group's latest hit, and play it over and over so that the band members could learn their parts. Coles asked the members of one group to stay late so that he could give them a few pointers. One of the teenagers looked him up and down: "Where's your record, man? You got a hit record?" He also took a group to see the Count Basie band so that the members could learn how to use amplifiers more effectively. When Coles started explaining Basie's setup, the group's leader quickly lost interest. "Yeah," said the young singer, "but man, he ain't got our *sound*." What these singers needed most of all was performance polish — and there to provide it was Cholly Atkins: "Some of the groups would see me practicing, and would ask for a few pointers on their acts. I'd show them some steps if I liked them."[20]

Starting in 1953 with the Cadillacs, Atkins was so successful as a coach that other groups eagerly sought his expertise. Atkins recalled that "every time anybody got a hit record they brought them to me." He taught the Moonglows, Heartbeats, Cleftones, Bow Ties, Teenagers, Dominoes, Solitaires, Turbans, and Satins. Stearns and Stearns have described Atkins as the "number one babysitter and scout master" for these groups. He taught them stage etiquette, along with specially tailored movements from vernacular dances (e.g., trucking, Charleston, boogie woogie, applejack, Suzy-Q, and the camel walk) that were suitable for the lyrics. A small number learned the time step, and Frankie Lymon even studied with Pete Nugent and Baby Laurence long enough to become a competent tap dancer. Atkins's skills were solicited by the Shaw and William Morris Agencies, and by 1962 he was teaching classes on Wednesdays and Saturdays at 53d and Broadway in New York City's Ed Sullivan Theater.[21]

One of his greatest successes soon came with Gladys Knight and the Pips. At an Ohio theater in the early sixties, Melvin Franklin of the Temptations was awed by the performance polish of this group: "Those Pips were so beautifully choreographed—Cholly was coaching them—they virtually ran us off the stage. We didn't even exist in those people's minds." Gladys Knight described Cholly Atkins as the group's "everything. . . . He taught us how to walk onstage, how to walk offstage, how to move—for me, surprisingly, how to be feminine. . . . The guys, he used to work them to death. We used to work from nine in the morning until nine in the evening, rehearsing." Performances by Gladys Knight and the Pips, in particular, personify elements of the class act tradition, minus the taps: precision, detached coolness, elegance, flawless execution, and dignity. Many of the leaning pull-ups, casual slides, and gliding turns so characteristic of performances by Coles and Atkins appear over and over in the Pips' arrangements. According to Atkins, Gladys Knight and the Pips were prime class material: "There are some people who have what we call inborn sophistication. . . . Even if they try to get funky they do it in a sophisticated way. And it just so happened that all of the members possessed that. Plus," he added, "they were willing to work hard."[22]

In the midsixties, while working with Gladys Knight and the Pips in Bermuda, Atkins was offered a job at Motown, by then nicknamed "Hitsville, U.S.A." For Atkins this was not only a steady job, paying $25,000 per year, but a chance to join a dynamic African American organization that was starting to exert a tremendous influence on America's music industry. Atkins recalled that "at the time we were very conscious of the Black movement, and to be a part of something destined to become a first and contribute to the future of Black artists was an opportunity."[23]

Detroit's Motown Records was founded by Berry Gordy, a third-generation descendant of a line of southern black entrepreneurs. In the early fifties, he had patted his feet to the rhythms of bebop played by a group of sophisticated Detroit musicians who had attended Cass Technical High School and Northeastern High School, both of which had exceptional music instructional programs in the forties and fifties. Those sessions inspired him to open the 3-D Record Mart, a jazz retail store. When that failed, he secured a job at the Ford factory and, as the story goes, he began humming tunes and matching them with lyrics during his work hours. Tapes in hand, Gordy made regular visits to the Flame Show Bar, the Paradise Theater, and the Masonic Temple—places where singers could be found. Eventually the Flame Show Bar offered him his first big break. In 1957, Jackie Wilson's agent was there looking for material and hired Gordy. In the ensuing three years, as a member of Wilson's "hit-making team," Gordy proved aggressive, ambitious, and highly skilled. With Billy Davis he wrote the Wilson hits "Lonely Teardrops," "Reet Petite," "That Is Why (I Love You So)," and "I'll Be Satisfied" and thus earned the reputation around town as one of the most talented tunesmiths. In 1959, his cowriter and friend Smokey Robinson persuaded him to start independently marketing their own music.[24]

According to the Motown historian Nelson George, "over the next three years, roughly 1960–1962, a community of administrators, musicians, and entertainers began coalescing inside 2648 West Grand Boulevard, motivated by family pride, marital ties, a sense of black unity, the chance to make music, and, of course, the desire to become rich and famous." Smokey Robinson, now a vice president of Motown, revealed Gordy's strategy for capturing a young white American audience: "Berry's concept in starting Motown was to make music with a funky beat and great stories that would be crossover, that would *not* be blues. And that's what we did. . . . We took it a step further to try and make melody and words memorable and a dance beat very, very audible." To ensure that the potential audience could find the backbeat, songwriters used devices like tambourines, foot stomps, hand claps, wooden blocks, ball points, and even snow chains for some songs.[25]

Although Gordy's immediate goal was to produce hit records, he felt that the groups' longevity would depend on the presentation of stylish live shows to crossover audiences. On an autumn day in 1962, five cars and a bus waited outside the headquarters of Hitsville, U.S.A., for forty-five anxious passengers: the Marvelettes, the Contours, Marvin Gaye, Mary Wells, Little Stevie Wonder, and the Supremes, the first *Motor Town Revue*. Gordy's model for this package was probably not so much the rock and roll revues of the fifties as the vaudeville format of the *Idlewild Revue*, which was staged at a black resort area in Michigan where Gordy often vacationed. The usual entertainment format in the black vaudeville tradition had a chorus line, singers, and dance acts. Elements of these shows made their way directly into later Motown acts, like the Supremes' classic hat-and-cane routine, choreographed by Cholly Atkins, done to "Rock-a-Bye Your Baby with a Dixie Melody."[26]

Among the many factors responsible for the overwhelming success of Motown are Gordy's own strength as a corporate leader, his stable of excellent songwriters and jazz musicians, and Motown's accessibility to Detroit's black community. But foremost in the overall equation was Motown's Artist Development wing, known among the artists themselves as "Motown U." "Artist Development's goal was to vanquish the unsophisticated, gum-cracking manners and attitude that so annoyed Bean Bowles [the saxophonist/arranger] during the first Motor Town Revue."[27]

Prior to 1964, Motown U existed as an ad hoc operation directed by Harvey Fuqua with the assistance of Gordy's two sisters, Anna and Gwen. Both women had studied cosmetology and modeling with Maxine Powell, the proprietor of a local finishing and modeling school. When Powell was persuaded to give up her own school and join Motown's ranks, Artist Development became a permanent institution. She constantly reminded the groups that they were being groomed for two places—the White House and Buckingham Palace. With such stages in mind, she insisted that singers be mindful that unacceptable onstage deportment included grimacing, closing your eyes, protruding your buttocks, hunching your shoulders, and standing with widespread legs.[28]

Harvey Fuqua, who had performed Atkins's choreography when he was singing with the Moonglows, knew exactly what was needed to change Gordy's streetwise hitmakers into successful "supper club" attractions. In 1965, Cholly Atkins became Motown U's staff choreographer, and Maurice King came aboard as the new musical director. During the second half of the forties, King had managed the International Sweethearts of Rhythm, a highly successful female dance band. Both men, from a rich tradition of black dance and music, had toured for many years, appearing on concert stages and in nightclubs throughout the world. While King paced the show and worked out the song order, Atkins offered "choreography sessions" in which the groups learned steps to match their songs. Atkins worked with the singers for two hours daily, starting with floor exercises that lasted forty-five minutes and ending with rehearsals of their routines.[29] Mary Wilson of the Supremes found Motown's rehearsal standards demanding and exacting even on the road: "We moved into a New York hotel, joined by Cholly, music director Gil Askey, and arranger Johnnie Allen. We would get so tired, but we'd snap right to whenever Gil would say, 'We have to work on this until we get it right.' Cholly was more blunt: 'I don't care if we work until we're blue in the face.' We'd go back to the hotel for a few hours, then we'd be back at rehearsal. We sang the same notes, made the same moves, recited the same lines hundreds and hundreds of times." The demure style that Atkins developed for the Supremes consisted primarily of stylized swaying hands, half turns, and across-the-shoulder glances, but it set the standard for numerous female groups of the sixties and beyond.[30]

Before joining Motown in 1965, Atkins already had worked briefly with the Supremes, the Miracles, and the Temptations. In fact, the Miracles' well-known routine done to "Mickey's Monkey" was choreographed by Cholly Atkins when he was freelancing during the early sixties. The movements in this routine had teenagers across the country doing the monkey. Although the original idea was songwriter Mickey Stevenson's, Atkins "exaggerated the movements, made them more visual, and generally speaking tightened the act."[31]

In *Nowhere to Run: the Story of Soul Music*, Gerri Hirshey insists that "in their prime, nobody could work a crowd like the Tempts. No one dressed as well; no set of voices could match their full-court give-and-go. And surely no one could outdance them. Even gravity was just a pissant nuisance to the Tempts. They popped, jerked, and flew their bodies, spun like a quintet of sequined gyroscopes that somehow always stopped at exactly the same second on the same spot." The Temptations' first choreographer was Paul Williams, the member of the group who developed the "Temptations' Walk." Williams worked out periodically with Peg Leg Bates, who passed on to the group "around-the-world" spins and other jazz movements.[32]

At Motown, Atkins made the Temptations' hits more sophisticated choreographically and helped prepare them for places like the Copa in Vegas and the Versailles in Cleveland: "What I did with the Temps was try to polish them up, like I did an old 'rain' medley—using rain tunes like 'Singing in the Rain' and using umbrellas. We used them like canes. It was almost like a tap dance, you know. We did it with British homburgs."[33]

Thanks to his expertise and exposure, Atkins managed to keep much American vernacular dance alive in the choreography of popular vocal groups. His superb "vocal choreography" might appear natural and effortless, but it is extremely difficult to execute. The body is always doing something that is rhythmically different from the voice. In the film *Watch Me Move*, Atkins explains what he was working toward with his early acts of the fifties and later at Motown:

> It was like Dixieland music, you know. Every instrument is playing and it sounds great, but everybody is playing what they want to play. That was the same thing with the vocal groups. Everybody was moving, but they were doing whatever they felt like doing. My object was to take it and organize it and put it in a form where it would be more precise. Now I used moves from modern jazz, balletic moves, or jazz tap moves without the taps—whatever I thought about doing I could do with the Cadillacs. I only had a few groups that I could do that with. The Cadillacs was the first, then later came the Pips.[34]

Atkins's choreography is characterized by precise visual polyrhythms. The movement is continuous: even when the backup singers are not in the mike area, they are still performing interesting steps derived from authentic jazz movements, especially black chorus line dancing of the twenties, thirties, and forties. Sometimes his work includes actual tap moves, like cross-steps, over the tops, and trenches done in a jazz manner. Although the physical aspect of "vocal choreography" is extremely important, Atkins cites the mental aspect as the one that determines the intricacy of a routine. Atkins sees the choreographic process as a mathematical one in which the singers have to move away from their mikes to dance, then get back by a certain time to sing. "If you don't *get out front* before the 'da de da ya,'" he declared, "you won't have time to shift for the 'doo de doo.'" At the same time, the steps that bring them back to the mike area must be designed with breathing in mind, so that they do not appear winded but look relaxed when they begin to sing.[35]

Within the context of vocal choreography, Atkins managed to capture two of the distinguishing hallmarks of rhythm tap: self-expression and individualism.

> I let the punishment fit the crime. I let my clients' talent dictate to me what to do with them, and that basically stops anybody from looking like somebody else. You go with the degree of talent you have to work with, and you try to get the best out of that. We all have certain moves, the standard things . . . the level to raise the arm, how far to step forward, how far to step back. Everybody's doing the same thing at the same time, but they're doing it in their own way so you let them retain the one thing that they will think is very important, their individualism.[36]

His position as the refining mentor for vocal groups has been an extremely advantageous one for a choreographer, because each time there is a new hit song, a new routine is needed. And Atkins seems to have an endless array of movement combinations. This is one of the keys to his professional longevity. The other key is the longevity of many of the groups he coaches—clearly a result of his ability to nurse them through fads while building them into standard acts. For Atkins, this essentially means changing ordinary singers into well-rounded performers who can deliver tunes in more than one style and who can carry on some of the variety act traditions that had been part of his performing career. He explained: "If someone had a flair for comedy, then we would put in some comedy thing. The Cadillacs had a character called Speedo. . . . Instead of just doing the song drylongso [in an undoctored way], I gave the lead singer a hat and cane although he was doing a rock-and-roll thing. I taught him how to twirl a hat and twirl a cane, and things of that sort that stopped them from being just a vocal group."[37] In discussing his career as a choreographer, which has spanned approximately four decades, Atkins said: "I get a bang out of servicing my clients and becoming involved with them, because they have made a transition in coming from one type of show business, which is black. On the other side is another type of show business, like with TV and smart supper clubs. I've had all the experience in the world in those fields, so I take R&B artists and teach, educate, and prepare them for that transition from the chitlin circuit to Vegas." He built all of Motown's groups into standard acts, taking them beyond the rock and roll of the sixties so that they could, in Atkins's words, "grow up with their fans."[38]

"In whatever shape and form Atkins's steps materialized on stage, they became immediately enshrined in the hearts of adoring teenage audiences. Thus these vernacular movements, simplified and reinterpreted, took on a new and widespread life." Television, the "ultimate drum," broadcast black American vernacular dances into American homes from coast to coast. At its peak in the sixties, Dick Clark's *American Bandstand*, with its rock-and-roll dance hall format that showcased singers as well as the latest dance crazes, was televised over 105 stations, reaching approximately 20 million teenagers. In the seventies and eighties, *Soul Train*, with its similar but all-black format, joined *American Bandstand* in continuing to keep millions of American youngsters abreast of the latest dance steps— performed both by singers and by the shows' hired dancing youngsters. Like the *Motor Town Revue*, these television shows, very often presenting Atkins's work (and its imitations), have helped keep black vernacular dance alive and in front of a growing audience. For over twenty years, black stars also have sung and performed Atkins's vocal choreography in international concerts and in films, spreading these dance steps to a worldwide audience. Meanwhile, back home, African Americans copied their idols' steps and "moves," adapting them for talent shows and house parties—reclaiming material that had come full circle back to its vernacular source.[39]

Footage of live performances from the fifties through the eighties demonstrates how vestiges of American vernacular dances—some done as early as the twenties—have been incorporated into singers' routines. These films include the Flamingos bouncing in half splits, then breaking into the fast footwork of the lindy hop, spiced with jazz tap turns. In another, Frankie Lymon and the Teenagers are doing a jazz/tap crossover step along with half splits and the Charleston. The Ronettes were filmed in performance doing the shimmy and the Charleston. Gladys Knight and the Pips slip into jazz tap slides, glides, and turns. Then they effortlessly shift into the shorty George and close a phrase by doing tap's falling off the log. Dancing the mashed potatoes (which has leg gestures that are similar to the Charleston's), the Temptations will then ease into jazz/tap slides and glides, while in another clip, the Jackson 5 peck and jump first into the Charleston and then into the shorty George.[40] Some of these groups learned their choreography from Cholly Atkins; those like the Jackson 5, who were not formally trained by him, were copying others who were.

The Atkins contribution to American culture has been extraordinarily significant. He not only made polished performers out of rock-and-roll singers who started with a hit single and raw ambition. He taught them to *perform* their music by doing dances that worked their magic not by retelling a song's storyline in predictable pantomime but by punctuating it with rhythmical dance steps, turns, and gestures drawn from the rich bedrock of black vernacular dance. In so doing, he virtually created a new form of expression: vocal choreography. Thoroughly versed in twentieth-century African American dance forms, from social dances like the lindy hop to street-corner (and then stage) sensations like rhythm tap, Atkins gave his singing groups a depth and appeal that was sometimes lacking in their tunes and lyrics. Without knowing it, popular groups of the sixties, seventies, and eighties were performing updated versions of dances of the forties, thirties, and twenties—classic black vernacular dances—and projecting them to a larger audience than ever before. Through the good offices of Cholly Atkins, even movements from tap, markedly out of favor in the sixties, were being taught to sixties rock-and-roll stars, who introduced them to the new generation in the United States and around the globe. That the style or body language of rhythm tap is so accessible to young African Americans today has to be due in part to these "underground" efforts of vocal choreographer Atkins.

Since leaving Motown in 1971, Cholly Atkins has freelanced in Las Vegas, where he lives with his wife, Maye Atkinson. At eighty-two "Pop" Atkins, as he is affectionately called by his clients, still choreographs and says that he will dance "until he dies." Through his workshops at American colleges, universities, and dance festivals, he is starting a new career as an educator and embracing the current generation of dance and music students. His legacy is one that bridges dance and musical genres and touches people of all ages.

Cholly Atkins, "the ageless hoofer," continues to choreograph and stage acts for the O'Jays, the Temptations, Gladys Knight, Aretha Franklin, and others. As of 1996 Atkins had worked with the Temptations for thirty-two years and with the O'Jays for twenty-two. Richard Street, a former member of the Temptations, put it this way: "He can dance as well as those kids on *Soul Train*. . . . I mean he was showing us how to moonwalk before Michael Jackson was doing it. And when you can be that age and outdance anybody . . . you're going to be around."[41]

"W'en de Colo'ed Ban' Comes Ma'chin' down de Street": From African Processions to New Orleans Second Lines

You kin hyeah a fine perfo'mance w'en de white ban's serenade,
An' dey play dey high-toned music mighty sweet,
But hit's Sousa played in rag-time, an hit's Rastus on Parade,
W'en de colo'ed ban' comes ma'chin' down de street.
—Paul Lawrence Dunbar, "The Colored Band"

It has been called "the Lena Horne of Bands," "the E.F. Hutton of Marching Bands," "the most imitated band in America," and "the marchingest and playingest band in America."[1] The Marching 100 of Florida A&M University can set any stadium on fire just by stepping onto the field. As the perennial show stealer at sports events across the country, FAMU's band has become a standard bearer for high school and college bands throughout the nation. The impact of this African American institution results not only from its superb musicianship and top-notch precision marching but also from its unparalleled dance ability.

Since the sixties black college marching bands like FAMU's have included American vernacular dance in their halftime shows, bringing onto the football field the tradition of cutting contests and battles of the bands. The Marching 100's magnetic halftime performances serve as visual and oral histories of the African American heritage in dance and music. Although FAMU's tradition of excellence in marching bands has been treated by the mass media as an isolated phenomenon, it is unquestionably part of a much larger cultural and historical context that includes jazz and rhythm and blues dancing musicians of the twentieth century and reaches back through turn-of-the century brass bands, minstrel bands, and military bands to the slave fiddlers and set callers on the farms and plantations of colonial America. There, the coming together of western and central African art forms with European dance and music produced uniquely African American stylizations that have influenced and shaped all of American culture.

Most activities of traditional sub-Saharan African cultures are connected in some way with dance and music. Ceremonies commemorating agricultural rites, reenacting historical events, and celebrating the installation of important political figures involved special music. Expert singers and instrumentalists provided music for the formal activities of their particular villages. Those attached to the courts of chiefs and kings, as well as independent musicians, were often virtuoso performers and professionals who were highly esteemed by members of the community.[2] In 1817, Edward Bowdich, a European traveler in Ghana, described an Ashanti ceremony:

> The king, his tributaries, and captains, were resplendent in the distance, surrounded by attendants of every description. . . . The sun was reflected, with a glare more supportable than the heat, from the massy gold ornaments, which glistened in every direction. More than a hundred bands burst at once on our arrival, [all playing] the peculiar airs of their several chiefs; the horns flourished their defiances with the beating of innumerable drums and metal instruments, and then yielded for a while to the soft breathings of their long flutes, which were truly harmonious; and a pleasing instrument, like a bagpipe without the drone, was happily blended. At least a hundred large umbrellas, or canopies, which could shelter thirty persons, were sprung up and down by the bearers with brilliant effect, being made of scarlet, yellow, and the most shewy [showy] cloths and silks.[3]

During colonial America's early years, black musicians provided much of the music for social gatherings. Northern black musicians played frequently for town balls, country dances, and for dancing schools. Northern slave festivities such as Negro Election Day in New England were celebrations that also called for musicians. "All over the South slaves played for the dancing of their masters at balls, assemblies, and special 'Entertainments' in the plantation ballrooms and 'palaces' of the colonial governors."[4] Although most were self-taught, black slave musicians occasionally were presented with opportunities for formal training on an instrument. These rare chances included plantation visits by music instructors during which watchful house slaves benefited; lessons from members of slaveholding families or other slaves; and, in such urban centers as Charleston, South Carolina, instruction by professional musicians. Students attending the College of William and Mary in Williamsburg, Virginia, were routinely accompanied by their slaves. The slaves lived in rooms with the students and probably, on occasion, attended classes.

Colonial newspapers provided numerous listings of slaves whose great value came from their possession of musical skills. Dena Epstein reports that "black fiddlers became as pervasive a part of the plantation legend as black banjo players. But there was more depth to the careers of black performers than the . . . plantation myth would allow. These obscure musicians at times achieved what would have been a professional status if their earnings had remained in their own hands." Owners of slave musicians often granted them increased geographical mobility as well as a chance to earn extra money and possess some material goods. These "musicianers" (as they were sometimes referred to by their fellow captives) occupied positions of great importance within the slave community. The slave musicians' roles as artists, teachers, and essential figures at celebrations and frolics placed them in the top ranks of the slave hierarchy and allowed them to achieve dignity through their music. They also gained status from their ability to transmit aspects of African American culture and facilitate functions that generated community solidarity.[5]

At the "Saturday night function," musicianers dressed in their finest clothes and stationed themselves prominently so that they could be seen and heard by all. A doorstep, woodpile, platform, or barrel might typically serve as an impromptu stage where they made their instruments "ring, sing or talk." A description of one slave musician's carefully planned entrance calls to mind the stylish presentations of such charismatic jazz musicians as Jelly Roll Morton and Willie "the Lion" Smith:

> Uncle Warrie, a fine performer, teased his listeners with delays in order to heighten their appreciation of his music. He knew when to make his entrance—only after a crowd had gathered—and when he appeared, it was to the gratifying shouts and exclamations of eager dancers. Once settled in his chair, he stalled further by tuning his fiddle in front of the anxious assembly. . . . According to Warrie, no affair could begin without his fiddle. . . . When the music began, the players were in control. Uncle Warrie recognized the power he had at social functions. "When I'd rawsum up dat bow and draw it crost de strings dey'd lessen!"[6]

In addition to playing for social gatherings, black musicians in colonial America also performed instrumental music with the militia. In 1738, the

Virginia legislature enacted a statute that required free mulattos, blacks, and Native Americans to serve in the military. They were not allowed to carry arms and instead served as trumpeters, drummers, or "pioneers." This practice soon spread to other colonies and black musicians became permanent fixtures in colonial military units. Every year, training days were scheduled during which soldiers practiced drills and paraded for inspection before public officials and military officers. These sessions, on public grounds, were followed by games, refreshments, and socializing to the sounds of white and black musicians.[7]

Colonial field music grew out of the military band music of early seventeenth-century Britain. In Europe, black musicians were limited to the trumpet and drums until Janissary music swept the continent during the eighteenth century. The powerful janissaries, or soldiers, who marched in Turkish regimental bands dressed in elaborate uniforms and played instruments that were novel and fascinating to Europeans.[8] By 1770, most European armies had adopted the kettledrum, cymbals, triangle, bass drum, and "Jingling Johnnie" (Turkish crescent), "a wooden pole surmounted by one or more metal crescents which were adorned with red horsehair plumes hanging from the sides." Many countries brought Turkish bands in to play with their military regiments, but "after the first wave of Turkish musicians had come into Europe, Africans were generally employed to play the Turkish music." In Great Britain, however, Turkish musicians were never used, so there the tradition of powerful African musicians came into sharp focus as soon as the Turkish practices were adopted.[9]

The music historian Henry George Farmer describes the lasting impressions made by black players of Turkish music:

> Dressed in high turbans, bearskins, or cocked hats, with towering hackle feather plumes, and gaudy coats of many colours, braided and slashed gorgeously and gapingly, they capered rather than marched. . . . Their agility with fingers, arms and legs was only equalled by their perfect time in the music. . . . It should not be forgotten that these negro drummers not only gave a tremendous fillip to regimental music a century and more ago, but it was their contribution in this so-called "Turkish music" that opened the eyes of the great composers, beginning with Mozart and Beethoven, to the possibilities of a new tone colour and fresh rhythmic devices in the wider realm of orchestral music.[10]

Black musicians were the rage in British military bands until the mid-nineteenth century: "Regiments vied with one another in obtaining black musicians and achieved status according to the number of blacks they employed." Since British-style army bands appeared in the colonies as early as the 1750s, African musicians no doubt played some part in establishing a longstanding tradition of African American drummers who performed antics with their drumsticks. "Modern cross-handed drumming on the bass drum" can be traced to African styles. Farmer describes tricks performed by African musicians "such as throwing up a bass drum-stick into the air after the beat, and catching it with the other hand in time for the next [or] shaking the 'Jingling Johnnie' under their arms, over their heads, and even under their legs."[11] During the twentieth century, numerous jazz drummers became famous for what the trumpeter Rex Stewart calls "drum stickery." The music critic Whitney Balliett describes the artistry of Big Sid Catlett: "Once in a while he would twirl his sticks over his head or throw them in the air, allowing their motions to silently measure off several beats. The effect was louder than any shout."[12]

Over 5,000 blacks served in northern and southern integrated military units during the American Revolution. In New England, however, the regiments of Rhode Island, Connecticut, and Massachusetts had such all-black companies as Col. George Middleton's "Bucks of America." The typical black martial company included at least two drummers and two fifers: "The martial music of the Revolutionary War period emanated primarily from fifes and drums; occasionally, trumpets were used. According to the Orderly Book of a Virginia general, each regiment was allowed a 'Fifer-major' and a 'Drummer-major,' whose duties were 'to practice the young fifers and drummers between the hours of eleven and one o'clock every day, and to take care that they perform their several duties with as much exactness as possible.'" Spirited marches were played by armed services musicians in the field and during parades. A number of wind bands were also formed during the American Revolution for the entertainment and pleasure of the Continental Army officers.[13]

During the War of 1812 blacks were initially excluded from the army so most entered the navy. Although the law governing this exclusion was reversed in 1814, records of black army musicians of this period remain sketchy. One of the few written accounts tells how Jordan B. Noble, called a "matchless drummer," "beat his drum during all and every fight, in the hottest hell of the fire, and was complimented by [General Andrew] Jackson himself after the battle." Despite the scant records, it is clear that a significant number of black musicians were active during the war. Once it had ended, many all-black brass bands appeared on the scene, particularly in sections of New England and in Philadelphia, New York, and New

Orleans. One such group, which had played for Philadelphia's Third Company of Washington Guards, was led by Frank Johnson.[14]

Born in 1792, Francis Johnson was an extraordinary figure in what might be termed the "invisible history" of American music. He was one of several early nineteenth-century black musicians who performed and composed music for such European-American social dances as cotillions, waltzes, and quadrilles.[15] Johnson and other black musicians of the 1800s collaborated with white "dancing masters." His "band was celebrated for its dance music up and down the Eastern Seaboard and was the favorite band of the Philadelphia aristocracy." At costume balls and affairs sponsored by public officials and civic organizations Johnson and other black musicians "played the music to which Americans in the cities danced. Black musicians and all-black dance bands were in the vanguard."[16]

Johnson's was the first American musical ensemble, black or white, to perform in Europe and the first to introduce "Concerts a la Musard" (promenade concerts) to the nation. Thousands attended these each night and hundreds were turned away. During his six-month stay in England, Johnson was awarded a silver bugle by Queen Victoria. As a black musician, he was the first to tour widely in the United States, publish sheet music, give formal band concerts, appear in integrated concerts, and receive wide acclaim in America and England. Johnson also created the first "school" of African American musicians.[17]

In his 1878 study *Music and Some Highly Musical People*, James Monroe Trotter described the impact of Johnson's band:

> Indeed, the novelty formed by such an organization,—all colored men,—its excellent playing, and the boldness of the enterprise, all combined to create a decided sensation wherever these sable troubadours appeared. It is said that sometimes, while the band was on this tour, many persons would doubt the ability of its members to read the music they were playing, believing that they performed "by ear," as it is called; nor could such persons be convinced of their error until a new piece of music—a piece not previously seen by them—was placed before the band, and by the same readily rendered from the printed page.[18]

For two decades, Frank Johnson's band performed in Saratoga Springs, New York, where, well over a century later, Frank Johnson Day was formally declared. A printed program from the festivities declared Johnson "leader of the Band at all hops and balls—public or private; sole director of all serenades and inventor-general of cotillions." When Johnson died in 1844, Joseph Anderson became the director of the Frank Johnson Brass and String Bands, maintaining their standards until the Civil War.[19]

When that war broke out, brass bands played at troop farewells, recruitment rallies, and virtually every major campaign. Although little is known about black musicians in the Confederate Army except that slaves served as fifers and drummers, much is known about the experiences of slaves who fought and served as musicians in the Union Army. Officials in that army began at the war's onset to procure music instructors and instruments for its black soldiers. Drills and evening parades were emphasized: the First Regiment of Kansas Colored Volunteers sometimes spent five hours a day drilling and then ended the day parading in full uniform.[20]

Accounts of army life among black soldiers appear in the journals, diaries, and letters of northern whites who served the Union. The most well-known accounts were written by Harvard-trained Col. Thomas W. Higginson, who was a minister, abolitionist, writer, and leader of an all-black regiment. Higginson described a scene that was complete with a kind of drum major:

> The little drum-corps kept in advance, a jolly crew, their drums slung on their backs, and the drum-sticks perhaps balanced on their heads. With them went the officers' servant-boys, more uproarious still, always ready to lend their shrill treble to any song. At the head of the whole force there walked, by some self-imposed pre-eminence, a respectable elderly female, one of the company laundresses, whose vigorous stride we never could quite overtake, and who had an enormous bundle balanced on her head, while she waved in her hand, like a sword, a long-handled tin dipper. Such a picturesque medley of fun, war, and music I believe no white regiment in the service could have shown; and yet there was no straggling, and a single tap of the drum would at any moment bring order out of this seeming chaos.[21]

During the Civil War, each black regiment had its own band, several of which developed into top-notch performing units. Holidays and periodic parades and drills brought them in contact with the general public. When the war ended in 1865, black army inductees numbered more that 186,000. Many remained in the service and played with regimental bands on the frontier, where typically they won wide acclaim for producing superior music. Others left to join town bands, road shows, and minstrel troupes, another major training ground and performance arena for black musicians.[22]

"Father of the Blues" W. C. Handy played with the Mahara Minstrels for several years: "It goes without saying that minstrels were a disreputable lot in the eyes of a large section of upper-crust Negroes, . . . but it was also true that all the best talent of that generation came down the same drain. The composers, the singers, the musicians, the speakers, the stage performers—the minstrel shows got them all." In 1896, Handy joined the Mahara Minstrels as the orchestra's cornetist. Not only did this provide him with the chance to travel; it provided the opportunity to "rub elbows with the best Negro musicians of the day." In time the management decided to add another band to the show, and Handy became director of forty-two musicians for night concerts and thirty for parades. The minstrel parade started shortly after 11:45 A.M., with the band playing spirited marches as the participants strutted through town.

> The parade itself was headed by the managers in their four-horse carriages. Doffing silk hats and smiling their jeweled smiles, they acknowledged with easy dignity the small flutter of polite applause their high-stepping horses provoked. After them came the carriage in which the stars rode. The "walking gents" followed, that exciting company which included comedians, singers, and acrobats. They in turn were followed by the drum major—not an ordinary drum major beating time for a band, mind you, but a performer out of the books, an artist with the baton. His twirling stick suggested a bicycle wheel revolving in the sun. Occasionally he would give it a toss and then recover the glistening affair with the same flawless skill. The drum major in a minstrel show was a character to conjure with; not infrequently he stole the parade. Our company had two such virtuosi; in addition to twirling their batons, they added the new wrinkle of tossing them back and forth to each other as they marched.[23]

Formed originally by Charles Hicks, the Georgia Minstrels was well known for its thirteen-piece brass band. Trotter cites the "high musical culture" of this particular group. He explains that four members were accomplished music teachers, one had played with England's best orchestras, several played two or three instruments, three could arrange and write music, and one played no fewer than twelve instruments. After a late nineteenth-century European tour, the company returned to the States, where songs and marches were cheered by a reviewer who noted that the musicians "possess a genuineness which no burnt-cork artists can fully imitate."[24]

In what some historians have described as an attempt to counteract the threat of black soldiers in the Union Army, white minstrel players began portraying Negro troops as cowardly incompetents, comically unable to perform the simplest maneuver or to obey the most elementary command. When told to "Fall in," the blacked-up minstrel soldiers jumped into a lake. Their ready response to "Eyes right" was *"I'se right too!"*[25] Versions of these "Raw Recruits" routines became standard features in black minstrel shows as well.

In 1877, for instance, Callender's Minstrels, a black group, developed a mock-military skit called the "Ginger Blues." This piece was based on a white variety house act that featured authentic black social and marching club steppers, "excellent marching units that took great pride in themselves, their uniforms, and the parties they threw." Billy Kersands was a smash hit in the lead role.[26]

When J. H. Haverly bought the rights to Callender's Minstrels, he added a brass band and the "Ginger Blues" skit was retained and renamed "Recruits for Gilmore" after Patrick S. Gilmore, a former Union Army band conductor. By 1886, Kersand's own minstrel company, known for its spectacular marching band, exuberantly headed the Mardi Gras parade in New Orleans. At that time he offered $1,000 to any unit that could out-parade or out-drill his minstrel marchers.[27]

According to William D. Piersen, it is highly probable that the use of mock military displays in minstrel shows was originally adapted from slave culture. "By 1750, muster, or Training Day as it was known, had become an important holiday assuming social as well as military significance. In Connecticut and perhaps elsewhere, black trainings also became a part of the holiday." During these performances, slaves lampooned white military practices. When commanded, for example, to "Fire and fall off!" the black troops "threw themselves from their horses." Piersen reminds us that throughout the Western Hemisphere slaves used satire and mimicry "just as they had done traditionally in Africa." By 1800, white muster trainings in New England had become farcical; at midcentury whites there were "consciously adopting a black satirical style like that utilized in black elections and trainings."[28]

Mock military displays were not limited to African Americans in northern states. William Cullen Bryant witnessed this same kind of activity among slaves at a corn-shucking dance in South Carolina: "From the dances a transition was made to a mock military parade, a sort of burlesque of our militia trainings, in which the words of command and the [bodily gestures] were extremely ludicrous." During the 1830s military burlesque parades flourished from Maine to Georgia.[29]

While the records cannot tell us for certain that the evolution of mock military displays followed the route suggested, we do know that they entered fully into the minstrel show and became "central to the entire range of 19th century self-entertainments." Classic burlesque, based in part on the minstrel show, featured mock-military production numbers as early as the 1860s. Drill performances including parodies and "regular army maneuvers" were also adopted for other traveling shows and musical theater. Tom Fletcher reported that the U.S. Ninth Cavalry performed regular army maneuvers in *Black America,* a late nineteenth-century show.[30]

From the mock military parades of slaves to the current step shows of black fraternities and sororities, drilling has become a permanent fixture in African American performances and celebrations. Various parades in cities and towns across America feature high-stepping marching units in which African American children combine military drilling with energetic vernacular dance movements.[31] Teen drill teams representing various mosques in the Nation of Islam meet annually in Chicago for their national competition.

Medicine shows, carnivals, circuses, and such touring shows as *In Old Kentucky* featured black bands along with the other performers. According to Tom Fletcher, who played for the "Pickaninny Band," a boys' musical group that was part of the *In Old Kentucky* lineup, "Our big hobby was, whenever we played the same town with a company that had a band, to get right behind their band and run them off the streets." Billboards for *In Old Kentucky* promised "Fifty Dollars to anyone that can stick us with any march."[32]

Numerous African American boys' brass bands came into existence during the late nineteenth century. Probably the most famous was the Jenkins Orphanage Band, organized in Charleston, South Carolina, by Rev. Daniel Joseph Jenkins. Under the initial tutelage of musicians P. M. "Hatsie" Logan and Francis Eugene Mikell, the first band was created to raise money for the orphanage.[33]

The first Jenkins Orphanage Band started performing in the 1890s on the street corners of its hometown; just after the turn of the century it was touring the country in "brightly coloured military-type uniforms, with the tiny drum-major heavily bedecked with shining braid." When subsidiary units were formed, the orphanage sometimes had as many as five groups on the road at once.[34] Dicky Wells was in Louisville, Kentucky in the twenties, when he saw one of the marching units:

> Briscoe was a short, tubby, left-handed guy and he used to throw his horn around and play louder than the whole band. All the kids followed him.

When he played dances he would sometimes put his right hand behind him, hold his horn with his left, then bend over and go along pushing and skidding the slide on the floor. . . . Briscoe would also take the horn apart and play with just the mouthpiece, then assemble it bit by bit until he had it all together again, playing all the while—a one-man show. He'd play with his foot in the slide, too.

Leonard De Paur, a conductor and composer, saw the band during his childhood and later described its leader as "somebody who could dance like hell."[35]

The band members' musicianship and dance stylizations set the stage for them to perform in Theodore Roosevelt's inaugural parade and in two Broadway shows, *Uncle Tom's Cabin* and *Porgy*. Their skillful playing took them to Paris, Vienna, Berlin, London, and Rome. The legacy of Rev. Daniel Joseph Jenkins has been carried forward by such jazz musicians as William "Cat" Anderson, Jabbo Smith, and Freddy Jenkins, who received their early training with his bands.[36]

The Jenkins Orphanage Band was born during the golden age of American brass bands, black and white. Patrick S. Gilmore and John Philip Sousa toured extensively, playing for loyal audiences. Arthur Pryor, an African American alumnus of the Sousa band, formed a group of his own that featured, as part of its repertoire, ragtime works, including tunes written specifically for cakewalking. The widely imitated Arthur Pryor Band outdrew Sousa in the Midwest.[37]

By the last decade of the nineteenth century there were approximately ten thousand bands in the United States, many of them marching bands. By 1908, the number had reached eighteen thousand. These bands were not only more popular among Americans than classical symphonic orchestras but they were also the nation's most popular source of musical entertainment. Most American towns actively supported a civic band: "Just as baseball was to become the sport of the people, bands were understood to provide the music of the people." With flashy uniforms, impressive soloists, and a measured beat, American brass bands were nothing if not entertaining. Band publicists also claimed the ability of the groups to "elevate" and enrich all classes of Americans. They even emphasized the potential health benefits of playing in such groups. Blowing horns and marching, they said, developed broad shoulders, strong lungs, and vigorous bodies.[38]

Business and community leaders alike could see other practical uses for marchers. By attracting crowds, these brass bands helped sell land, publicize commodities, and promote amusement parks. They underscored the can-do philosophies of various social, political, and religious organizations. They enlivened military drills and parades and accompanied couples on dance floors throughout the country. According to the *Minneapolis Tribune* of 1875, the bands represented democracy in action: "These concerts are the contribution of art to the people, to be enjoyed by the occupant of the humblest cabin and by the master of a mansion, and harmonizing all classes in the democracy of music." These marching bands seemed to embody America as it liked to see itself—cocky, stepping to a proud beat, ready for any change.[39]

Although bands were spread across the country, one of the main centers, especially for black brass bands, may well have been New Orleans. The city's balmy climate made outdoor events and ceremonies possible all year, so not surprisingly, by the turn of the century black New Orleans featured dozens of brass bands, dance orchestras, and strolling groups of music makers—all responding to that city's extraordinary demand for musicians. Nowhere is the importance of music to the Crescent City better expressed than in Sidney Bechet's autobiography, *Treat It Gentle*: "New Orleans, that was a place where the music was natural as the air. The people were ready for it like it was sun and rain. A musicianer, when he played in New Orleans, was home; and the music, when he played it, would go right to where he sent it. The people there were waiting for it, they were wanting it."[40]

In this city that gave the world Louis Armstrong, Jelly Roll Morton, and Sidney Bechet, there was a broad tradition of excellent musicianship among blacks. Since the early years of the nineteenth century, opera, chamber music, and other European forms had flourished in New Orleans. Creoles of color, who lived primarily in the downtown French-oriented section of the city, absorbed a rich mix of Franco-American cultural elements. Their children were routinely sent to music tutors and sometimes to conservatories in Paris. Sons of Creoles often studied with musicians from the French Opera Company and also played in the string trios, brass bands, and dance orchestras of the downtown district.[41]

Although many African Americans, who lived uptown, also received European musical training, they were more strongly influenced than downtown Creoles by the vocal music of black churches, field hollers, work songs, and the rhythms of Congo Square. The uptowners formed numerous brass bands that reflected the more African and distinctively African American culture of that community. When a strict segregation code was enforced in the 1890s and downtowners were forced to move uptown, the best musicians of both groups played together in bands, enriching one another by exchanging musical ideas.[42]

Another key influence on the New Orleans music scene was self-taught country musicians, who brought into the city the sounds of the spirituals, jubilees, early secular songs, and chants. The mixing of the by-ear playing and improvising of these country musicians with that of the reading musicians of the city enriched the musical environment immeasurably. This rich gumbo gave New Orleans its distinctive sound.[43]

An important training ground for New Orleans black brass bands was created by the white politician Henry Clay Warmouth. Warmouth retired from politics in 1874 and founded the Magnolia Plantation, which housed a large sugar-producing industry. Magnolia also maintained several black brass bands, whose playing and marching, Warmouth was convinced, gave incentive to his workers. Warmouth hired James Humphrey to tutor these musicians, some of whom went on to become top performers.[44]

Born in 1859, Humphrey was a brass band teacher and a professional musician. According to one historian, Humphrey "played in the brass bands, he played in the string bands, and he played in the classical orchestras of his time. His bands played for parades, dances, concerts and also weddings and birthday parties."[45] As a teacher who was well-versed both in the American vernacular and in the European classical idioms and who insisted that his students read music well, "Professor Humphrey" had a far-reaching impact on New Orleans jazz musicians.

Boarding the train each week in his swallow-tail coat, Humphrey taught at Magnolia and other plantations along the Mississippi River. Typically, he gave his students syncopated rhythms as exercises, which, when added to standard ragtime arrangements, produced what was called "swinging a piece of music." A former band member elaborated on Humphrey's teaching technique and his particular emphasis on the drum as the band's "foundation":

> The first way he'd do, he would get the band on its foots, you see, and then he'd commence with his trumpet, and then, again, he'd get 'em all straight first, you see. But the first thing he would do, that battery [drum]—that's the first thing he would get straight first, that battery . . . that's the bass and the trombone and the drum and everything—after he'd get all that straight first, and then he'd jump on the trumpets, you see, and he'd get them. Because that battery, that's the foundation of the band, you see. And so when he'd get that straight, then

after that, the trumpets, you see—he'd get on them. And then, when he'd get them straight, all right, he'd say, "Come on, let's go; everybody."

When the city needed additional bands, or on special days such as Mardi Gras, Humphrey would bring his groups into New Orleans. Humphrey's marchers were tightly drilled, but they were still swinging to the ragging beat of the "battery."[46]

During the 1880s and 1890s, two of the top New Orleans black brass bands were the Excelsior Brass Band and the Onward Brass Band, of which James Humphrey was a member. The Excelsior's reputation reached beyond New Orleans. It toured through the East and North, performing in Baltimore, Philadelphia, New York, Boston, and other cities. In New Orleans these bands played for dances, picnics, parades, concerts, and funerals and were supported by black funeral homes and burial societies.[47] Those who danced behind the bands when they paraded—spurring them on as they were spurred on by the music—were called the second line.

The second line is characteristic of most New Orleans parades, and many great jazz artists were recruits from its ranks. One was little Louis Armstrong, who carried the horns of King Oliver and Bunk Johnson with great pride. Another was Sidney Bechet: "When I was just a kid, I used to get in on a lot of those second lines, singing, dancing, hollering—oh, it just couldn't be stopped." Frederic Ramsey Jr. describes the relationship between dance and the black brass bands:

> From the beginning, the music of Negro brass bands, both in New Orleans and Alabama, seems to have been related to dancing. This alone would not distinguish them from the earliest white bands known in Alabama or elsewhere; but it is unlikely that white audiences indulged in the sort of loose-hipped dancing which accompanies both the New Orleans or Alabama bands' music. One can see this sort of dancing flowing along in the Second Line that follows a funeral band in New Orleans today; and its counterpart can be seen when the Lapsey or the Laneville-Johnson play for Negro audiences in Alabama. In New Orleans, the bands have played, traditionally, for festive occasions, and for funerals. In Alabama, they do not play for funerals, but they are on hand for all outdoor "good times": barbeques, picnics, baseball games. The rhythm set up by these bands is not a tight, regular march step; it is more of a flowing, anticipatory emphasis and counteremphasis, ideally suited to [an improvised] style of dance.[48]

A firm tradition of trained municipal and self-trained provincial bands was established in the New Orleans musical milieu prior to 1900. But by

1910, many of the former brass band musicians had become dance band leaders, participating in the creation of what was later called jazz.[49]

Many of these dance band leaders were sidetracked once the United States entered World War I in 1917. When the war ended, more than 200,000 African Americans had served in the U.S. Army, ranking (according to the limits of segregation law) from privates to captains. Most black units maintained bands, and several of those bands won distinction throughout Europe for their superior music and generous efforts to raise the morale of soldiers. Two renowned black military bands were Tim Brymn's 350th Infantry and Will Vodery's 807th Infantry. Willie "the Lion" Smith marched with one of these bands: "We had Tim Brymn's brass band in our division. They got to be known all over Europe as the Seventy Black Devils of the U.S. 350th Field Artillery. Their nickname came from the Senegalese soldiers in the French Army, who fought next to us at the front. . . . I had the honor of being the drum major for the Black Devils' band when we were marching. But when we were resting someplace I would play the piano, if one could be found, and some of the horns from the band would join me in a sort of early jam session."[50]

The most famous of all the World War I black military bands, however, was the 369th Infantry "Hellfighters" band, led by James Reese Europe. Composer, violinist, pianist, and band leader, Reese was born in 1881 to a Mobile, Alabama, family of musicians. After his family moved to Washington, D.C., Europe studied violin with Enrico Hurlei (assistant director of the U.S. Marine Corps Band) and later theory and instrumentation with Hans Hanke (former member of the Leipzig Conservatory of Music), and with Harry T. Burleigh (black classicist).[51]

During the early 1900s, Europe left Washington for New York City and found his way to the newly established center of black artistic life, West Fifty-third Street, the location of the black-owned Marshall Hotel, which served dinner and provided music to extremely well-dressed crowds. The black artistic elite, including writers, dancers, composers, musicians, actors, and well-paid vaudevillians, all flocked to the Marshall. On any Sunday evening, the clientele might include Williams and Walker, Paul Lawrence Dunbar, Will Marion Cook, Ada Overton, Ernest Hogan, or Will Dixon.[52]

Europe worked as a cabaret pianist for a year before he started writing the music for a variety show produced by the comedian Ernest Hogan. The Memphis Students, Hogan's group of dancers, singers, and musicians, were a resounding success at Hammerstein's Victoria Theater in New York City in 1905. James Weldon Johnson describes this group as "a playing-sing-ing-dancing orchestra, making dominant use of banjos, mandolins, gui-tars, saxophones, and drums in combination, and was called the Mem-phis Students—a very good name, overlooking the fact that the performers were not students and were not from Memphis. There was also a violin, a couple of brass instruments, and a double-bass."[53]

This group pioneered several jazz band features including the singing band and the dancing conductor. Will Dixon, a composer, conducted the band: "All through a number he would keep his men together by danc-ing out the rhythm. . . . Often an easy shuffle would take him across the whole front of the band. . . . The whole band, with the exception, of course, of the players on wind-instruments, was a singing band . . . that is, a band singing in four-part harmony and playing at the same time." A third feature that greatly added to the appeal of the show was the trick trap drum-ming of Buddy Gilmore, who performed juggling and acrobatic stunts "while manipulating a dozen noise-making devices aside from the drums."[54]

After Europe's association with the Memphis Students ended, he worked as musical director and composer for several musical comedies including shows produced by Williams and Walker and Cole and Johnson. By 1910, he was one of black musical theater's major directors and com-posers. With the sudden deaths of George Walker, Ernest Hogan, and Bob Cole, opportunities for work in downtown theaters became scarce. But hotels and cabarets still needed dance orchestras. To fill this need, Europe joined Ford Dabney, Joe Jordan, Will Vodery, and William Tyers to set up the Clef Club, which offered the services of orchestras of any size, available day or night. Furnishing music for most of New York's cafes and elite private parties, his group cornered New York's "entertainment band" market.[55]

The Clef Club's crowning artistic and showbiz achievement came at a concert held at Carnegie Hall in 1912. On that evening, 125 musicians filled the stage with cellos, drums, double basses, saxophones, cornets, clarinets, banjos, guitars, mandolins, and ten upright pianos. James Wel-don Johnson was in the audience: "When the Clef Club opened its con-cert with a syncopated march, playing it with a biting attack and an in-fectious rhythm, and on the finale bursting into singing, the effect can be imagined. The applause became a tumult."[56]

James Reese Europe's significance to American dance music is difficult to overestimate. He was "a central figure in the [social] dance craze" that swept the United States between 1912 and 1916. Urban whites began dancing "in new ways to new rhythms, borrowing steps from black Americans" and adapting them to their own cultural style. Such European-American dances as the schottische and the waltz were rapidly eclipsed by a series of black vernacular dances including the shimmy, Texas tommy, turkey trot, and fox trot. White ballroom and cabaret exhibition dancers became twentieth-century "dancing masters," rigidifying, diluting, and codifying the dances to make them acceptable to white "high society." These hybrid dances, popularly known as "modern dancing," were performed to syncopated music that was a cross between ragtime and pre-jazz. Black dance music was in demand.[57]

Europe's response to the call of the times was to organize the Tempo Club, offering dance orchestras for hire. Around the same time he began a fruitful association with Irene Castle and Vernon Castle, the premiere white ballroom dance team at that time. Europe's Society Orchestra provided music for their tours and dance salons and accompanied them in private homes, cabarets, dance halls, and on film. Dabney and Europe helped make the Castles famous by composing special music for their dances and by recommending specific dances to them.[58] One dance suggested by Europe was the foxtrot: "Mr. Castle has generously given me the credit for the fox trot, yet the credit, as I have said, really belongs to Mr. [W. C.] Handy. You see then that both the tango and the fox trot are really negro dances, as is the one-step. The one-step is the national dance of the negro, the negro always walking in his dances."[59]

When the United States became involved in World War I, Europe enlisted in the black New York regiment and was later asked to organize a military band to equal the Clef and Tempo Club groups. Egbert Thompson, bandleader of the 367th "Buffaloes," helped train the musicians; the songwriter Noble Sissle became the drum major. Europe's band won spectacular fame throughout France and was invited in 1918 to play in Paris at the Théâtre des Champs-Elysées: "Before we had played two numbers the audience went wild. We had conquered Paris. General Bliss and French high officers who had heard us insisted that we should stay in Paris, and there we stayed for eight weeks. Everywhere we gave a concert it was a riot, but the supreme moment came in the Tuileries Garden. . . . We played to 50,000 people at least, and, had we wished it, we might be playing yet."[60] In a 10 June 1918 article that appeared in the *St. Louis Post-Dispatch*, Noble Sissle vividly described the band's first presentation of jazz to a French audience:

It seemed, the whole audience began to sway, dignified French officers began to pat their feet, along with the American General, who, temporarily, had lost his style and grace. . . . His [Europe's] body swayed in willowy motions, and his head was bobbing as it did in days when terpsichorean festivities reigned supreme. He turned to the trombone players who sat impatiently waiting for their cue to have a "jazz spasm" and they drew their slides out to the extremity and jerked them back with that characteristic crack. The audience could stand it no longer, the "jazz germ" hit them and it seemed to find the vital spot loosening all muscles and causing what is known in America as an "eagle rocking it." . . . Among the crowd listening to that band was an old woman about 60 years of age. To everyone's surprise, all of a sudden she started doing a dance that resembled "Walking the Dog." Then I was cured, and satisfied that American music would some day be the world's music.[61]

Returning home from the war, the 369th Infantry Regiment, drums up front, and with drum major Bill Robinson leading the way, were the first troops to march through the New York City Victory Arch. A *New York Times* reporter believed that James Reese Europe had produced a group that "all Americans swore, and some Frenchmen admitted, was the best military band in the world."[62]

Europe's idea of how to make music drew from his own vernacular experience and from his training in the European classics. Both his Society Orchestra and his Hellfighters band stood for "precision and control associated with 'strictly written' music, combined with a new improvisatory freedom and directness."[63] Although Europe's bands did not dance per se, they certainly did make others dance—not just with their music but with their syncopated marches and with the rhythmical body movements that accompanied their playing.

Many African American musicians developed their artistry by composing and playing in several different, but mutually enriching arenas, including black minstrel bands, military bands, dance bands, marching bands, and bands that performed in traveling shows and musical theater. This extensive cross-fertilization benefited all: "Many minstrel men joined army bands and the army bands in turn gave to the minstrels better musicians. Everything was on the upgrade musically speaking."[64]

Many of these musicians, professional or military, took their skills into black educational institutions. Some of their students became leading figures in American music. Writings on numerous jazz musicians mention the contributions of Maj. N. Clark Smith, the most legendary of these great teachers with a World War I background.[65]

Before starting his teaching career, Smith traveled internationally with minstrel companies and also directed several military bands. In 1907 he joined the military faculty at Tuskegee Institute, where he organized ensembles, bands, and choral groups. This paved the way for Capt. Frank L. Drye, who had been a band conductor with the Tenth Cavalry. At Tuskegee, Drye taught scores of musicians, including Shorty Hall, who later became Dizzy Gillespie's teacher in North Carolina. Smith later joined the faculty at Wendell Phillips High School in Chicago, where he taught many future jazz musicians, including Ray Nance, Milt Hinton, Nat Cole, and Eddie South. Clarke Terry was one of his students in St. Louis.[66] As a young boy, Lionel Hampton studied under Smith in the *Chicago Defender* Youth Band. According to Hampton, Smith

> always carried himself like a military man and sometimes dressed in military clothes, with a hat and a cape, and wearing medals. . . . He was kind of portly and had a handlebar mustache. . . . When he wasn't wearing military clothes, he always wore a vest, morning suit, striped pants. He had both flop tails and the short-tail coat for dress. . . . Walter Page and all those great musicians from Kansas City studied under him, including a couple of guys who later joined Jimmy Lunceford's band. . . . Major N. Clark Smith taught all those great jazz musicians, but he never taught jazz. The only time we'd play jazz was when Major N. Clark Smith wasn't in the room. He'd throw a stick at you in a minute. He taught harmony and reading, playing what you see. He taught you to play all kinds of instruments. He was a demon, about the greatest musician I guess I have ever known.[67]

During the first decades of the twentieth century, southern black academies and colleges, established by the American Missionary Society, were the training grounds for most black youth in the South. Many of the colleges maintained outstanding music programs staffed first by whites trained in European music. As racism forced African American artists to retire from the concert stage, many joined the music faculties of black colleges.[68]

In addition to their excellent choral ensembles and marching bands, black schools were the incubators for such dance bands as the Alabama State Collegians, led by Erskine Hawkins. Often the same students who played in the school's dance band also played in the marching band, resulting in a rich cross-fertilization. Many jazz musicians merged their vernacular training with the education they received from women and men schooled in European music: "One of the good things about the division of musical culture in Afro-America is that there have always been musicians trained in European styles and techniques, who pass it on to youngsters who opt for jazz." Ralph Ellison, who played in the bands at Tuskegee Institute in the early thirties, always credited his experience in music as providing the discipline he would later apply in his work as a writer.[69]

The relations between jazz and the black marching band is magnificently articulated in Ellison's description of his boyhood in Oklahoma City during the twenties:

> You see, jazz was so much a part of our total way of life that it got not only into our attempts at playing classical music but into forms of activities usually not associated with it: into marching and into football games, where it has since become a familiar fixture. A lot has been written about the role of jazz in a certain type of Negro funeral marching, but in Oklahoma City it got into military drill. There were many Negro veterans from the Spanish-American War who delighted in teaching the younger boys complicated drill patterns, and on hot summer evenings we spent hours on the Bryant School grounds (now covered with oil wells) learning to execute the commands barked at us by our enthusiastic drillmasters. And as we mastered the patterns, the jazz feeling would come into it and no one was satisfied until we were swinging. These men who taught us had raised a military discipline to the level of a low art form, almost a dance, and its spirit was jazz.[70]

During the years leading up to World War I, Florida Agricultural and Mechanical College was organizing its very first marching and concert band. The Marching 100's current extraordinary level of musicianship, its precision marching, and its stop-the-show dance stylings are extensions of an abundantly rich African American cultural heritage in music, song, and dance. The 329 members play with the technical skill of Frank Johnson, march with the snap and precision of the James Reese Europe regiment, and dance with the ebullience of a New Orleans second line on the last leg home.

Chapter Nine

The FAMU Marching 100:
From Ballpark Bleachers to
the Champs-Élysées

> Everything in our repertoire has expanded. . . . But we know what the
> music of our people is; and that's important. We know that they look
> at drills and all that kind of thing. But we know that our people like
> dances. And we don't cheat them.
> —Interview with Julian White

The African American drill sergeants of World War I who introduced
both melody and foot-stomping syncopation into military cadence
counting permanently altered the standard Western marching call that had
been in place for centuries.[1] This transformation in marching style is seen
and felt as well as heard: the body language of musicians in the black
marching band has always been distinctly different from that of their white
counterparts. While white American soldiers of World War I ardently strove
to march like well-oiled war machines, like battle-ready robots, the members of James Reese Europe's black 369th Regiment stepped to the beat
of a different drummer.

Distinct differences in cultural style between white and black are apparent today in this country's college marching bands, but the dividing
lines are blurring slightly as white bands work harder to pick up the black
style. Florida A&M University's Marching 100 not only captures the halftime spotlight wherever its musicians perform but it also serves as a model that black and white collegiate bands across the country try to emulate.

What audiences and other bands respond to is the tradition that goes
with the FAMU Marching 100's motto: "Perfection in music, highest quality of character, and precision in marching."[2] And what bands find hard-

est to imitate is the ingredient that gives the band its universal appeal and renown: its stop-the-show, jazz-spirited dances. FAMU's is the *dancing* marching band. Its legacy extends back to the far reaches of the African and African American past; it is the band that nobody can outdance.

The Marching 100 does not use female dancing groups or majorettes in its halftime presentations. The band members are their own dancers; they "strut their stuff" in specially designed uniforms with tough fiber expandable crotches constructed to accommodate half splits. When FAMU's 329 pacesetters step on the field, anything can happen: barrel turns, backbends, hitchkicks, swivel turns, pelvic thrusts, pelvic rotations — they glide, they slide, they slither and skitter. They even drop to the ground and roll onto their backs so that they can shake not just one but both legs to the pulsating rhythms of the percussion section.

With flawless timing, jaggedly syncopated facings, and level changes, the high-stepping women and men play on audience expectations. Drum majors ease into the slithering FAMU "rattler," weaving in and out with wave-like fluidity, then just as quickly slip back into a standard marching step. Underlying the appeal of these gestures are the moves not made explicit, but expressed through what Zora Neale Hurston calls *dynamic suggestion:*

> Negro dancing is dynamic suggestion. . . . Every posture gives the impression that the dancer will do much more. . . . *It is compelling insinuation.* . . . The Negro is restrained, but succeeds in gripping the beholder by forcing him to finish the action the performer suggests. . . . His dancing is realistic suggestion, and that is about all a great artist can do.[3]

Audience teasers, in the form of danced interludes, break up FAMU's halftime presentation. Even during the concert selections, drummers lean their torsos back and between beats execute carefully designed arm gestures that are similar to those done by black vocal harmony groups of the 1950s and 1960s.

But the appeal of this band is rooted in something more than its dance routine choreography, musicianship, and precision marching. The choreography of its entire presentation is ingeniously structured. At one point, for example, the band may use "divided-band technique" to create four groups: woodwinds, upper brasses, lower brasses, and percussion. Along with five drum majors and a flag corps (known as the Dirty Dozen), the instrumental divisions perform as independent units which at the same time are interdependent parts of the whole. The audience cannot focus on just a few performers, however, for over all the football field there is eye-catching activity, which simultaneously involves all of the interdependent sections.

Angularity and *asymmetry* are prominent throughout the Marching 100's dance repertory, which consists primarily of authentic jazz movements drawn from the rich storehouse of American vernacular dance. In the band's routines, we catch glimpses of the Charleston, birdland, boomerang, mashed potatoes, shorty George, monkey, chicken hop (from rhythm tap), twist, shimmy, and the Temptations' Walk. These dances, which flourished from the twenties through the sixties, are interspersed with the eighties' snake, gush, and funky-butt and the nineties' Tootsie Roll, butterfly, and bankhead bounce. Like no other, this band has an endless array of dance steps, and its particular way of accenting and syncopating the movement keeps spectators in rapt anticipation.

Excellence in Florida A&M's marching bands is not a phenomenon of the eighties and nineties; its tradition for excellence stretches at least as far back as the twenties, when the band traveled with the FAMC president J. R. E. Lee and served as the school's primary vehicle for recruiting students. Former band member Julian C. Adderley Sr. glowed with pride when he recalled the band's rivalries with minstrel bands, which served as the early training grounds for many of this country's best black musicians: "Talk about the Marching 100, 200, 2000 and all that kind of stuff. Well, they couldn't compete with us, oh no, because we were the best there was at that time and the only bands that could compete with us were the minstrel bands. . . . The band under Arnold Lee was one of the finest black bands anywhere. The Florida A&M band was recognized and rivaled."[4]

The Florida State Normal School for Negroes opened its doors in 1887, with Thomas DeSaille Tucker, born in Sierra Leone the grandson of a king, as the school's first president.[5] Some time later, legislation was pushed through to establish the school as a land-grant college under the Morrill Act of 1890, a federal mandate providing grants of land to state colleges that specialized in agriculture and mechanical arts.

Participating states that refused to admit blacks to their land-grant colleges could not receive money unless separate schools were set up for Negro students and the funds equitably divided. Thus, in 1909, the Florida State Normal School for Negroes became Florida Agricultural and Mechanical College (FAMC). By 1953 the institution had evolved to university status, and its popular name became FAMU. In its early years the college suffered severe shortages of support staff, supplies, laboratories, and equipment, for state officials illegally funneled most of the federal money to Florida State University, Florida A&M's all-white neighbor.[6]

Almost from the beginning, Florida State Normal School gave special attention to its music program. In 1892 P. A. Von Weller, an excellent German musician, began his tenure as the school's director of instrumental and vocal music, but at that time there was not enough money to support a band. Former students remembered Von Weller as quite an effective teacher.[7] When he left in 1898, the college music program continued to operate, though its money problems were, if anything, worse than before.

During those years, the school might have had a concert band. According to the school's official history, "the college had a band only when students owned their own instruments and only when the administration could find among faculty members someone who could give instruction." One such faculty bandleader was Herman Spearing of Jacksonville, who staged outdoor concerts, conducted music exercises in the chapel, and provided services to the military organizations on campus.[8]

Thus in 1910, when Nathaniel Campbell Adderley organized the first marching and concert band, the school already had a tradition of providing good musical instruction. He accepted the invitation of N. B. Young, the school's third president, to study tailoring at the college while putting together a band from whatever talent and equipment he could find. According to N. B. Young Jr., son of the president and a member of that first sixteen-piece band, Adderley "gave incentive and furnished motivation to many budding musicians on campus, some of whom developed into professionals."[9] Young recalled the creative interplay between the college band's playing "by the book" and its imitation of the highly syncopated black minstrel bands:

> The minstrel bands were super-musicians and the amateurs would follow behind them and watch them. And they began to learn and imitate what the minstrel bands did. . . . In the last three years we were beginning to use syncopation. But in the early days we played straight band music from the books put out by the Germans. Of course the black musicians put in curls and did things, especially with the trombone. So the moment they started to play, they put in personal touches. You could tell whether it was a black band or a white band in the early days. . . . The minstrel shows came in and they influenced us. The black school bands were playing more like minstrel bands as the time went on.

Under Nathaniel Adderley until 1915, the band played for the cadet daily dress parades, for special occasions during the week, and for chapel on Sundays. Throughout the year, it also participated in celebrations of the local towns and accompanied the baseball and football teams on trips all over the state: "The band played going to the games. They'd shout and yell. There was no such thing as a band playing a game in those early days. Between halves they just sat down, they didn't think about having music during a game. . . . The band was just a thing of itself."[10]

Nathaniel Adderley began a family tradition when he enrolled at the school. His brother Quentin and his sister Myrtle soon matriculated too. In 1923 Julian Adderley enrolled and began playing in the band. After him would come his two sons, the alto saxophonist Julian "Cannonball" Adderley and the trumpeter Nat Adderley. Julian Sr. joined the band as a high school student at a time when there were only eight to ten students enrolled in the school's college department. According to James D. Anderson, Julian Sr.'s situation was common: "Before 1920 southern black public secondary education was available primarily through private institutions. The total number of blacks enrolled in public and private secondary schools in 1916 was 20,872. Of these, 11,130 were enrolled in private high schools, 5,283 in public high schools, and 4,459 were in the secondary education departments of the twenty-eight land-grant and state normal schools and colleges." As a high school student who stayed on to attend the college program, Julian Adderley Sr., like many others, had quite a long tenure with the band. In turn his son Nat started with the band at age eleven and stayed with it for nine years.[11]

In 1923 the Florida State Board of Education tried to appoint a new president to the school who was reputed to be a poor administrator and weak leader. This effort sparked a student uprising that began with the burning of several dormitories and ended with several students in jail and all the others shut out of classes while the institution was closed under martial law. The disputed candidate's name was dropped from consideration, and several months later a former Tuskegee Institute professor, J. R. E. Lee, was appointed. One of the golden periods in FAMC's development was about to begin. President Lee had taught under Booker T. Washington and came to FAMC intent on patterning its growth after that of Tuskegee, whose outstanding band was led by Capt. Frank Drye, a veteran of James Reese Europe's 369th Regiment and the best known black college band director of the twenties. President Lee appointed Arnold W. Lee, one of Drye's former students, as the first salaried band director. According to Julian Adderley Sr., it was under President Lee's leadership that the FAMC band became known throughout the state of Florida:

> Actually it is through President Lee and the tone that he set and the things that he did that Florida A&M is what it is today. He believed in his band and he'd take us around everywhere. We'd go recruiting and trying to encourage blacks to send their kids to school. . . . He'd get up on the rostrum and tell about the opportunities and he'd tell lies on the band boys and we'd sit up there and enjoy it. . . . He'd say, "You don't have to have a lot of money; you come with what you got and let us work with you. See that Adderley boy over there? That boy with the horn setting up there? He came to school; he didn't have anything. Sometimes he didn't have money to get socks, he'd wear socks so long that they'd stand up like boots![12]

One summer President Lee hired the band director and the entire band to dig ditches for laying pipes on the campus, which not only provided employment and promoted a sense of familyhood among the band members but also allowed them to continue practicing and rehearsing together through the summer. During Lee's presidency, FAMU's band was the first black band to play for the Gasparilla (the traditional white state fair modeled on Mardi Gras) in Tampa, Florida, and the first to broadcast over Florida radio stations. It also performed during the Florida state centennial festivities.[13]

In the midtwenties a small dance orchestra called the FAMC Collegians was established, whose nucleus was drawn from FAMC's band and included Julian Adderley Sr. and Leander Kirksey. The football coach and two professors seem to have started the group by putting together the Casgoblacks, which staged a minstrel show at the college to raise money to purchase instruments for the school band. The musicians who played for that show stayed together as the FAMC Collegians, one of the nation's first black college dance bands.

When Arnold Lee left FAMC in 1928, Capt. W. Carey Thomas, another Tuskegee alumnus, took over the band, and under his leadership it continued to flourish. By 1930, one of its own alumni, Leander Kirksey, was ready to take over the position of band director. A master of the violin, Kirksey was the grandson of a slave who made fiddles and son of Leander Kirksey Sr., the ex-slave who founded Florida's first high school for blacks. His mother was an FAMC alumna of 1900 who had studied with P. A. Von Weller and who had been invited to tour Europe with Fisk's Jubilee Singers.

During Kirksey's fifteen years at FAMC, the band and the Collegians reached new heights. He established a scholarship program for band members, helped to organize the FAMC undergraduate program in music, and started the first instrumental music program for black high school students in Florida. His accomplishments at FAMC were wide-ranging in significance:

> In 1942, Kirksey went to Indianapolis, Indiana to the National Music Convention where he conceived the idea to start a program for black students in instrumental music in the public schools of the State of Florida. This notion of course created the possibility for the colleges, particularly Bethune-Cookman and FAMC, to have two hundred piece bands. Kirksey's initiatives were influential and indelible in that graduates from the department of music who majored in instrumental music under his tutelage became band directors in the state. At one time, every black band director in the State of Florida was a pupil of a pupil of a pupil of Kirksey.[14]

Leander Kirksey's FAMC band did not dance per se, as later bands did, but its marching and playing during halftime shows had an unmistakably syncopated snappiness. The Kirksey band continued playing for daily chapel meetings, Sunday vespers, and Wednesday night prayer meetings. Because of these performances, along with the regular rehearsals, Nat Adderley believes that band members received a great deal of personalized instruction:

> Mr. Kirksey was a very well-rounded man. We played more of a variety of music within the marching band tradition. We didn't really play jazz music, but Mr. Kirksey played in the Collegians with us—which of course made for a better relationship. And it also made for a lot more instruction again because we were getting instruction while we were playing. He was there playing alto [saxophone]. My brother [Cannonball] played first alto and he [Kirksey] played third alto in order to give him the experience of playing first. And a lot of us came out of there with a lot of experience because he was with us.

Under Kirksey, the Collegians toured every summer, not only in Florida, but also outside the state, traveling as far as Kentucky and Oklahoma.[15]

World War II drained FAMC's male population and put a severe strain on the band program. But by 1945 men were returning from the war and well-trained musicians were coming out of the public schools. When Kirksey left in 1945, J. Richmond Johnson served as band director for one year until the arrival of William Patrick Foster, known among students as "The Law." Foster's assistant, Lancelot Allen Pyke, had earned his master's degree in music at the University of Michigan, where he had played in the band under that famous trainer of band members William Rivelli.[16]

Foster obtained his professional musical training at the Kansas City Conservatory of Music and the University of Kansas, but he cites his years with the Sumner High School Band as the ones that provided the greatest inspiration for his future work at Florida A&M. Before going to FAMU in 1946, he had served as a band director at Lincoln High School in Springfield, Missouri (1941–42); as an assistant professor of music at Fort Valley State College in Georgia (1943); and as director of the band and orchestra at Tuskegee Institute in Alabama (1944–46).[17]

Nat Adderley, a member of the band during Foster's first five years of service, calls Foster "a strict disciplinarian kind of man [who] came with L. Allen Pyke. They brought this fast marching and these formations and making turkeys on the field and having legs come off at Thanksgiving. We'd heat it up by Lee Auditorium going down to the old football field and the very tempo of the music would have the football fans in a frenzy because it was all new and very exciting."[18] Foster is a highly skilled organizer who made it his business to fine-tune the group's structure. He also rehearsed the band and conducted all of the one-on-one instruction, while Pyke assisted him in developing the marching formations, writing parts for the band's various sections, and helping with the other myriad tasks involved in keeping such a group going.

It was Foster's dream, from the start, to build a band of one hundred marching musicians. By 1949 that dream was realized, and although numbers increased over the years, the Marching 100 became the band's permanent name. According to Foster, "the name was so strong, we couldn't change it." During those years the band was not a dancing band. But the syncopation was there, as a signature, and when the band played and marched at a quick, percussive clip, "the spirit was that of jazz." Although the group concentrated on standard band pieces like those of John Phillip Sousa, many of the players were involved in jazz dance music after hours, and the feeling came through. The drums, for example, did not play straight march rhythms but loosened up into what Nat Adderley later learned were "swing beats." "At the time I just thought they were hip beats. . . . The drum section played what Pyke and Pat Foster told them to play or what they wrote for them to play. It was always different and the rhythm was somehow different from what standard marching bands did."[19]

After three years Pyke left FAMU for Bethune-Cookman College and was succeeded by William Penn, another University of Michigan alumnus. Then in 1958, FAMC hired Leonard C. Bowie, the first in a series of A&M band directors who had played under Foster as students.[20]

With a solid foundation to build on, the FAMU band developed steadily through the fifties and sixties, starting many practices that are now traditional. One of the most significant changes came in the early sixties when dance steps were added to the band's halftime shows. FAMU may not have been the very first school to have a dancing band at halftime, but it certainly was among the first. Beverly Barber, a professor at FAMU and the director of the school's dance company, choreographed the band's first dance routine to the popular song "Walk on the Wild Side." Julian White, FAMU's associate director of bands who was a student when the dancing band first stepped out, calls Barber's choreography "eye catching and appealing. . . . She put dancing on the map. We had the vehicle but she gave us the impetus, she gave us the steps that were really appealing to the people."[21]

Thomas Lyle, former director of bands at Alabama State A&M, served as an assistant to William Foster from 1960 to 1964. In 1962 he began to work closely with Beverly Barber and probably persuaded Foster to include dance in the halftime performances. Barber explained how she and Lyle "would listen to the music and talk about what I had in mind. I tried steps out on him because they were concerned about the angles of instruments and he wanted to make sure they could do whatever we decided on without losing that speed, that angle for various instruments and without losing their lines." After a couple of years, the band staff took over the choreography, and, soon after, students began to choreograph. The idea of student participation at this level probably originated in one of Lyle's band pageantry or instrumental technique classes, in which students would come up with ideas for creating shows and then present them to the staff. Lyle was more than willing to have the students participate in the choreography. For one thing their direct involvement would keep the routines up to date: "We didn't want them to do the jitterbug. That's what I was doing when I was in high school and college, and really, I was too old to do the twist."[22]

In 1963 Foster set up the student Dance Routine Committee. Chaired by Lyle, it helped to bring versions of the latest social dances into the band's choreography. They started cautiously. "We did the twist in a stiff way," Lyle maintains, "because we were afraid of criticism and because the twist was thought to be vulgar." Stiff though their twist might have been, they were a knockout with the fans: "The 36,284 fans, now in a frenzy, went wild as the . . . band 'walked on the wild side' to the jazzy tune of the same name and made its exit while playing the 'All Sports March.' Nearly four-fifths of the huge crowd remained for the marchers' trip to Birdland for the post game show. The loyal fans came to their feet as the bandsmen did the 'Twist' from the formation of a pair of dark glasses while playing Ray Charles' 'Unchain My Heart.' "[23]

The current organizational structure of the Dance Routine Committee was established in 1973 by Julian White, who joined the band staff after serving for ten years as band director at Raines High School in Jacksonville, Florida. For White, that high school directorship was a perfect prelude to his position at FAMU because Kerna McFarland, the principal and a former student of Leander Kirksey, had been his high school director and provided the administrative support at Raines that enabled White to cultivate one of the nation's leading high school bands. Returning to FAMU was also a homecoming for White since he had been a drum major at FAMU ten years earlier.

The head of the five-member Dance Routine Committee is one of the most sought after and revered positions in the band. For ninety minutes each week that person is completely in charge. Even the drum majors are subordinate. Starting in early May, after the academic semester has ended, committee representatives are charged with scouting out the best new dances from the avant-garde of the vernacular dance scene: black American teenagers at parties back home.

About the second week of June, the committee begins to meet with White twice a week to scrutinize new dances, view films of them, and discuss which ones would be best for the band. After the steps are selected—along with the music that will show them off best—the piano score is prepared by the band's arranger, Lindsey B. Sarjeant. A jazz pianist and composer, Sarjeant has worked with Nat Adderley, Archie Shepp, Slide Hampton, and many other notable jazz figures. His newly arranged score is given to the students on the committee and they use it to prepare the routine.[24]

It is when they present their work to the band staff that the most intense scrutiny begins. The staff has to be careful about how the material is altered: taking out too much can kill the morale of the band, while leaving in too much that is new or "risqué" can shock or offend some of the fans. Matching the newly arranged score with the appropriate steps is seldom an easy process.

On one occasion the student body found out that a popular dance called "the gush" was being edited out of the band's dance routine. The next day the student newspaper's headline asked, "Is the Gush Dead?" During an interview of White by a staff member of the paper, White stated, "There'll be no more gushing in the band. We want to satisfy everybody, but also maintain the dignity of the organization and the integrity of the football stadium." Yet the students finally prevailed when the original choreography was restored after the audience responded in a cool manner to the revised steps.

As soon as the dance routine is set, Sarjeant uses the piano music to arrange a score for the band. Meanwhile, the Dance Routine Committee works out how the steps should be taught to the band, where the teachers and microphones should be stationed, and other such details. Not until the band's dance is choreographed is the music brought on the scene and aligned with the movements.

The playing marchers must master and then memorize the score before they can learn the dance. The highly organized preparations pay off richly. The Dance Routine Committee shows the steps to the marchers. Then the band staff takes over the fine-tuning of the performance, straightening the marchers' lines, and angling their instruments just so. In the final stages of rehearsal the band members go over the dance steps and perform them to the music. As one band staff member put it, "We teach them every aspect of the dance routine, just as if we were teaching them a drill or a piece of music."[25]

White explains the logic behind the band's dance component: "People enjoy things that they can identify with, and they enjoy mass movement. And that's what our dance routines are about. They're about massive movement. You have all of this energy channeled in the same direction, and that is what people like. . . . It has high emotional impact and content, and bands are moving in that direction."[26]

The Orange Blossom Classic in Miami, founded by J. R. E. Lee Jr. in 1933, is the most spectacular event in black college football annals. Many fans attend just to watch the halftime show. At the Orange Blossom Classic of 1964, the Marching 100 was the main attraction in a parade and halftime tribute to Olympic gold medal winner Bob Hayes. According to one reporter, "it was like John Philip Sousa doing the Watusi. Workers even came out of the manholes to watch (they could HEAR it down there) and hundreds of Miamians lined downtown streets to see the 160-piece Florida A&M University band. . . . Christmas shoppers stopped. Salvation

Army kettles didn't clink. 'That's the only band I ever saw march on its hips and shoulder blades,' said one parade fan."[27]

Although the high knee lifts and fast stepping (about 260 steps per minute) originated at the University of Michigan, these quick maneuvers look very different when performed by the FAMU musicians. The style of the Marching 100 is based on extremely high energy levels. Whereas most college marching bands use the glide step, the FAMU band marches with "points" and "drive." That is, each band member picks up one leg and then expends the same amount of energy to put it down, thus creating a pistonlike action between stationary points. Then a high knee lift and a 180-degree instrument swing are added, making each band member look like a drum major.[28]

Accenting all of the band's movements are dramatic haltings of all movement, which Foster calls "stopping points": no matter how fast the band marches, it almost always has some stopping points. True to its African and African American tradition, this stop-start pulsing in the band produces a very compelling percussiveness and dynamism. The swinging of instruments also involves "points": rather than waving them continuously, FAMU's band members move their instruments with startling quickness—up, down, and across their upper bodies—between stationary points.[29]

This movement of instruments along with the stylized shifting of the torso is called "instrument upper body flash." When this technique, accented by the straight lines and triangles of the high knee lifts, is added to the pulsating drive of the drummers, the visual effects are electrifying. The band staff tries "to have the percussion section *felt* rather than prominently heard, except when playing cadences or accents in support of the musical performance."[30]

The deeply felt thunder of the band's drums can rock a huge stadium from foundation to rafters. Moving through the great beams of sound created by the drummers and the highly percussive horns, the Marching 100 adds visual flash to standard maneuvers. The Marching 100's left face, for example, is executed with a danced snap that separates it from by-the-book military moves. Here is efficiency with flair. According to Julian White, quickness, precision, and unity are the keys: "We try to get all the instruments together, get all the arms together and I tell them I want all fingers going in the same direction; and that really gets them. I say, you know what? If you're going to blink your eyes, I want everybody to blink their eyes together or else everybody do twenty-five sit-ups.' They say I'm crazy, but they like extremes because it lets them know that we're going after perfection."[31]

Unlike other bands, the FAMU musicians never put their instruments down to dance, although at times they tease their audiences by starting to put them down, but then they quickly break right back into their routines. Other stylistic elements of the shows include deceptive facing movements, "neon flash" (quick change) formations, four-dimensional figured formations, and "kaleidoscopic patterns and dance steps interwoven into one concise routine." They also do all they can to make the transitional steps between formations just as eye-catching as the final patterns.[32]

At the Pro Play-Off Bowl in 1964 at Miami's Orange Bowl Stadium, the band presented "Television Showcase," which Foster regards as his best halftime show. The first animated formation, performed to the "Ben Casey" theme, was of a syringe, the injection of serum from it, and the word OW, which was formed after the needle descended. This was followed by a picture of the scales of justice, which tilted to "The Defenders' Theme." Since the back and front overlays of the musicians' uniforms were contrasting hues, the scales changed color as they moved up and down. The final formation, a sunburst, was done to a swing version of "You Are My Sunshine."[33]

According to Foster, *relevance* is the key word that identifies the band. The band staff tries to find ways for the band to project images of the current American lifestyle and of its current social, political, and otherwise newsworthy events, everything from the astronauts walking on the moon to Michael Jackson's moonwalk. White explains:

> The techniques that we have, they're good for us, they work. We've experimented with a lot of different kinds of half-time shows, but we always come back to the basic philosophy of doing shows that are relevant, that people can relate to. We try to play music that people can identify with. Everything in our repertoire has expanded. We play classical music and everything, but we know what the music of our people is; and that's important. We know that they look at drills and all that kind of thing. But we know that our people like dances. And we don't cheat them.[34]

At the 1986 Circle City Classic in Indianapolis, Indiana, a routine to the music of Janet Jackson stopped the show. The word NASTY took shape on the field, and the group bounced from side to side in an ironically "Holy Ghost" rock, each performer's free arm waving high "in testimony." Finishing a complete turn, and using leg kicks reminiscent of the lindy hop, the band members fell into half splits, rotated 360 degrees on their bottoms, and ended stretched out on the ground, legs crossed, elbows propped, the picture of nonchalant confidence. Their body language read, "*Ain't we bad?!*" The band's own halftime announcer intoned coolly: "Let's set the record straight: *Nobody* can outdance the Florida A&M Marching 100."[35]

Members of the Marching 100 keep their shows relevant for their audience by staying on top of current dance styles and also by expressing their African heritage. When the five drum majors take their classic stance on the field, they are assuming an adaptation of a bodily gesture that Robert Farris Thompson has traced to central Africa. Among the Bakongo, *télama lwimbanganga* (left hand on hip/right hand forward) was a pose reserved for persons of authority. "In Kongo," contends Thompson, "placing the left hand on the hip is believed to press down all evil, while the extended right hand acts to 'vibrate' the future in a positive manner."[36]

This angulated pose became a signature stance for the dancing baton twirlers or major joncs associated with Haitian rara bands and was presumably brought by Haitian slaves to New Orleans, where North American blacks adapted it to their needs:

> *Télama lwimbanganga* became *pose Kongo* in Haiti, then *pose Kongo* became the drum majorette pose in the United States. Almost all the early baton twirlers in and around New Orleans were black, or so it has been asserted by informants in New Orleans. But the commanding, strictly chiseled, crisp quality of the pose was too powerful, evidently, for whites to resist. Today the world center of baton twirling is said to be Mississippi—just east of Louisiana and not far removed from the influence of New Orleans.[37]

According to Thompson, John Szwed argued as early as 1971 "that baton twirling—now considered all-American and even Anglo-American—might conceal deep African roots." That same point of view was maintained twelve years later by Szwed and Roger Abrahams in their introduction to *After Africa:* "It seemed amazing to us as folklorists and ethnographers that such black cultural innovations as baton twirling, cheerleading, jug bands, broken field running in football, the North American cultivation of rice, okra, yams, and sweet potatoes, the terms *OK, wow, uh-huh and unh-unh, daddy* (as a term of endearment and respect between unrelated males), and *buddy* were not recognized as such."[38]

Many movement patterns, gestures, and stylizations of the FAMU dancing musicians have obvious African roots. For example, the use of angulated, asymmetrical patterning in their piston-like movement style echoes the segmenting of body parts and "playing of the musculature" in traditional African sculpture and dance. The artful stick twirling and attitudes of the FAMU drummers and the skillful hand movements of the cymbalists bring to mind descriptions of African percussionists in European military bands as well as the long tradition of drumming antics practiced by black American jazz musicians. When the drum majors break into their showstopping dances they become modern-day versions of Tricky Sam Robert's and Charley Randall's eight strutting drum majors, an act that Bill "Bojangles" Robinson joined in 1901. At the turn of the century, a fancy stepping drum major was often used to open cakewalk contests in Madison Square Garden.[39]

On the stadium field and in the bleachers, the Marching 100 is a repository of elements that link African and African American performance styles: cutting contests, propulsive rhythms, call and response, the drum as a force driving the band, the merging of visual and aural by featuring "dancing musicians" and "singing musicians," and "getting down," or moving closer to the earth during the most virtuosic dance moments.[40] Control, dynamism, coolness, and compelling insinuation are present in all of the band's shows. The ability of the Marching 100's staff to combine significant African American rituals of affirmation with relevant contemporary themes has won the band loyal fans who return to the college year after year just to see the halftime shows.

These loyal fans are particularly evident at homecoming. The festivities present FAMU as "the zenith of black colleges. . . . The parade through Frenchtown is like a Mardi Gras," reports White. Over 30,000 people and thirty-four bands, led by many FAMU Marching 100 graduates, showed up in 1988. Florida A&M's homecoming weekend is much more than an occasion for past graduates to reunite and pay tribute to their alma mater. It is a community ritual that draws people from throughout the state of Florida, many bordering states, and beyond. Former FAMU student Barbara Wynn shares her feelings about this important gathering: "Homecoming games strengthen the communal ties that bind FAMU alumni, students and friends. It's like uniting, sharing what's going on and continuing our history and tradition. A lot of kids come to the games now. That's good. They see positive role models, and that lets them know that they can be successful and high achievers—and it all starts here."[41]

"Homecoming '90—Rattler Venom More Potent Than Ever" was the theme of the 1990 celebration, which featured dance in many of the scheduled activities, especially the homecoming concert. "They're about to put the venom in 'em" blared from the loudspeakers as Pretty Poison, a squad of fifteen female dancers, thrilled the crowd of three thousand at the homecoming preconcert show. Next came the Strikers, twenty-four dancing men and women, followed by the Rattlerettes, FAMU's dancing cheering squad. The preconcert show ended with three brief presentations by amateur rap groups: Ratini on Ice, Rap Sensation, and the South MC's. All three featured back-up dancers.[42]

Dance was also the highlight of "Battle of the Bands," a field competition that included twenty-five high school bands from Florida, Georgia, and Alabama. Many looked like miniature Marching 100's as they high stepped and "California wormed" before a panel of judges that included the Florida A&M band staff. Those same bands marched in the homecoming parade the following day and were part of the twenty-five hundred musicians that played "The Star-Spangled Banner" on the field of Bragg Memorial Stadium for the opening of the homecoming game.

At all games, the real excitement starts to mount as soon as the university's 329 musicians leave the bleachers. Showtime begins, not on the field, but the second the band approaches the sidelines. For FAMU's band and for most black college marching bands, getting onto the field is itself a ritual. The Marching 100 forms lines along the sides of the field, makes an L-shape, then starts to move at an extraordinarily slow pace (20 steps per minute — 1 step every three seconds) known as the "death cadence." Then they explode into a spine-tingling pace of 360 steps per minute (6 steps per second). This spectacular entrance is followed by a drill or picture formation, a concert selection, the dance routine, and a flashy exit, during which the tuba players leap into the air and hit the ground so hard the stadium seems to shake.[43]

At FAMU's home games — and indeed whenever the band appears at a halftime show — concessionaires say that the peak selling period comes not at intermission but at the start of the third quarter. Julian White says, "There's a special thing at our football games. Halftime, everybody stays in the stands and it's going to have to be a heck of a football game to keep most of them in the stands during the third quarter because over on the student side they come down the stairs, under the bleachers and talk to band members. Some places we go they [band members] mingle and sign autographs."[44]

This special feeling the band generates remains long after graduation. Band members often cite their participation in the Marching 100 as the most significant aspect of their college years. Col. Bernard D. Hendricks, head of the FAMU ROTC unit, explains: "I learned more from Dr. Foster and the band staff about achieving a standard of excellence, and about the importance of completing a mission, than from any other experiences, courses, or activities that I had in college. The closeness and camaraderie of the band members seemed much deeper than even those of fraternity brothers. We were family. The friendships I formed then have stood the test of 22 years." As a builder of character, pride, self-respect, leadership, and—as the record shows—academic excellence, the Marching 100 is unparalleled on FAMU's campus. The organizational structure of the band is designed to give members an extremely active role in the preparation and perfection of halftime shows. The key positions of drum major, section leader, rank leader, and head of the Dance Routine Committee are cherished ones for which band members compete with great energy. Foster points out: "Band members are expected to be leaders as well as to strive for perfection in music and precision in marching. And they must dedicate themselves to service. . . . Get the emphasis off 'I' and onto 'we.' "[45]

This commitment to excellence compels Florida A&M's student body to take tremendous pride in the Marching 100 and great interest in its activities. Friday evening rehearsals draw scores of spectators, more than the practice sessions of the football, baseball, or track teams combined. Even the band's internal "politics" make news all over campus; for example, auditions for drum major—once the field of applicants has been cut to ten finalists—are public spectacles and enormous social events: "People would die to be a drum major in the band. Some try out for the position three times. The audition is like a production in itself because you have 500 people out there. They have to conduct, march, and show ability on the field with 500 people watching. You talk about putting yourself on the line. Some are not ready and you can't legislate how those 500 people will treat somebody who's out there."[46]

Like Friday night rehearsals and drum major auditions, the ten-day "pre-drill" session for freshman draws spectators from all over the city. Early each morning the aspiring band members meet for an eight-to-ten-hour work session on "The Patch," an outdoor practice area the size of a football field that has been worn bare by years of marching feet. The climax of this training session is called the "shaking of the tree," a ceremony in which freshmen are chosen to join the ranks of the band.[47]

Before 1974 there were no women in the Marching 100. According to

White, getting the first two female applicants accepted was "like trying to integrate the public schools." Band members complained that "girls couldn't keep up and that they wanted an all-male band." "Now women play a prominent role in the band," White added, "and we wouldn't have the quality band that we have now, if we didn't have women in it."[48]

The administration takes great pride in the quality of the Marching 100 as well. Just as President J. R. E. Lee used the band to attract students in the twenties, FAMU presidents have kept the numbers of admissions high by showing off the band throughout the year. According to Julian White, the band is the single most important recruiting tool for the university.[49] Showing off the band is easy considering the national and international exposure it has received. The Marching 100 made its national debut in 1963 in Miami's Orange Bowl Stadium. Since then the band has marched for football halftime shows on national television thirty-four times. In 1984 it performed for the Summer Olympics in Los Angeles. It also has appeared in three films, four national television shows ("20/20," "60 Minutes," "P.M. Magazine," and a Disney special), and three television commercials.

Each year the band receives hundreds of invitations to appear throughout the United States, South America, and Europe—many more than it can possibly accept. In 1989, the Marching 100 did accept an invitation to participate in France's bicentennial celebration of Bastille Day, which was broadcast to over eighty countries. The idea of inviting the Marching 100 to Paris came from Jean-Paul Goude, artistic director of the Bastille Day Parade. Included in his fourteen-scene "opera ballet" were 150 Senegalese drummers, 200 British military bagpipers, China's Peking opera dancers, Russian ice skaters, and many other groups from around the world. But occupying the most coveted position in the parade was FAMU's Marching 100. Having seen the band on "60 Minutes" in the early eighties, Goude was convinced that it was *the* group to represent America.[50] He was looking for a band that could reflect "world music" with a strong beat—music that is influenced by such artists as James Brown: "I have been to China, Russia—all over the world. No matter where I've gone, black music permeates. The reason why I selected Florida A & M's Band was because it is the epitome of black music. This band has virtuosity and the unique ability of combining dance with music." At Goude's request, the band performed Brown's music while they moonwalked and California wormed down the Champs-Élysées.[51]

The Paris streets were filled with people during the early morning parade rehearsal on 13 July. When FAMU's dancing musicians suddenly stopped playing their version of James Brown's "I Feel Good" and broke into an exuberant "BABY, BABY, BAYBEE . . . BABY, BABY, BAYBEE . . . ," the crowd of spectators "erupted." The responses to the band were such that French officials moved the Marching 100 from seventh place in the parade to last, the most honored spot.[52]

On the day of the parade, the Marching 100 was framed by six floats that "were built like bleacher seats topped with stadium lights . . . flag waving cheering section, pompon girls and all."[53] Their ebullient, angular dancing and musical arrangements swept Paris off its feet. The three-mile route from the Arc de Triomphe to the Place de la Concorde lit up as spectators clapped their hands, shook their heads, and danced to the pulsating rhythms of the "Godfather of Soul." "Thousands of young Parisians poured into the Champs-Élysées, breaking through all police cordons."[54] Edward Thomas, a senior trumpet player, recalled the excitement when the Marching 100 brought up the rear of the parade: "I remember looking back at one point, and people were just marching along behind us, dancing, singing for miles. It looked like they all wanted to be in the band, too." Another student said that he wondered if Parisians worked: "It seemed like they were all out in the streets, marching alongside us."[55]

In the world of college bands, FAMU's influence has been powerful. In 1985, the Marching 100 received the John Philip Sousa Foundation's Sudler Trophy, called the Heisman Trophy of the marching band world, a distinction given to the bands of only three other schools: the University of Michigan, Ohio State University, and the University of Illinois. Appropriately, Leander Kirksey also received the award as a tribute to his role in the development of the band and of musical education throughout Florida. Two white Florida schools, Florida State University and the University of Florida, are adding dance routines to their halftime shows thanks to FAMU. The University of Michigan and Ohio State University have requested videotapes of FAMU's Marching 100 and may soon put dancing bands on the field. FAMU alumni have served as band directors at Tuskegee University, South Carolina State College, Prairie View State University, Central State University, Hampton University, Alabama State University, Florida Memorial College, and Texas Southern University. And many Florida high school principals clamor for Marching 100 graduates to direct their bands.[56]

Alumni and tradition remain important to the band. In 1996 the staff was made up entirely of FAMU band alumni. Foster supervises a team of four men who have established reputations for excellence in the United

States and abroad. Julian E. White, Lindsey B. Sarjeant, Charles S. Bing (assistant director of bands), and Shaylor L. James (director of percussion) have worked together for over twenty years. White, often called the "drill sergeant" by students, explains how the staff works: "We are responsible for the nuts and bolts of the operation . . . for the overall coordination, designing, music writing, and implementation. We operate as a team, and Foster oversees it all."[57] From 1979 through 1989 Foster and his staff were also in charge of the McDonald's All-American High School Band, which marches annually in the Macy's Thanksgiving Day Parade in New York City.

Since the early twenties, the Florida A&M marching band has been recognized for its excellence. As a carrier of tradition, its high energy and spell-binding shows evoke African processionals, minstrel parades, and Caribbean carnivals. FAMU's Marching 100 is at the cutting edge of American college marching bands, cutting back to its rich heritage in African and African American music and dance, slicing into the future as the avant-garde band of the nineties.

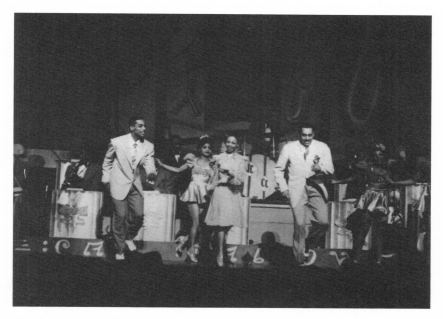

Cholly Atkins and Dottie Saulters with the Cab Calloway Revue (1943). Front row (*left to right*): Cholly Atkins, Dottie Saulters, and Cab Calloway. (From the Cholly Atkins Collection, courtesy of Cholly Atkins)

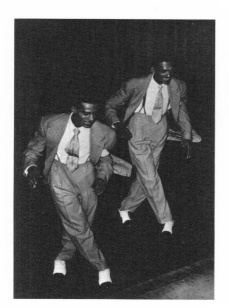

The classiest of class acts, Coles and Atkins, onstage (1940s). *From left:* Cholly Atkins and Honi Coles. (From the Cholly Atkins Collection, courtesy of Cholly Atkins)

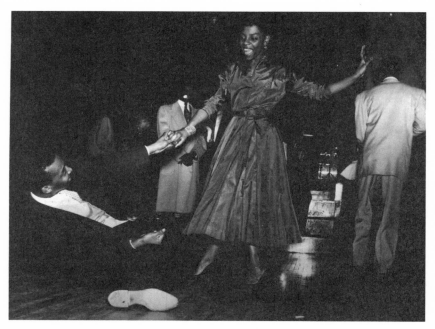

Stomping at the Savoy, 1953. (Courtesy of AP/Wide World Photos and the Photographs and Prints Division, Schomburg Center for Research in Black Culture, the New York Public Library, Astor, Lenox, and Tilden Foundations)

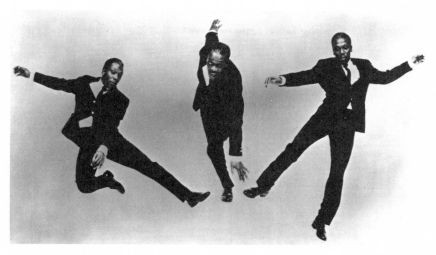

Baby Laurence, tap dancer. His body shapes and rapid-fire taps comprised an eloquently expressive language (1961). (Courtesy of the Dance Collection, the New York Public Library for the Performing Arts, Astor, Lenox, and Tilden Foundations)

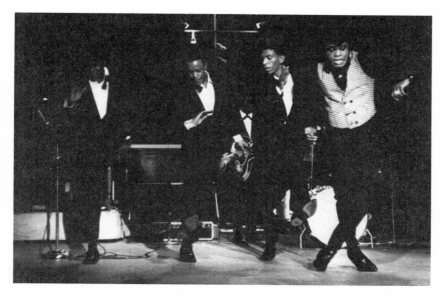

James Brown (*right*), the Godfather of Soul, and his Famous Flames thrill the audience in the 1965 Teenage Awards Music International Show. (From the Frank Driggs Collection, courtesy of Frank Driggs)

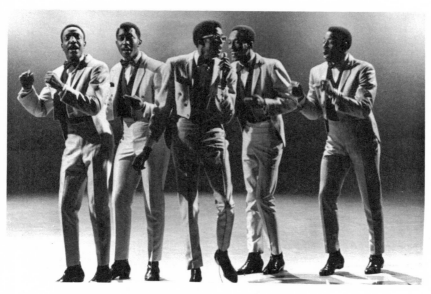

In concert, the temptin' Temptations, for whom Cholly Atkins has choreographed smooth, precise steps and turns for thirty years (circa 1966). (© Motown Historical Museum, from the collections of the Motown Historical Museum)

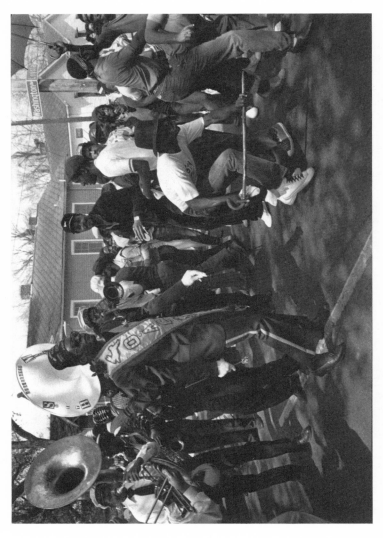

Olympian Aid Club's annual parade, New Orleans, Louisiana (1983). (Courtesy of Michael P. Smith)

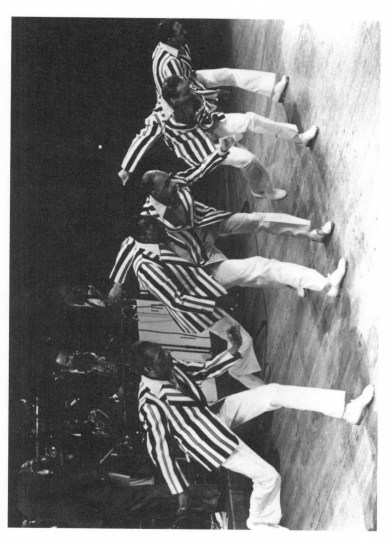

The swinging Copasetics in performance. These expert dancers were among the leaders of the rhythm tap resurgence that began in the seventies and inspired young hoofers worldwide (1979). *From left*: Honi Coles, Phace Roberts, Charles "Cookie" Cook, Bubba Gaines, and Buster Brown. (Courtesy of LeRoy Myers)

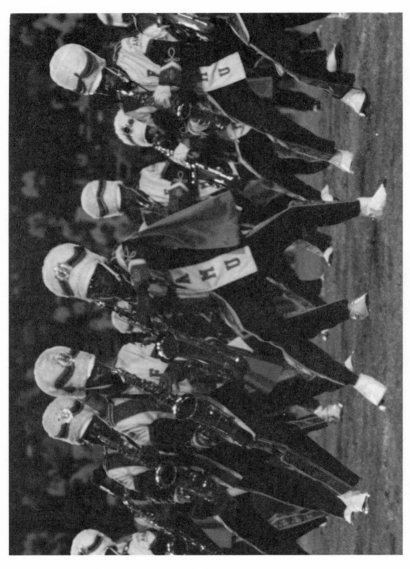

FAMU Marching 100's dancing saxophonists rock the stadium (1989). (Courtesy of William P. Foster)

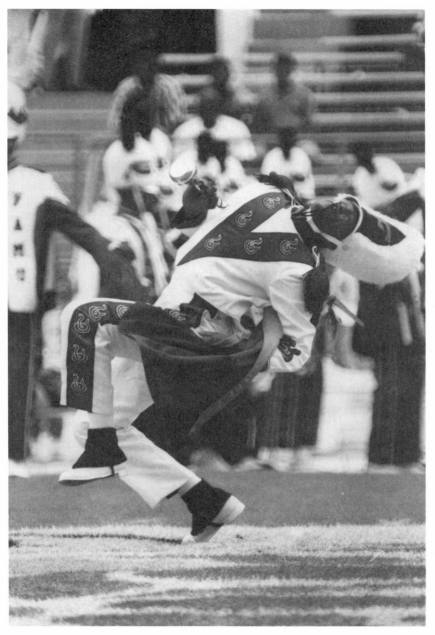

A Florida A&M drum major prances into action (1989). (Courtesy of William P. Foster)

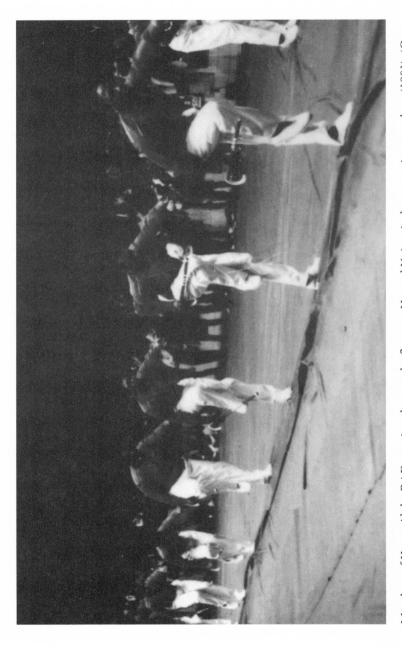

Members of Kappa Alpha Psi Fraternity take over the floor at a Howard University homecoming step show (1981). (Courtesy of the Moorland-Spingarn Research Center, Howard Unversity Archives, Photo by S. Devonish and W. Jackson)

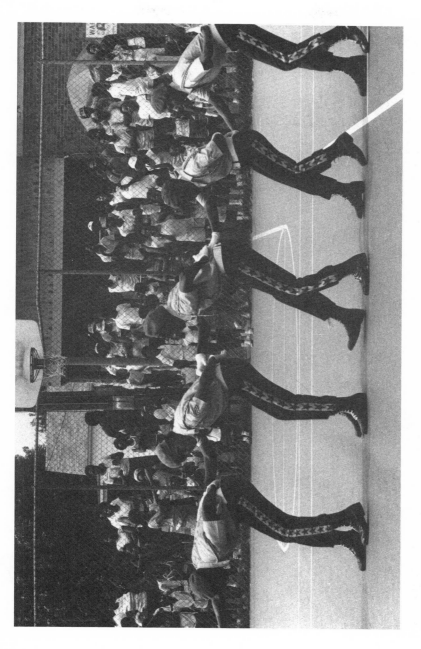

Drill team from the Earle C. Clements Job Corps Center of Morganfield, Kentucky, thrills the crowd at a 1982 Emancipation Day celebration. (Copyright © 1982, the *Courier-Journal*. Reprinted with permission)

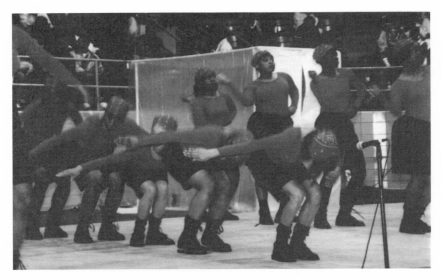

"Got to get down!" The Delta Sigma Theta stepping team of Howard University competes for the first place women's trophy at the Black Arts Festival Step Show (spring 1994). (Courtesy of Paul Woodruff)

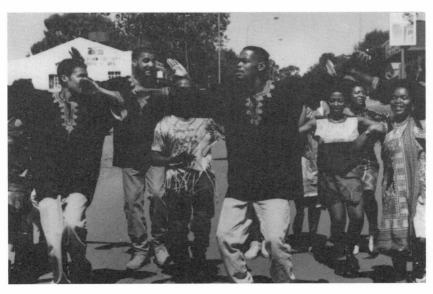

"Dancing in the streets." Members of Alpha Phi Alpha, Beta Chapter, demonstrate stepping in Johannesburg, South Africa (1994). Front row (*left to right*): Matthew Watley, Paul Woodruff, and Sydney Hall. (Courtesy of Paul Woodruff)

African American Mutual Aid Societies: Remembering the Past and Facing the Future

> They furnish pastime from the monotony of work, a field for ambition
> and intrigue, a chance for parade, and insurance against misfortune.
> Next to the church they are the most popular organizations among
> Negroes.
> —W. E. B. Du Bois, *Economic Co-operation among Negro Americans*

Although many historians have explained the prevalence of secret societies in African American life as an antidote to racism in the United States, that is only part of the story. African Americans of the eighteenth and nineteenth centuries were *culturally predisposed* to creating and joining mutual aid societies. As early as 1936 Carter G. Woodson identified the connection between African secret societies and African American secret societies. Woodson suggested that a comparative study of western African mutual aid associations with the most prominent African American ones would yield significant findings.[1]

African American Greek-letter sororities and fraternities, among the most prevalent mutual aid organizations in the black community today, were indeed founded in part as alternatives to European American sororities and fraternities, which excluded blacks. Yet the historical importance of these groups to black Americans, their evolutionary development, and the purposes they have served are all linked directly to the eighteenth- and nineteenth-century black self-help organizations that were grounded in western and central African patterns of mutual aid and economic cooperation. These widespread African cultural precedents paved the way for the pervasiveness of eighteenth- and nineteenth-century fraternal, sororal, and benevolent societies among blacks in the United States.

Between 1890 and 1910, sometimes called the "golden age of Negro secret societies," African Americans, systematically excluded from the general fabric of American social and economic life, created thousands of organizations that provided insurance and other benefits and that also offered opportunities for leadership and recreation. These societies, celebrating numerous holidays with colorful parades that owed their style at least in part to Africa, also were agencies of remembrance.

Alpha Phi Alpha, the first intercollegiate black fraternity, and Alpha Kappa Alpha, the first intercollegiate black sorority, were founded during the first decade of the twentieth century. At the same time, a wave of black activities aimed at economic cooperation and racial solidarity for political, economic, and social advancement was sweeping the country. During these years, many black banks, insurance companies, and retail businesses were formed by mutual aid organizations and secret societies.[2]

W. E. B. Du Bois delineated the function of mutual aid and fraternal and sororal associations in the early twentieth century: "They furnish pastime from the monotony of work, a field for ambition and intrigue, a chance for parade, and insurance against misfortune. Next to the church they are the most popular organizations among Negroes."[3] Du Bois and most other scholars, however, have failed to address the unique style of these organizations and how their development influenced African American music and dance. Throughout America, they provided halls for public dances, made available rehearsal spaces for musicians, and hired black bands for their various activities. In some cases they established their own bands. Black mutual aid groups have particular significance in New Orleans, where fraternal and sororal organizations provided the springboards for the black brass bands that helped give rise to the birth of jazz music and nurtured the jazz-spirited dance that influenced and was influenced by the music.

African American Greek-letter societies have, since their inception, provided jobs for black musicians and given support and special recognition to black performing artists. Undergraduate members of Greek-letter organizations have continued classic traditions in black dance, music, song, and language through "stepping," a multilayered dance genre that evolved from their song and dance rituals. Although most white Americans in the eighties and nineties learned about black sororities and fraternities through this nationally recognized dance style, they are unaware of the groups' rich history and the philanthropic dimension of their activities. The media has been more than eager to overlook the fact that African American Greek-letter sororities and fraternities are, first and foremost, service organizations.

Born in a climate of social and economic self-help, they were destined to eventually become service-oriented agents of social change. In the 1990s these organizations sponsored programs that addressed such problems as illiteracy, teen pregnancy, homelessness, health care, employment, drug abuse, AIDS, adoption, hunger, juvenile delinquency, and care for the elderly. They also made significant contributions to the United Negro College Fund, the National Urban League, and the National Association for the Advancement of Colored People. Indeed, much of the behind-the-scenes money that helped support the civil rights movement during the fifties and sixties was provided by black sororities and fraternities.

Numerous African American women and men have gained access to a college education through scholarships provided by these internationally recognized organizations. Unlike their white counterparts on American college campuses, many black Greeks maintain their memberships after college by affiliating with graduate chapters in the United States and abroad. At the end of the twentieth century, the memberships of the eight major African American sororities and fraternities—Alpha Phi Alpha, Alpha Kappa Alpha, Kappa Alpha Psi, Omega Psi Phi, Delta Sigma Theta, Phi Beta Sigma, Zeta Phi Beta, and Sigma Gamma Rho—totaled well over 700,000 with the numbers still increasing. With chapters in Africa, Asia, Europe, and the Caribbean, these organizations are involved in philanthropic and charitable work, not just in the United States, but worldwide.[4]

Origins

African slaves brought to the Americas were taken from areas where voluntary associations and secret societies flourished. From Senegal to Angola, these organizations functioned as powerful agents of social regulation that addressed political, economic, and religious concerns along with a range of other ones. Music, song, and dance were essential to their activities and many held annual festivals that included dances and processions.

Close parallels to African American lodges and benevolent societies of the late nineteenth century and the early twentieth existed in Dahomey. The *gbe*, organized for mutual aid, was one type of association that served as a permanent insurance society, providing members with money for funerals. Each society had a banner and ritual secrets, and through processions publicly displayed its resources and power, especially when walking in a large body to funeral rituals. Because the African worldview that life must have a proper ending was maintained by slaves brought to the

Americas, burial insurance became a central feature in North American black benevolent societies.[5]

Among the Ibo, "mutual aid was recognized as a moral obligation." The Ekpe, or Leopard Society, functioned as a governing body that recovered debts, judged important cases, made and enforced laws, and protected its members' property. In a region called Upper Guinea (Gambia, Senegal, Liberia, and Sierra Leone), life was, to a great extent, controlled by secret societies and voluntary associations. In Sierra Leone, the all-male Poro and its parallel women's society, Sande, conducted long sessions of training for youth who had reached puberty. Late fifteenth- and early sixteenth-century accounts of life in Sierra Leone underscore the importance of Poro councils: "They presided over matters of peace or war, the exercise of justice, the enforcement of penalties, the market price of yams and other goods, or the organization of dances and other public fun. . . . Membership was indispensable to self-respecting adulthood."[6]

Robert Farris Thompson has written pointedly about the Ejagham Ngbe Society of western Cameroon and southeastern Nigeria, "an all-male brotherhood devoted to the making and keeping of law, the maintaining of village peace, the hearing of disputes and, above all, the pleasurable dancing in public of secret signs of magic prowess." Membership is tested by sign language battles based on a secret gesture language called *egbe*.[7]

Most Africans brought to North America were from societies that exercised some form of initiation. Among the Bakongo, initiation was designed to strengthen society and ensure its preservation. Initiatory schools transformed adolescents into full-fledged community participants through training that involved music and dance on a large scale: "In the enclosures of the initiatory schools, dancing was performed for the benefit of supernatural powers which were embodied in sculptured figures or objects which served as snares for 'spirits'. The symbolism of form and of gesture constituted a language and an instrument which bound man to the whole of the Creation. They provided him with roots in the universe and in a past which opened with 'the time of the beginnings.'"[8]

In many parts of Africa from which slaves were taken to the Americas, there was a tradition of organized economic endeavor and cooperative mutual aid efforts. This tradition of organization and discipline provided a strong foundation for the spirit of cooperative endeavor that Africans kept alive through the establishment of secret societies, self-help groups, and a community approach toward group labor that was nurtured by the very nature of the plantation and farm systems in the colonies:

The tradition of cooperation in the field of economic endeavor is outstanding in Negro cultures everywhere. It will be recalled that this cooperation is fundamental in West African agriculture, and in other industries where group labor is required, and has been reported from several parts of the slaving area. This tradition, carried over into the New World, is manifest in the tree-felling parties of the Suriname Bush Negroes, the *combites* of the Haitian peasant, and in various forms of group labor in agriculture, fishing, house-raising, and the like encountered in Jamaica, Trinidad, the French West Indies and elsewhere. This African tradition found a congenial counterpart in the plantation system; and when freedom came, its original form of voluntary cooperation was reestablished.[9]

Charles Joyner has commented on the adaptation of a "basic African work orientation" or the imposition of a group consciousness on the work habits of slaves in South Carolina's All Saints Parrish, where African Americans hoed side by side to work song rhythms.[10] On Hilton Head Island off South Carolina, similar forms of cooperative work existed right after slavery: "Neighbors might help each other even when they were not ill, working first in the fields of one family and then in the fields of the other. . . . The societies such as Mutual Friendly Aid would come out without being asked to help a member who fell behind in his work."[11] Nineteenth-century Cuban cabildos were mutual aid organizations with direct African precedents. On Dia de Reyes, or Black Carnaval, they paraded to show their power and solidarity. One such group was formed by members of the Abakuá Society, a brotherhood "originally established by Efik and Ejagham (Ekoi) slaves from the region of Calabar and the Cross River of Nigeria-Cameroon."[12] Mutual aid societies that function like credit unions have been identified in several Caribbean countries. In the Bahamas this kind of institution, called *esu*, is believed to be a direct descendant of the Yoruba institution *esusu*.[13]

In his immensely important article "Early Black Benevolent Societies, 1780–1830," Robert L. Harris Jr. makes the point that late eighteenth- and early nineteenth-century African American benevolent societies were primarily responsible for laying a foundation for the establishment of such key institutions in black American life as independent churches, schools, insurance companies, and credit unions. They were instrumental in creating a feeling of community across state lines for urban free blacks. The earliest societies had strong links to African practices and frequently used *African* in their names. Such groups as Newport Rhode Island's African

Union Society (1780); Philadelphia's Free African Society (1787), the parent organization of the African Methodist Episcopal church; Boston's African Society (1796); Newport's African Benevolent Society (1808); and the New York African Society for Mutual Relief (1808) all worked to improve social, economic, and political life for free blacks and slaves in the North American colonies. What these and other black benevolent societies shared were ancestry, historical experiences, cultural affinities, and grievances.[14]

Many members had been born in Africa or were one generation removed from the continent. Thus it is not surprising that some of the major concerns of certain types of western and central African associations were sustained in early black benevolent groups: proper burial, good conduct, and moral training. "The free black benevolent societies resembled both the scope of African [voluntary associations] and the communal nature of African life. It could be that because of their communal experience, Africans in the New World had a greater tendency toward mutual cooperation. Moreover, their well-ordered and hierarchical social systems might have provided a greater propensity for organization."[15]

Although black benevolent societies in North America were culturally informed by an African heritage, they were not transported without change from western and central Africa. In addition to moral conduct and proper burial, to adapt to the new problems in a new environment benevolent societies addressed such additional concerns as education, charity, insurance against sickness and disability, credit unions, and pensions for the families of deceased members. Many formed discussion groups debating such questions as emigration or associating with the Underground Railroad. Membership was quite selective and those who violated established codes of good conduct were quickly expelled.[16]

By 1837, benevolent societies were the most widespread form of organization among free blacks in New York, New Jersey, Rhode Island, Massachusetts, and Pennsylvania. In addition to burgeoning numbers of national fraternal organizations, such as the Galilean Fishermen, Nazarites, and Good Samaritans, early black benevolent societies were directly responsible for the founding of independent black churches in Boston, Philadelphia, and Rhode Island. By 1830, when the first national convention of African Americans convened in Philadelphia, there was a well-established tradition of mutual cooperation among urban free blacks, especially in the North.[17]

The creation of self-help groups in the South, especially the deep South, was much more difficult than in the cities of the North. In many parts of the South, slaves were forced to hold secret religious services, which became a source of internal mutual aid organizations. Indeed, the church was the fundamental institution for African American self-help. "Benevolent and burial societies, it appears, were . . . numerous among the slaves. An account of mutual aid societies among the slaves in Virginia says that in every city of any size there existed organizations of negroes having as their object the caring for the sick and the burying of the dead. In but few instances did the society exist openly, as the laws of the time concerning negroes were such as to make it impossible for this to be done without serious consequences to the participants." Religious meetings also served as forums for designing insurrectionary activities. Public gatherings of African Americans were closely guarded in the South, especially in areas where uprisings already had occurred. But despite tremendously high risks, slaves and free blacks worked together to develop plans to liberate people of color in North America.[18]

One such plan involved Rev. Moses Dickson, the organizer of a group called the Knights of Tabor, twelve young men who joined forces in 1846 to create a liberation army throughout the South. Within ten years, over 40,000 men were recruited from all slaveholding states except Missouri and Texas. Their plan to attack Atlanta in 1857 with 150,000 troops was canceled when it became obvious that the Civil War was imminent. According to some slave accounts, the recruits, known as the Knights of Liberty, formed a network that assisted fugitive slaves. After the Civil War, Dickson founded the Knights and Daughters of Tabor, a benevolent society to commemorate the original twelve organizers.[19]

Southern free blacks maintained benevolent societies more successfully in the upper South, although there is some evidence that there were openly organized societies in New Orleans and Charleston. Some organizations included members who were slaves. For example, Frederick Douglass joined the East Baltimore Improvement Society while still a slave.[20]

In Lexington, Kentucky, free blacks formed the Union Benevolent Society in 1843. Its stated purpose was to bury the dead, care for the sick, and provide support for orphans and widows. Whites who aided the society permitted the formation of a lodge among the slaves in 1852. What the white patrons did not know was that this society also encouraged industry and education among free blacks and cooperated with Kentucky Underground Railroad agents in helping slaves to escape.[21]

Charleston, South Carolina's most successful benevolent societies among free blacks were the Brown Fellowship Society (1790) and the Humane Brotherhood (1843). Both groups "considered the care, education and apprenticeship of deceased members' children an important responsibility."[22] Among the most successful benevolent societies in the upper South were the Burying Ground Society (1815) and the Beneficial Society (1815) of Richmond, Virginia, and the Resolute Beneficial Society (1818) of Washington, D.C.

A widespread pattern of mutual aid continued to grow in secret and in the open in both the North and the South during the years preceding the Civil War. By 1848, Philadelphia had 106 black societies with approximately 8,000 members. Before the Civil War, Baltimore was the home of at least twenty-five beneficial societies. The Daughters of Jerusalem, Star in the East Association, and Friendship Benevolent Society for Social Relief in Baltimore had substantial savings accounts. John Hope Franklin suggests that many societies in the South continued to be secret, despite their numbers:

> In other cities there were benevolent associations of mechanics, coachmen, caulkers, and other workers, suggesting that blacks were organizing themselves into unions at about the same time as whites. In the deep South these organizations were frowned upon by most whites and were outlawed altogether in many communities. They persisted, however in some places. As late as 1860 they were being organized in New Orleans, where the Band Society, with a motto of "Love, Union, Peace," had bylaws requiring its members "to go about once in a while and see one another in love" and to wear the society's regalia on special occasions.[23]

In addition to forming their own associations, African Americans did begin to make inroads into all-white secret societies during this period. When Freemasonry lodges were formed in the American colonies in 1730, African Americans were excluded from membership. But an English regiment near Boston initiated fifteen black men into its Masonic lodge in 1775. Nine years later, Prince Hall, an abolitionist, a former slave, and a member of that first group of black initiates, secured a warrant for African Lodge no. 459. In 1842 African Americans were similarly refused membership in the International Order of Odd Fellows on the basis of race. But Peter Ogden, a black member of the Grand United Order of Odd Fellows of England, obtained a charter for a black lodge a year later. That secret order also grew rapidly.[24]

After emancipation, mutual aid societies mushroomed in the South.

Many of the groups that were formed before the Civil War blossomed during these years and numerous new groups were started. Aside from the church and the Freedmen's Bureau, these were the organizations to which the newly freed slaves turned for guidance. "Every southern city found itself filled with a myriad of groups with enchanting names such as the Galilean Fisherman, the Samaritans, or the Knights of I Will Rise Again." These benevolent and secret societies played a major role in helping freed women and men readjust to emancipation's changes. The Knights of Pythias and the Knights of Tabor vied for members. Black women joined the Sisters of Calanthe and the Order of the Eastern Star. Such local beneficial and insurance societies as the Young Mutual Society of Augusta, Georgia, the Workers Mutual Aid Association of Virginia, and the Beneficial Association of Petersburg, Virginia, collected weekly dues and provided business training for members. The Grand United Order of Galilean Fishermen was founded in Baltimore in 1856 but was not legally incorporated until 1869. W. E. B. Du Bois reported in 1907 that it had more than five thousand members, owned real estate worth $250,000, ran a bank in Hampton, Virginia, and was one of Maryland's most influential beneficial societies.[25]

Louisville, Kentucky, is the home of the United Brothers of Friendship, organized in 1861 by "a few young men, free and slave, being desirous of improving their condition." The United Brothers of Friendship began as a benevolent order, but later became a secret order, although the focus remained the same: burying the dead, administering to the sick, taking care of widows and orphans, and acquiring real estate. By 1905, the organization had over 63,000 members, including women, in fifteen states and in Liberia. Female members were known as the Sisters of the Mysterious Ten.[26]

Maggie L. Walker of Richmond, Virginia, brought the Independent Order of St. Luke (IOSL) to national prominence in the first decades of the twentieth century. The IOSL was established in 1867 to bury the dead, care for the sick, and encourage racial solidarity and self-help among African Americans. By 1899, when Walker became executive secretary, she was faced with a dwindling membership of 1,080, a treasury of $31.61, and numerous unpaid bills. Within six years, she established a bank, a newspaper, and a large department store. The bank financed 645 black homes by 1920. In addition, an educational loan was set up for prospective college students. During the late twenties the IOSL had over 100,000 members spread over several states, a $70,000 emergency fund, a $100,000 building, and 200 employees. It taught self-help to more than 20,000 children who participated in thrift clubs and attended special classes designed to teach hygiene, morals, and frugality.[27]

The Mosaic Templars of America was organized by fifteen women and men in 1883 in Little Rock, Arkansas. Although it was set up as a benevolent organization to serve blacks in Little Rock, it expanded to twenty-six states, Panama, Central America, and the West Indies. The principles of the society stemmed from readings of the life of Moses: "The Mosaic Templars was designed from the very beginning as an organization of love and charity and also as a medium of giving protection and leadership to members of its race as did Moses to the children of Israel." Its original purpose was to provide aid for burials and sickness, but its overwhelming success led to the development of a building and loan association, a Uniform Rank Department to train youth in drilling and calisthenics, and a newspaper, the *Mosaic Guide*. The Mosaic Templars purchased real estate in many states, contributed liberally to the U.S. government during World War I, and provided business training for African American youth.[28]

The most extraordinary African American organization at the turn of the century was the Grand Fountain of the United Order of True Reformers, organized in 1881 by an ex-slave, Rev. William Washington Browne, from Habersham County, Georgia. The True Reformers began as a joint stock corporation of women and men to provide "mutual beneficial insurance for its members." Over a period of twenty years, Browne developed a bank; a building and loan association; a printing office; a financial, agricultural, and industrial newspaper called the *Reformer*; a hotel; and a children's department. The organization bought fifteen halls, two residences, and three farms and opened several grocery stores and a home for the elderly. From 1881 to 1901 national membership skyrocketed from 100 to over 50,000.[29]

Benevolent and secret societies gave black Americans opportunities for cooperative enterprise, leadership, and social camaraderie. They fostered the development of community solidarity and gave valuable training that led directly to the evolution of black-owned insurance companies and banks. These organizations had characteristic styles that were manifested in the way the members dressed, presented themselves in public, and celebrated holidays and special occasions.

Given the importance of personal style in African American culture, it is not surprising that an organization's appearance in public and its uniforms and regalia would play a role in attracting members. Many small burial societies required special attire. One such society founded by a Baltimore woman fined members who did not appear at funerals in the designated outfit: "black dress, shawl and gloves, with lead colored bonnet and trimming, and white cuffs."[30]

Hundreds of mutual aid societies were formed in Virginia during the late 1800s. According to one source, "regalia of all kinds were worn and the society having the greatest amount of regalia was the most popular." Throughout the country, society members displayed carefully selected caps, robes, hats, buttons, collars, badges, tassels, swords, and spears. The dress of secret society members was in part adapted from the uniforms and brilliant regalia of black state militia during Reconstruction.[31]

The founder of the True Reformers, William Washington Browne, understood the relationship between member enrollment and pomp and splendor: "With a full white beard, a flowing black cape, and a huge flat-brimmed hat which shielded his piercing eyes, he captured the masses and added an air of the supernatural to the order. To many he appeared as a black John Brown. He took good advantage of this image and imposed a solemn ritual along with lavish regalia upon the members, and he added to that an annual convention which provided Richmond with its largest and most colorful annual parade." The anniversary parade of Baltimore's Galilean Fishermen was one of the most celebrated events in the city. On that great day, more than a thousand members marched in full regalia. The parade included "the Bishops commandery, the Gideonites commandery, the Priesthood of twelve persons, representing the tribes of Israel, each bearing a white stone in which the name of the tribe was cut, and 500 Virgins of the Ascension, with white dresses and veils, and with purple streamers about the waist, with the Ark of the Covenant in their midst."[32]

Secret societies offered an opportunity for black Americans to step out in style and march through the streets of America with resounding titles, including "supreme," "grand supreme," "honorable," "master," and "grand president." Among the ranks of the marchers were those designated as marshals, inspectors, legal advisers, orators, writers, secretaries, vice presidents, counsellors, inner and outer sentinels, chaplains, and wardens.[33]

Because military drilling was an especially important part of the training administered in juvenile departments, numerous societies developed crack drill teams. In Mississippi, Howard Odum discovered that most communities sponsored children's societies that met monthly to play, talk, sing, and drill. The Uniform Rank Department of the Mosaic Templars routinely featured drill contests for its male and female youth.[34]

The Improved Benevolent Order of Elks of the World, established in 1899, was especially noted for parades that featured dynamic drill teams in military uniforms. In 1895, the United Brothers of Friendship and Sisters of the Mysterious Ten held a grand parade in Kentucky that ended with a concert, speeches, and a drill competition.[35]

Throughout America, parades hold special meanings in black communities. In the early decades of the twentieth century, parades by fraternal and sororal organizations in Harlem garnered special attention and appealed to everyone:

> Harlem is also a parade ground. During the warmer months of the year, no Sunday passes without several parades. There are brass bands, marchers in resplendent regalia, and high dignitaries with gorgeous insignia riding in automobiles. Almost any excuse for parading is sufficient—the funeral of a member of the lodge, the laying of a corner-stone, the annual sermon to the order, or just a general desire to "turn out." . . . A brilliant parade with very good bands is participated in not only by the marchers in line, but also by the marchers on the sidewalks. For it is not a universal custom of Harlem to stand idly and watch a parade go by; a good part of the crowd always marches along, keeping step to the music.[36]

Numerous societies established their own bands or hired local bands for parades, dances, and other activities. W. C. Handy directed a Knights of Pythias band in Clarksdale, Mississippi. Indeed, many biographies and autobiographies of African American musicians reveal that secret societies provided work, rehearsal spaces, and early training for large numbers of musicians. Elmer Snowden, an early Duke Ellington Orchestra alumnus, had played with Eubie Blake's band at one of the many Pythian Castles during the teens. The hall had a dance floor where a male dance instructor ran an operation similar to a dancing school.[37]

Duke Ellington ruled the teens' dance space called Room Ten in Washington, D.C.'s True Reformers' Hall, "the meeting ground for young aspiring musicians and their coterie of admirers."[38] At the age of thirteen, Harry Carney, another Ellington band member, received early musical training with a Boston Knights of Pythias band: "They had an instructor who taught all the instruments in the band, and he taught me for the very nominal rate of fifty cents a lesson, the band furnishing the instrument." At fifteen, Dizzy Gillespie sat in with professional musicians at the Elks' Hall. Gillespie later applied for membership in the Masons. This secret society listed Ben Webster, Milt Hinton, Willie "the Lion" Smith, Garvin Bushell, and other jazz musicians on its membership roll.[39]

Jay McShann's band and many other musicians in the Southwest routinely played for club and fraternal dances. In cities across the nation, Saturday night was the ideal time to stomp the blues to the tunes of top jazz bands that played in such ballrooms as those of the Masonic Temple, Elks' Lodge, and the Odd Fellows' Hall. Mahalia Jackson recalled the Saturday night dances held in New Orleans during her childhood: "Down the street from our house was the Pride of Carleton dance hall. They had jazz music there for lodge dances every Saturday night. The children in the neighborhood were allowed to go and dance from eight until nine while the band was warming up and the people coming in. I was always dying to go but Aunt Duke never let me near that hall." Nowhere is the connection between black American music, dance, and mutual benefit societies more pronounced than in New Orleans, where in the 1990s social aid and pleasure clubs continue to strut through the streets to the music of brass bands.[40]

Mutual Aid Societies in New Orleans

> This is a music that you play for people. And when you're trying to reach people, you have to be genuine, you have to really express what you feel to them. See a lot of people don't really understand that, they think that if you just . . . play a lot of notes, then you make the job or you play to impress the musicians . . . But I believe that this music was made for people, it was made for that interaction. . . . Something beautiful happens, something beautiful transpires between the musician and the listener or the musician and the secondliner, or the musician and the dancer.
> —Michael White, *Liberty Street Blues*

New Orleans boasts a long-standing tradition of dance and music. From the time that this culturally diverse city was first established as a French colonial outpost, dancing was by far the most popular recreational activity among both blacks and whites. The first sustained musical activities, including concerts and opera, were supported by dance. Most documented accounts of life in New Orleans during the early nineteenth century point to the importance of dance in the day-to-day lives of the city's residents. One visitor during the nineteenth century wrote, "In the winter, they dance to keep warm, and in the summer they dance to keep cool."[41]

By 1806 there were at least fifteen public ballrooms; thirty additional dance sites were established between 1836 and 1841. Free blacks in New Orleans used some of the same ballrooms for their dances as whites did. Every evening in taverns and cabarets, black residents, free and slave, mingled freely with white residents. Most accounts of dancing among black New Orleanians emphasize activities at Congo Square, but slaves also attended public balls despite the many attempts by government officials to stop them. Numerous halls sponsored large dances and almost all private parties ended with dancing. According to Henry A. Kmen, "negro dancing in New Orleans was at once more complex and more widespread than the legend implies." They danced on the levee, in stores, in large rooms, and on city streets; they strutted along behind parading bands that might appear at any time of the day.[42]

In New Orleans, where residents were always ready for a parade, picnic, dance, excursion, or public ritual, brass bands were ubiquitous. By 1865, "a brass band tradition was firmly rooted in the black community." After emancipation even the politicians were indirectly promoting the bands. The black Reconstruction leader P. B. S. Pinchback urged blacks to organize in order to improve their social standing: "Form Societies of Benevolence, hold meetings at least once a week to debate the questions of the day, that relate directly to us, thus keeping the masses posted in what is going on." These benevolent societies were the springboards for black street bands.[43]

A few black benevolent associations were formed as early as the 1780s in New Orleans, but by the early 1860s, social and beneficial clubs were central to African American life. From the late nineteenth century through the early decades of the twentieth, many of these organizations hired bands to play for funerals, dances, annual parades, and various other club-related activities. Over 226 African American societies were active between 1862 and 1880. The wide range of groups included racial improvement societies; lodges of the Odd Fellows, Masons, Knights Templar, and Eastern Star; social and literary clubs; baseball clubs; rowing clubs; militia companies; religious societies; orphan aid associations; and benevolent associations.[44]

During Reconstruction, these societies were vital to the black community, building halls, acquiring real estate, establishing bank accounts, offering financial assistance in times of need, and providing communal recreation for all ages. African American societies sponsored train and steamboat excursions to other cities in and outside of Louisiana. These trips provided employment for bands that typically entertained about 900 people. Large picnics were held at Oakland Riding Park, the fairgrounds, and the city park. Blassingame reports that "this was one of the most important forms of com-

munal recreation encouraged by schools, churches, and social organizations." Participants enjoyed baseball games, shooting matches, military drill
competition, foot races, band music, sack races, fencing matches, croquet,
buggy races, raffles, and, of course, competitive dancing.[45]

Aside from churches, black societies furnished almost all social activities for African Americans except such commercial entertainment as theatrical productions and traveling shows. Important events were celebrated with giant parades and huge gatherings; Congo Square and Lafayette
Square were the sites of mass meetings. By the final decades of the nineteenth century, approximately four-fifths of the city's population belonged
to mutual aid societies. With the exception of the church, more blacks in
New Orleans were members of benevolent societies than of any other kind
of voluntary association.[46]

Typically, the benevolent societies acted as social organizations and
insurance agencies. Members paid dues in exchange for sick benefits, the
privilege of attending social affairs, and funeral coverage. "The tradition
of funeral parade music in New Orleans dates back to the 18th century,
when slaves, under the French, were permitted to bury their dead with
music." Although military and state funerals featured martial music in
Louisiana during the eighteenth and nineteenth centuries, the ceremonies were European in prototype. According to New Orleans newspapers
of the 1850s, whites used brass bands at funerals. They played in the form
but not in the style that became associated with black funerals.[47]

What became known as the New Orleans jazz funeral is probably a
combination of western and central African funeral rites with eighteenth-
and nineteenth-century martial music. Although whites eventually rejected
the brass band funeral form, blacks continued to find it perfect for the
expression of their culture.[48]

Black funeral processions in New Orleans are led by the grand marshal,
who walks in front of the band and wears a dark suit and white gloves. A
group of dancing enthusiasts, called the second line, brings up the rear
of the processional. After the church and burial services are completed,
people on foot regroup and wait for the parade to start. Zutty Singleton, a
former band member, recalled the typical funeral scene: "Right out of the
graveyard, the drummer would throw on the snares, roll the drums, get
the cats together and light out. The cornet would give a few notes and then
about three blocks from the graveyard they would cut loose."[49] One observer described this ebullient cutting loose at the burial service:

Tension loosened, sorrow gives way to a lighter mood. The band strikes up "Oh, Didn't He Ramble!" The grand marshals change to a quick and lively strutting, with second liners following suit. Some begin to dance. . . . Suddenly, open umbrellas of every size, color and shape appear, some fantastically adorned with bells, feathers, flowers and ribbons. The rejoicing is exuberant and general. Musicians and spectators want to give the deceased a good send-off—which he is indeed getting, probably just the kind he would have ordered, as a member of one or more of the numerous benevolent and burial societies. The deceased had probably looked forward, during his lifetime, to just such a grand *demise*. As one second-liner said: "Your proudest day is when they lay you away!"[50]

The high-spirited stepping of the second line underscores the interrelatedness of dance and music in New Orleans. The support for brass bands that was provided by the societies, clubs, and fraternal organizations not only kept the music alive and fostered its evolution but also helped initiate the close connection between dance and jazz music that reached its peak in African American culture during the 1930s. William J. Schafer, author of *Brass Bands and New Orleans Jazz*, sees a marriage of dance and music in the street parades of black New Orleanians: "The dance feeling is one of the strongest elements of the New Orleans streetband sound, an element permeating the music and communicating itself to the second liners following the band. The followers never march in four-square fashion; they shuffle and strut. And the dance impulse is the fabric of the music."[51]

The traditional jazz clarinetist and native New Orleanian Michael White has asserted that he is at his creative best when playing in parades because "brass band music offers the closest link to the true spirit, nature, and harmony between musician and listener."[52] Second-liners who follow the parades do the same thing with their bodies that musicians do with their instruments. Just as the musicians enjoy a kind of call and response with each other, they also converse with the second-liners. This form of communication is conversational although it does not involve words:

You are not saying actual words or expressing actual words, but you are expressing genuine emotions—you laugh, you cry, you sing, you shout, you dance sometimes with the music. . . . All those emotions that you express musically are also being expressed by the dancers and that's what we see in their movement. . . . We see in their movement what we're playing. We see the same emotions being expressed nonverbally through dance that we are expressing musically. . . . We are doing an audio thing and they're doing a visual thing but it's expressing exactly the same emotions for the same reasons and there's a mutual understanding.[53]

Second-line dancing is largely improvisational so no two people do it the same way. Although different generations incorporate the social dances of their eras, there is a characteristic style that is unique to black New Orleanians. The most important thing, however, is to move to the rhythm of the music. Black New Orleans parades generate a kind of renewed spirit among the bands' followers during celebratory peaks. The combination of exciting music and exuberant dancing has a healing, almost magical effect on the second-liners: "Walking canes and crutches that almost never leave the ground are suddenly hoisted high in mock imitation of the grand marshall's umbrella. Elderly faces that often express a tiredness and hopelessness in the struggle against death, now glow. Bodies that have been bent by decades of hard times now straighten out, twist, and gyrate with renewed vitality, and say that they will continue dancing 'until the butcher cuts [them] down.'"[54] Initially second-line dancing served as "a parallel to the jazz tradition that offered the spectator a chance to participate on the same level as the musician and that's exactly what happened at dances and street parades."[55]

The ongoing presence and significance of New Orleans street parades is frequently explained as an outgrowth of the rich cultural mix of the city and its beginnings as a French colony. While those factors are certainly part of the story, the importance of western and central African processions is often underplayed, even though African Americans have had the greatest and most enduring influence on the character and continuity of street parades in New Orleans. The overwhelming presence of Kongo and Kongo-related cultures in New Orleans played a major role in the continuation of street parades by black social aid and pleasure clubs, the modern-day offshoots of black benevolent societies. "Bakongo and their neighbors formed the majority population in New Orleans, the people who named Congo Square, who gave that place its Kongo dance, and lent their minds to the formation of new creole styles which eventually reverberated all the way to Broadway and the entire world."[56] Among the Bakongo, parading was a serious matter: "Bakongo believe that ritual processioners ideally carry fortune and spiritual rebirth to a village that they circle." They further believe that hidden problems can be mystically healed and that their environment can be cooled by circling gestures of good faith and felicity. Among the Yoruba, it is believed that the ceremonial visitation of Egungun maskers rolls away evil and bad luck and brings on good fortune.[57]

Processions, carnivals, and street parades play a central role in the black communities of South America, the Caribbean, the United States, and elsewhere. Contrary to the opinions of many metropolitan critics, festival arts are highly structured events with cultural influences that are centuries old. What critics also fail to recognize is the value of "the procession as a choreographic form." Rex Nettleford, a choreographer and the artistic director of Jamaica's national dance company, considers this form significant: "Mobilizing masses of people in marches, with their feet keeping a basic rhythm while the upper parts of the body in polyrhythmic counterpoint carve myriad designs in space, produces a different kinesthetic quality and visual impact than that of the American Modern Dance or the European classical ballet, both of which are rooted in the cultural realities of their respective habitats."[58]

Michael White calls African American parades in the Crescent City moving parties that collect people. He has commented insightfully on the "unique spiritual and musical connection" that exists between New Orleans and parades and the functional role that brass band music has always played in New Orleans: "This music was fun, but it was serious at the same time. It had conviction, it was about something. It wasn't done as entertainment or for money. You always had the sense that the end result of playing, the reason for playing was the music."[59] The music's spirit transcends the kind of things that normally divide people; it expresses a cultural bond and makes participants feel that they are part of an extended family. White explains that joining a New Orleans moving party is "a way of achieving freedom on a spiritual level":

> You're doing what you want to do, you're feeling free, you're expressing your whole life—the good part, the bad part, the hard part, what the white folks are doing to you, what your own folks are doing to you, your happiness, your celebration, and it's your time and your chance to attain true freedom. . . . This freedom . . . it transcends everything. It transcends your social condition, whether you think you're a Creole or a Negro or whatever you want to call yourself; whether you come from educated, uneducated, literate, illiterate, or what have you. You're all on an equal plane and you have your time to express yourself and you have your time to create and say what you want to say.[60]

K. Kia Bunseki Fu-Kiau is the founder of the Kongo Academy in Bas-Zaïre. His explanation of the meaning of parades among the Bakongo dovetails nicely with Michael White's views and gives further credibility to the acknowledged influence of Kongo philosophy on black New Orleans processions: "Festivals are a way of bringing about change. People are allowed to say not only what they voice in ordinary life but what is going on within their minds, their inner grief, their inner resentments. They carry peace. They carry violence. The masks and the songs can teach or curse, saying in their forms matters to which authorities must respond or change. Parades alter truth. Parades see true meaning."[61]

According to White, the sound of the bass drum in a New Orleans black neighborhood can still draw literally hundreds of people out of their homes in anticipation of an opportunity to dance along the streets behind a brass band. He has identified four kinds of parades in New Orleans: church parades, jazz funerals, miscellaneous community parades, and club parades, those sponsored by black social aid and pleasure clubs. Louis Armstrong felt the excitement of club parades during the early decades of the twentieth century: "To watch those clubs parade was an irresistible and absolutely unique experience. All the members wore full dress uniforms and with those beautiful silk ribbons streaming from their shoulders they were a magnificent sight. . . . The members of the club marched behind the band wearing white felt hats, white silk shirts (the very best silk) and mohair trousers. I had spent my life in New Orleans, but every time one of the those clubs paraded I would second-line them all day long." Social aid and pleasure clubs of the nineties do not provide the same degree of financial assistance as the earlier benevolent societies did, but they have continued other important aspects of the tradition: jazz funerals, balls, and annual parades.[62]

Club parades, held annually on Sunday afternoons from September through December, represent a rich and colorful festival tradition. They typically draw larger crowds than other African American street parades. Brass bands are hired on the basis of their ability to generate energy and spark excitement in the parade.

Each Sunday afternoon during the festival season, communities eagerly anticipate the club members' display of elegance in dance and dress. Style, innovation, and creativity are of supreme importance, and although some clubs buy expensive outfits and rent limousines, performance is the most important aspect of these events. The display of wealth is always secondary to the club members' desire to demonstrate distinctiveness and unity through music, dance, and artistic sensibility. Club members see their parade day as an opportunity for individual expression in dance and a chance to "strut their stuff" for friends, relatives, neighbors, and competing clubs.[63]

Parades of the late nineteenth century and the early twentieth helped increase community pride and social consciousness by demonstrating strength and unity among African Americans. Black New Orleans street parades of the 1990s grow out of that rich history; they provide a way to celebrate and keep alive a cultural tradition that reaches back to western and central African processions. Kept alive largely by African American sororal and fraternal organizations, black street parades in New Orleans offer much more than diversions from daily life; they offer freedom, fellowship, and spiritual rebirth.

The importance of mutual aid and sororal and fraternal organizations to African American life since the eighteenth century cannot be overstated. Black Greek-letter fraternities and sororities inherited a rich tradition of mutual aid and cultural reinforcement. Their belief systems and rituals do more than keep alive values that perpetuate social, political, and economic advancement for blacks. Through stepping and other social activities they affirm and extend African American cultural style in music and dance. They are among the modern-day versions of early black benevolent societies. They help provide a way for African Americans to face the future and remember the past.

Stepping: Regeneration through Dance in African American Fraternities and Sororities

> Good glory, give a look at Sporting Beasley
> Strutting, oh my Lord.
>> Tophat cocked one side his bulldog head,
>> Striped four-in-hand, and in his buttonhole
>> A red carnation; Prince Albert coat
>> Form-fitting, corset like; vest snugly filled,
>> Gray morning trousers, spotless and full-flowing,
>> White spats and a cane.
> Step it, Mr. Beasley, oh step it till the sun goes down.
>> —Sterling Brown, "Sporting Beasley"

"Regeneration of Soul" is the homecoming theme at Howard University, where hundreds line the bleachers of Burr Gymnasium at the largest fundraiser of the week-long celebration: the annual homecoming step show. A halftime guest appearance by the Muslim Girl Training and General Civilization Class, Nation of Islam is ending as the drill team of young women marches off the floor. The gymnasium starts to buzz with excitement in anticipation of the show's second half, a battle of Howard's fraternities in stiff competition for the first place trophy.

All eyes are riveted on the gold, black, and silver sphinx painted on a canvas pyramid that stands in one corner of the gymnasium. The Alpha step team announcer begins: "Ladies and gentlemen, good evening. For us as a people of African descent, the turn of the century brought darkness. But all hope was not lost. For in the year 1906, seven bright lights stood upon the Nile to guide us to peace. From that vision, from that dream, in 1907 Beta was made. And the vision is a reality, a reality that started off very small."[1]

Rap music blares from the speakers as ten African American boys (ages six to nine), burst through the front flaps of the pyramid and perform their versions of the latest hip hop steps. The crowd is ecstatic. When the music stops, the ten boys freeze in angulated stances, proudly displaying the Alpha Phi Alpha hand signal. After their exit, the announcer sets the stage for the Alpha step team: "But now, ladies and gentlemen, that small dream is a reality. And now, the brothers from Beta are here to make it happen. To the Howard University Homecoming step show theme, 'Stepping in Sequence,' showtime proudly presents 'Standing Room Only, the Brothers of Alpha Phi Alpha.'"[2]

The "aesthetic of the cool" swings into operation when, one by one, the twelve Alphas emerge from the pyramid. For this year's show they've chosen a Boyz II Men look: black Bermuda shorts, black baseball caps, white long-sleeved dress shirts with ties, black socks, and heavy-soled black shoes.

The men of Alpha Phi Alpha strut, glide, and pimp across the floor as they slap five, coolly acknowledge the crowd, exchange hugs with their brothers, and "profile" their way to center stage. In the words of the vernacular, they are "dead up in the tradition." With heads bowed, feet firmly planted in a wide stance, and arms crossed, each member waits for the first call from the step leader. It is unquestionably *show time*. They are about to perform one of the most exciting dance forms to evolve in the twentieth century: stepping, a complex multilayered dance genre created by black American Greek-letter fraternities and sororities.

Spike Lee's 1988 film *School Daze* provided the first widespread exposure for this ritual dance form, which began on college campuses. Since that time it has been featured on such television shows as "A Different World" and the "Arsenio Hall Show," in music videos, in television commercials, at regional dance conferences, and in a one-hour documentary produced by Jerald Harkness. In January 1993, the Alpha Phi Alpha step team of Howard University performed on the Mall in Washington as part of President Clinton's inaugural celebration. During December 1994, the Alphas were invited by the Soweto Dance Theater to Johannesburg, where they performed, taught stepping, and took classes in South African dance forms.

Stepping features synchronized, precise, sharp, and complex rhythmical body movements combined with singing, chanting, and verbal play. It requires creativity, wit, and a great deal of physical skill and coordination. The emphasis is always on style and originality, and the goal of each team is to command the audience with stylistic elements derived primarily from African-based performance traditions. Even though the choreography is prearranged, competition ensures an element of surprise and helps keep standards high, not an easy feat when the onlookers are aficionados who understand all of the codes of the genre and eagerly look forward to something new and unique at each performance. Their enthusiastic participation is what gives a step show its dynamic quality. "The spirit of stepping," writes dance critic Sally Sommer," is what I would wish for all dancing."[3]

A step, which usually lasts from one to five minutes, is defined as a complete choreographed sequence or series of movements. It can be verbal, nonverbal, or a combination of the two. Women and men perform on separate teams, and at Howard University fraternities and sororities are judged separately, although they appear in the same shows.

What we call stepping today grew out of song and dance rituals performed by Greek-letter chapters as a way of expressing loyalty toward their organizations. Over a period of approximately fifty years, this constantly changing dance form has evolved and absorbed many cultural influences, including military drilling, black social dances, African American children's games, cheerleading, vocal choreography, martial arts, the precision marching of historically black college bands, South African "gumboot" dancing,[4] music videos, acrobatics, and American tap dancing. Like many other vernacular forms, stepping has the ability to assimilate almost anything in its evolutionary path and still retain its distinctive character.

Because the most characteristic movements and body stances of stepping are based on traditional western and central African dance styles, many practitioners of the form believe that it "came from Africa." But this is a somewhat misleading point of view, especially when one considers how cultural transference takes place. It would be more accurate to view stepping as a uniquely African American dance genre that was created in the United States but is, in the words of Roger Abrahams, "animated by the style, spirit, and social and aesthetic organization of sub-Saharan Africa."[5]

In a step show, we see all of the five traits of western African dance and music: dominance of a percussive concept of performance, multiple meter, call and response, songs of allusion/dances of derision, and apart playing and dancing. What we notice first and foremost in contemporary stepping is the sound of the drum. According to Francis Bebey, "the drum is, without question, the instrument that best expresses the inner feelings of black Africa. . . . Even when the drum itself is physically absent, its presence is reflected by hand-clapping, stamping, or the repetition of certain rhythmic onomatopoeias that are all artifices that imitate the drum beat."[6] At step shows, however, drums are not played. Rather, the body becomes an instrument, and through clapping, foot stamping, and intricate slapping of the hands against various body parts, multiple rhythms are produced. One of the most interesting aspects of stepping is that the older it gets, the more African it looks.

A Zairian scholar initiated in traditional Bakongo culture, K. Kia Bunseki Fu-Kiau responded in the following way after seeing footage of a Howard step show: "When I just opened the film I said, 'I can't believe this is passing; that this is being done at Howard University. And my question was: 'Who is the trainer of these young people?' Because this person could not lead them to do this without going to the Kongo area."[7] According to Fu-Kiau, crossing the hands underneath the thighs and above the thighs (as performed by the Howard step teams) is typical Kongo play, especially among young girls. The Ki-Kongo name given to games and play done with gestures of the hands and feet is *nsunsa*, and there are specific songs that are associated with that movement. *Nsunsa* also gave rise to maroon *susa*, a Suriname sparring dance.

Fu-Kiau reports that the foundation of the slicing arm and hand movements done by step team members is called *mbele* in certain areas of lower Zaire. *Mbele* literally means "knife" and it consists of moving the hands in a cuttinglike fashion, similar to fighting. *Mbele* includes circling and turning around one's playmate, which reenacts the movement of the stars. The children involved chant songs as they move from one spot to another. This kind of play can be seen currently in the cities and villages of Kinshaasa among young people. It is also typical play in Jamaica, where Ki-Kongo words appear in the songs that accompany the play.[8]

Robert Farris Thompson tells us that women and men with shared Kongo beliefs created related dance patterns throughout the Black Atlantic World. Thompson contends that

> the bumping of waists to end a dance, Kongo *bakana*, became Afro-Cuban *vacunao* and Afro-Brazilian *umbigada*; that Kongo *tiénga*, circulatory hip motions, became the Kongo grind in U. S. jazz dance and *gouyade* in Haitian choreography; and that the thigh-and-chest slapping dances imparting confidence and self-spirit in Kongo *kamba* evolved into nineteenth-century North American patting juba, twentieth-century black-Brazilian *bate coxa* (literally "slap thigh" dancing), and twentieth-century hambone in the black United States. Further expressions—the

conga lines of Afro-Cuba and the ring shout of the Deep South Old
Time Religion—brought back the circling "altars in motion" not only
of Kongo play and worship, but before them, of San and Pygmy styles
of reverence by the fires of God and the forest.[9]

Since the early nineteenth century hand patting and foot stomping have
been mentioned in writings on African American performances from slave
festivities to traveling shows, vaudeville, musical theater, and rhythm tap
dancing. Slave literature is replete with references to the rhythmical patterns produced by blacks. Cultural heritage, according to Gerhard Kubik,
can be transmitted unconsciously from generation to generation:

> In a time of slavery and oppression some specific cultural traits may be
> forced to disappear among their carriers. They do not really disappear.
> They only *retreat* to a safer area of the human psyche. For example, if
> you prosecute drumming in an African community and even burn all
> the drums of the people, what will happen? The drums will perhaps
> really disappear and the drum patterns will not be sounded again, but
> they will still remain—in a silent shape. The drum patterns will just
> retreat into the *body* of the people. And there inside they will remain
> like on micro-film. This has nothing to do with genetics, because the
> transmission is cultural, through human interaction. The drum patterns
> will be transformed into a set of *motional behavior;* they will go back to
> their source. In this form they will continue to be transmitted from
> mothers and grandmothers to their children, from father to son during
> work, non-verbally, as an *awareness* of a style of moving. When a favor-
> able moment in history comes, the drum patterns surface again, perhaps
> on some other instruments. Some young people suddenly "invent"
> something new.[10]

Vigorous hand and foot interplay among slaves was referred to as "patting." The former slave Solomon Northup explains in his narrative that
"patting is performed by striking the hands on the knees, then striking the
hands together, then striking the right shoulder with one hand, the left with
another—all the while keeping time with the feet, and singing."[11] Although
many scholars who have written about dance during slavery maintain
"patting" was an activity created by slaves because drumming was discouraged in many areas, it is, as Fu-Kiau and Thompson have pointed out, an
African tradition. Hitting the body with the hands or "using the body as a
drum is fundamentally Kongo." Some Dahomean women's societies accompany their songs with a unique sound produced by beating the chest
with a clenched fist or open hand.[12]

While doing research on corn shucking ceremonies among slaves in North America, Roger Abrahams found substantial evidence to support the view that African Americans preferred to dance on planks rather than the bare ground because they acted as sounding boards for the complex rhythms that were produced.[13] What we see in stepping is a 1990s version of the same practice. Most step teams prefer using hard-soled shoes on wooden surfaces in order to amplify the sound.

Sorority and fraternity members also use canes and sticks as percussive devices. The use of canes, staffs, and sticklike objects has been noted in the dances of many traditional African cultures. Among such nomadic groups as the Mbuti, who have no drums, sticks and other implements are carried for musical purposes and used in conjunction with rhythmic stamping, hand clapping, complex body movements, and vocal techniques. Dancing with sticks is not usually seen in the Kongo area, but in northern Zaire and Sudan, where the martial arts are very popular, the use of sticks is coupled with dancing and chanting. Sticks are used for dancing by the Zulu, in South Africa, and among various cultures in Zambia and Mozambique.[14]

Slaves brought to North America commonly used sticks to beat time on the floor. In African American dance acts of the 1920s through the 1940s, canes were often used to add flare and variety to stage presentations. The Berry Brothers were internationally famous for their acrobatic strut and cane dancing. In a display of perfect rhythmical timing and incredible agility, they could twirl their canes with lightning speed, bounce them off the floor, slide them down their arms, and throw them in the air, while tapping or performing flashy spins and knee drops.[15]

Although Kappa Alpha Psi is reputedly the most skillful at using canes, several of Howard's step teams have adopted this practice. Through the use of canes, sticks, or the hands and feet, large step teams sometimes separate into three or four carefully spaced sections and function like drum choirs, each performing a different rhythm at the same time. Multiple meter is present in the body movements of the individual performers as well. Usually they dance at least two rhythms simultaneously, although at times three rhythms are played, particularly when canes are used. At the 1991 Howard University homecoming step show, the University of Virginia Kappas coordinated sharp head turns with three different rhythms: one with their canes, another with their feet, and a third with their left hands pounding against their chests.

Call and response between the step master or whoever gives the first

call and the other members of the team happens on a verbal and nonverbal level. As an introduction for a step that is done blindfolded, the Alphas of Howard moved to the following call-and-response pattern:

> Leader: Brothers!
> Team: Ice!
> Leader: A Phi
> A Phi A
> Uh, get *down!*
> Team: Got to get down!
> Got to get down!
> Leader: Get *down!*
> Team: Got to get down!
> Got to get down!
> Leader: Get *down!*
> Team: Got to get down!
> Got to get down!
> Leader and Team: A Phi A Alpha Brothers
> have *got* to get down! . . . Uh, you know![16]

There is a continuous call-and-response pattern between spectators and
dancers. Audience members spring to their feet with the exuberance and
enthusiasm of a football stadium crowd, and during the most virtuosic
movements, the steps evoke verbal support and encouragement: "Break
it down, y'all!" "Get it, girl!" "All right!" "Work it out!" "Go, Sherri!" "Get
down, Chris!" Whistles, yells, barks, and numerous other verbal incanta-
tions almost drown out the performers. When teams don't quite meet the
mark, a Howard step show audience can be as tough as the Apollo Theater crowds of the thirties and forties. Moving off beat, dropping props, or
forgetting choreography can mean instant defeat for any competing team.[17]

The special connection between the step show audiences and performers at Howard grows out of a shared knowledge of language and gesture
that constitutes what Gerald Davis calls an *aesthetic community*, "a group
of people sharing the knowledge for the development and maintenance
of a particular affecting mode or 'craft' and the articulating principles to
which the affecting mode must adhere or oppose" in performance.[18] The
audience members become both participants and observers, and the entire presentation of each team is designed specifically to elicit as much
positive response as possible.

While the audience's reaction depends greatly on the movement skills
of the performers, speech—witty speech, chanting, and verbal play—holds

a crucial role in the overall presentation. Steppers can trace the traditions of eloquence in speech to sub-Saharan Africa.[19] Ethel M. Albert's study of speech behavior in the traditional kingdom of Burundi is, according to Abrahams, characteristic of writings on African peoples:

> Speech is explicitly recognized as an important instrument of social life; eloquence is one of the central values of the cultural world-view; and the way of life affords frequent opportunity for its exercise. Sensitivity to the variety and complexity of speech behavior is evident in a rich vocabulary for its description and evaluation and in a constant flow of speech about speech. Argument, debate, and negotiation, as well as elaborate literary forms are built into the organization of society as means of gaining one's ends, as social status symbols, and as skills enjoyable within themselves.

When African slaves arrived in North America, they brought with them a "sensitivity to a wide variety of speech activities and a highly systematic sense of appropriateness in regard to content, formality, and diction."[20]

Many observers of slave life have commented on the African American everyday use of proverbs, speeches, and movement nuances. The leaders of such slave festivities as cornshucking ceremonies were selected for their ability to rhyme and improvise in a witty manner. Cornshucking captains and set callers at dances seized these opportunities to engage in social commentary: "The notion of employing song or rhyme for making oral commentary came directly from the various African cultures from which the slaves were taken."[21]

In keeping with the traditions of their ancestors, the festivities of slaves were occasions to celebrate through the use of song, dance, music, and language. This winning combination is maintained at step shows, where oral commentary and verbal play are central to the overall success of the event. The rhymes, however, are not improvised, but rehearsed in advance and are delivered more often by a group than by an individual.

Because stepping is rooted in a traditional African worldview that values communication that is interactive and interdependent, the language of stepping must be entertaining as well as functional. The forms of discourse used at Howard step shows grew out of a much larger system of terms or figures of speech that are present in the verbal play of African American communities throughout the Americas. Among the most widely used terms in the United States are *woofing*, *playing* (as in playing the dozens), *marking*, *sounding*, *signifying*, *shucking*, *jiving*, *cracking*, *rapping*, and *joning*. These "ways of talking" function as floating terms that to some degree vary in definition depending upon the community in which they are used. Abrahams insists that "many of the names for these ways of speaking change constantly from time to time and place to place, but the patterned interactions and the relations between the types of situated speech remain essentially constant."[22]

Although the patterned interactions were present in the step shows, most of the students did not describe their actions with these terms. For example, none of the students used the terms *signifying* ("to imply, goad, beg, boast by indirect verbal or gestural means"), *sounding* (a verbal dueling strategy that involves direct taunts), or *marking* (when a speaker, through direct quotes, reproduces the words, voice, and mannerisms of the targeted person or group). The umbrella term used by Howard's stepping community to cover all three verbal dueling strategies is *cracking*. Geneva Smitherman defines *cracking* as a way of "putting down" someone or showing disrespect for them, either in fun or seriously.[23]

Usually fraternities crack on other frats, and sororities limit their cracks to rival female groups. In this practice we see a close link to the songs of allusion/dances of derision of African music and dance styles. By diminishing the status of their opponents through witty verbal surprises, sorority and fraternity members draw cheers from the audience. As Smitherman points out, "excellence and skill in this verbal art helps build yo rep and standing among yo peers."[24] Delivered with just the right amount of rhythmical punch, a successful crack can bring the house down. In the following combination of marking and rapping, the Deltas of Howard parody the trade steps of the AKAs and Zetas:

> Leader: What is a Delta?
> Team: It is a serious matter . . . (performed in the song
>   and dance style of AKAs)
> Leader: That is definitely not a Delta!
>   Sorors, what is a Delta?
> Team: Woo-pee-dee, Woo-pee-dee . . . (performed in a
>   Zeta style)
> Leader: That is not a Delta!
>   Sorors, *what* is a Delta?
> Team: Devastating, captivating, oh so fine
>   My soul stepping sisters gonna blow your mind.
>   Many are called, but the chosen are few.
>   Delta Sigma Theta's gonna rock it for you![25]

Saluting, a term coined by the fraternities and sororities, is a way of paying tribute to another group. Through a combination of movement, song, and speech, fraternities salute sororities and vice versa. In a seven-minute salute to fraternities at the Howard 1991 homecoming step show, the Delta Sigma Theta twenty-two-member team captured the character-istic stepping styles, calls, and hand signals of the Kappas, Alphas, Sigmas, and Omegas. The step leader began the call as the Deltas prepared to stomp their way into a marching-band-like formation:

> Leader: Here's what you've been waiting for—D S T
> Team: Here's what you've been waiting for.
>   We are that mighty, mighty Delta squad!
>   Here's what you've been waiting for.
>   We are that mighty, mighty Delta squad!
>   Here's what you've been waiting for.
>   We are that mighty, mighty Delta squad![26]

Positioned in four sections across the gymnasium floor, they took turns performing takeoffs on the stepping style of each fraternity. The longest and last segment of the salute was preserved for the Delta soul mates, Omega Psi Phi:

> Leader: I said my D, my D, My D
> Team: S T
>   My Q, my Q, my Q
>   Psi Phi
> Leader: I said my Q, my Q, my Q
>   Psi Phi
> Team: My Q, my Q, my Q
>   Psi Phi
>   (continue chant until they change formation)
> Leader and Team: All of our love and peace and happiness,
>   we want to give to Omega.
>   All of our love and peace and happiness, we want to give to
>   Omega Psi Phi.
>   Repeat
> Leader: Sorors!
> Team: Yes!
> Leader: I said, my sorors!
> Team: Yes!
> Leader: I said, how do you feel about Omega Psi Phi?
> Team: I like to roop, roop
>   roop, roopity, roop.[27]

With hard-pumping body language, the Deltas broke into a series of typical Omega-like movements. The stands exploded with barks, cheers, and stomps, leaving no question about who would take home the women's first place trophy.

To understand the dominant role that Howard University has played in the evolution of black fraternities and sororities, it is necessary to examine the beginnings of these organizations during the first decades of the twentieth century and their impact on extracurricular activities. When Howard received its charter in 1867, black Greek-letter organizations were nonexistent. At that time black institutions of higher learning were in a stage of infancy, and although many were called colleges, they actually functioned more like preparatory schools for a newly emancipated people. Howard took on a different character from many of its rural counterparts further south. It was designated an integrated "university" for the liberal arts and sciences, where men and women could freely choose their majors from a diverse number of departments. And because it was located in Washington, D.C., students had firsthand exposure to speeches and discussions that addressed the nation's most pressing political issues.[28]

At evolving black colleges, the cultivation of morality, piety, and Christian virtues was the primary concern of the founders and the northern missionaries who held most of the faculty positions: "The Negro college was thrust into the roll of creating moral awareness and exercising moral control over those within its jurisdiction—a role which has been continually identified with its reason for existence. The presidents, both white and black, of the early Negro colleges were usually ministers."[29] These men invariably believed that blacks lacked morals and that they needed stringent guidelines established or they would not be able to follow correct rules of conduct, especially of sexual conduct. Rules for women were particularly stringent. An 1885 regulation for young women at Howard stipulated that "students [were] not to take rides, or walks, correspond, or engage in out-of-door games, with those of the other sex without permission from the proper authority."[30]

Dancing was prohibited by many administrators during the early years of black college development. When music was played at the formal socials of some schools, neatly dressed couples were allowed to march in unison under the watchful eyes of strict chaperones. After the "march," a carefully planned system of rotation limited conversations between couples to five minutes.[31]

The earliest extracurricular clubs at black schools were literary or debating societies. Their purpose was to nurture student intellect through debates, skits, speeches, and plays; some sponsored journals and magazines and a few helped establish private library collections. At Howard University between 1890 and 1903, music, art, literary, dramatic, and debating clubs were not as popular as oratorical contests, drilling, and athletics. Class associations were very important during the years preceding World War I. Each class selected a motto, colors, and a flower that it proudly displayed at interclass debates, oratorical contests, and athletic battles. Competition between classes, particularly the Sophomore-Freshman Flag Rush, generated intense rivalries.[32]

The emergence of Greek-letter organizations at black schools did not occur until the first decade of the twentieth century, but they developed at white schools much earlier. Although Phi Beta Kappa, begun in 1776 as the first American intercollegiate Greek-letter society, is now an honorary society, it started as a secret social and literary organization. Most societies at white schools were literary in nature before 1825, when the first characteristically social fraternities and sororities were established.[33]

At the beginning of the twentieth century, more African Americans were economically able to send their children north to attend white colleges and universities, but among the problems the students faced were segregated housing and social isolation. Black students at white schools were routinely denied the resources and environmental supports available to white undergraduates. Although some held part-time jobs in fraternity or sorority houses, they were systematically denied membership in these organizations.[34]

To combat racist practices at Cornell University in Ithaca, New York, eight African American male students formed a mutual support group. After meeting for a year to discuss the direction that the group would take, Alpha Phi Alpha, the first black American intercollegiate Greek-letter fraternity, was founded on 4 December 1906. Black Americans in northern colleges, writes Charles Wesley, "were not only nearest to the source of fraternity practices, but because of their isolation as a group, they were the first to feel the pressing need of close acquaintance and companionship." The records of the organization's early years reveal that the original purpose of the fraternity was to promote scholarship, build character, and provide mutual assistance and social activities for black students.[35]

In general, the authorities at black colleges and universities were adamantly opposed to the creation of secret societies among their students. Missionary educators preferred "a community of professing Christians." Their other equally important concern was the belief that fraternities and sororities were clannish, snobbish, undemocratic, "and tended to promote artificial caste and class distinctions among black undergraduates."[36]

Because the federal government began making annual appropriations to Howard as early as 1879 (a practice that became law in 1928), the situation there was somewhat different. Students were free of the many constraints that came with donations from church boards and organized white philanthropy. Thus, the emergence of Greek-letter organizations at Howard University began in 1907 when Alpha Phi Alpha fraternity initiated nineteen male students into Beta Chapter, the first Greek-letter fraternity chapter at a black institution of higher learning.[37] The presence of the Alphas started a campus trend at Howard that resulted in the addition of six more Greek-letter chapters over the next thirteen years.

Inevitably, the establishment of Beta lent support to the idea of creating a Greek-letter organization for women: "The original desire and inspiration for a women's sorority originated with Ethel Hedgeman of the Class of 1909 at Howard University. Her interest in a Greek-letter organization was stimulated by her friendship with George Lyle, president of the Chapter of Alpha Phi Alpha fraternity, recently established on campus." In 1906, the school's international student body was required to attend noon chapel on class days, but the weekend was a time to enjoy football games and matinee dances held by various student clubs. There were only two dormitories on campus, one for men and one for women.[38] All female students, ages twelve to twenty-five, were housed in Miner Hall until 1907, when "the ten or twelve college level women were given rooms together in a separate wing of the building. Thus the stage was set for the beginning of Alpha Kappa Alpha." In January 1908 Ethel Hedgeman and eight other students started Alpha Kappa Alpha sorority, the first intercollegiate Greek-letter organization founded at a black institution of higher learning and the first organization of its kind established by African American women.[39]

The evolutionary pattern of Greek-letter fraternities and sororities at Howard mirrored that of other American schools: differences in ideals, tastes, background, and social status among students ultimately gave rise to new groups. During the fall term of 1911, three inseparable male students met regularly in the office of Ernest E. Just, a biology professor, to discuss the structure for a national fraternity that would "enrich the social and intellectual aspects of college life." "Friendship is essential to the Soul" was the slogan adopted by the founders of Omega Psi Phi, begun at Howard University on 17 November 1911.[40]

This fraternity, based on the principles of "manhood, scholarship, perseverance, and uplift," was the first African American fraternity founded at a black university. Because the faculty and administration did not want the organization to expand beyond Howard, they granted approval under the condition that the newly formed group would remain local. Undaunted, the founders posted signs around campus announcing the formation of a national fraternity. The following day President Wilbur P. Thirkield announced at the noon chapel assembly that no such organization existed at Howard. After a long series of meetings with the faculty and administrators, Omega Psi Phi won the battle: "When the news came, brothers shook hands, threw up their hats, and some cut capers."[41]

By 1912, Howard was developing a new focus. A change in administration helped produce a "rising tide of Black consciousness at the university." Outside of the campus, the women's movement was gaining momentum and Washington, D.C., had become a center of black social and intellectual development.[42] Alpha Kappa Alpha sorority consisted of two opposing groups: young students who were caught up in the vibrancy of the times and older graduates who did not necessarily share the values of the younger members.

Convinced that a new focus was needed in the sorority, the younger members began developing a plan to restructure Alpha Kappa Alpha and change its name, motto, symbols, and colors. Several of the women had close relationships with some of the founders of Omega Psi Phi fraternity, who may have challenged them to organize a group like the one that they had established. After a reorganizational effort was successfully blocked by the graduates in Alpha Kappa Alpha, the twenty-two dissenting undergraduates began their appeal to the board of trustees for the establishment of a second sorority on campus. Delta Sigma Theta sorority received its charter on 13 January 1913. Chaperoned by T. Montgomery Gregory, a drama professor, the newly formed association marched in the 1913 woman suffrage parade.[43]

"Culture for service, service for humanity" was the motto adopted by the founders of Phi Beta Sigma fraternity, the second fraternity organized on Howard's campus and the brainchild of A. Langston Taylor from Memphis, Tennessee. Taylor conceived of starting the fraternity before enrolling as a student at Howard:

> One dull summer day in 1910, I was on my way home from downtown and paused for a while at Bumper's Beale Street Grocery to pick up the

latest news from the Squash Center, which usually held afternoon sessions there. I engaged in conversation with a young man recently graduated from Howard University, and since I had already decided to go to Howard, I was very much interested in what he had to say about the University. He dwelt at length on the activities of Greek-letter fraternities there. His talk gave me an idea, and from that day on, *Phi Beta Sigma* was in the making.

Taylor entered Howard in November 1910, but did not select a partner to help execute his plan until the latter part of 1913. The original twelve organizers of Phi Beta Sigma structured a plan for a national organization on 9 January 1914, and three months later Howard's board of deans granted a charter to the new group.[44]

Phi Beta Sigma was the only fraternity at Howard that actively participated in the establishment of an affiliated group for women. Initially two members of Phi Beta Sigma, Charles Robert Samuel Taylor and A. Langston Taylor, worked closely with Arizona Cleaver to swing the plan into action:

> When Zeta Phi Beta Sorority had its beginning at Howard University, Washington, D.C., in January 1920, the first World War had not been long ended. Woman was still kept on a pedestal; the chaperone was in vogue; the cigarette belonged only in the male realm; the tap room was unheard of, and no "lady" entered the "Women's Entrance" of the old-fashioned saloon. Curse words did not pass her lips, and even a bit too much make-up made her character questionable. . . . One day against the above background, a member of Phi Beta Sigma Fraternity, in the person of Charles Robert Samuel Taylor, while moving about the campus at Howard University in the company of Arizona Leedonia Cleaver, asked her if she would endeavor to establish a sister organization to Phi Beta Sigma. . . . Permission was secured from the authorities of the University to have another sorority on the campus, and a Zeta Constitution was formulated, based upon Sigma's Constitution. Thus, Zeta Phi Beta Sorority and Phi Beta Sigma became the first Greek-Letter Sister and Brother Organizations.[45]

Kappa Alpha Psi fraternity did not join the ranks of Howard's Greek-letter groups until December 1920, when Xi Chapter was established on campus. Although the fraternity was founded at Indiana University in 1911, the Howard University influence cannot be overlooked since two of the leaders of this effort, Byron K. Armstrong and Elder Watson Diggs, were recent Howard transfer students who had declined offers to pledge during their year in Washington, D.C. Most of the black students at Indiana "knew nothing about fraternities except the camaraderie they witnessed as waiters."[46]

Kappa Alpha Psi's beginning resembled that of Alpha Phi Alpha: it started as a mutual support vehicle for black students who found themselves ostracized and discriminated against in a predominantly white environment. African American students at Indiana University rarely saw one another on campus, were not allowed to use recreational and entertainment facilities, and were denied participation in contact sports. The administration's indifferent attitude toward blacks only added fuel to the fire. After sizing up the situation, nine young men met to discuss the formation of a fraternity. Out of that group Alpha Kappa Nu evolved; in 1915, the official name was changed to Kappa Alpha Psi.[47]

Like Kappa Alpha Psi, Sigma Gamma Rho sorority was also founded at a midwestern white university. It was originally formed (12 November 1922) as a "professional sorority for teachers" by seven students attending Butler University in Indianapolis and the Normal School at Terre Haute, Indiana. "Greater Service, Greater Progress" was adopted as a slogan in the midtwenties, and in keeping with that theme, the Articles of Incorporation were changed in 1929, making it a national college sorority. Howard gained its fourth and last sorority chapter when the Alpha Phi Chapter of Sigma Gamma Rho was established there in 1939.[48]

Greek-letter organizations dominated extracurricular activities at Howard by the midtwenties. What sororities and fraternities appear to have added to the social and intellectual life of the university is an ironic combination of enrichment and divisiveness. Between the early twenties and the early fifties, they sponsored interfraternal athletic games, lectures, forums, conferences, tutorial sessions, and essay contests. Some groups awarded scholarships to deserving students and presented programs that featured nationally and internationally known speakers.[49]

When the activities of the graduate chapters became more service-oriented, undergraduate outreach programs increased. Such national programs as Phi Beta Sigma's celebrated "Bigger and Better Business Week" and the Omega's "Negro Achievement Week" were adopted by Howard's undergraduate chapters. The wellspring of political and cultural activists invited to speak at Howard were constant reminders to the students that they had a responsibility to African Americans. Such speakers as Marcus Garvey, W. E. B. Du Bois, Nnamdi Azikiwe, and Mary McCloud Bethune made them aware of what was happening to black people internationally.[50]

During the early decades of the twentieth century they also received guidance from faculty members who were involved with cultural and political movements outside of Howard. For example, Alain Locke, a major voice in the Harlem Renaissance, was an honorary member of Phi Beta Sigma, as was T. Montgomery Gregory. Carter G. Woodson became an honorary member of Omega Psi Phi.[51]

Despite the contributions of sororities and fraternities to extracurricular activities, serious complaints about the Greeks were voiced in the *Hilltop*, Howard's student newspaper, as early as the twenties. Non-Greeks complained that members were chosen on the basis of color, popularity, and family background. Some students objected to hazing and other activities related to pledging. But what enraged the student population most was the creation of "Greek" political machines that prevented non-Greeks from holding such top-level positions on campus as editor of the *Hilltop* and homecoming queen. That system was brought to an abrupt halt in 1953, when the student council set up a new election process that limited political maneuvering.[52]

Even in the midst of controversy, Greek social activities continued unabated. A close reading of seven decades of the *Hilltop* makes clear that dance played a prominent role in the most frequently held social activities of the undergraduate chapters. From the twenties through the fifties, sororities and fraternities sponsored house parties, proms, coronation balls, semiformal balls, and special holiday dances.[53] A 1924 *Hilltop* article reveals that Howard University students were right in the swing of things when black social dance made its first great impact on America: "'Jazz' music and 'jazz' dancing dominate the social atmosphere of all localities. This is hardly less true of our own university than of the city of Washington, which is well known to be one of the greatest 'jazz' centers of America."[54] By the midthirties, annual proms became some of the most popular events on campus: "Trailing long streams of confetti, dodging multi-colored balloons, trucking, waltzing, and baudidling to the strains of Pete Moss's syncopated rhythms, the Kappa Alpha Psi Scrollers and their guests opened the season for public fraternal proms."[55]

Fraternity members also danced on Howard's upper quadrangle, the main outdoor gathering space known as "the Yard." The earliest *Hilltop* account of probates jitterbugging in the Yard was written in the late thirties: "The two weeks immediately preceding the Thanksgiving festivities were, if not exactly 'Hell Week,' at least a fortnight of Hades. . . . Omega Psi Phi had its men in the traditional dark suits with white shirts and white shoes, canes, dog collars and leashes. Any day at noon these poor 'dogs' could be seen rug cutting, pecking and big-appleing at the Omega Sundial,"[56] which was placed on the Yard in the thirties by Howard's Alpha Chapter. Between the thirties and the late fifties, fraternities and sororities established the practice of meeting to sing and dance on the Yard each Friday afternoon. According to Dean Vincent Johns, who came to Howard in the fifties, each fraternity and sorority had a designated spot, marked by a particular monument: "It was sacred ground and you did not *mess* with it. And if they showed up on Friday and you were in that spot, they would move you, literally. . . . That is still maintained today, even though they don't gather there on Fridays to sing and step." When song and dance rituals were made an official part of the pledging program, "probate shows" developed. On the last day of probation, each pledge group, or "line," was required to perform publicly.[57]

Numerous accounts of dancing and singing in the Yard appear in the *Hilltop* during the sixties. During those years fraternities and sororities waned in popularity, fewer people pledged, and the *Hilltop* became a battleground for verbal duels between Greeks and non-Greeks. As blacks became more involved with the civil rights movement and as African American identification with Africa increased, many students at Howard viewed Greek-letter fraternities and sororities as counterrevolutionary, elitist groups that threatened campus unity and had little to do with the African American struggle for social, economic, and political equality.

Non-Greeks were also outraged by the mental and physical abuse that pledges had to endure, the selective membership process, and what they viewed as a lack of community involvement. Unfortunately, the sorority and fraternity community service programs were invisible to the larger campus community: "Believe it or not, they [Greek-letter chapters] were sponsoring many good programs. But what the students saw were the shows, the dancing and singing on Friday, the parties that they had. This is what they *saw*. They never saw the tutorial programs, the clothing drives, the voter registration drives, and other major social action programs. Students never saw that. So they thought that the groups did nothing but sing, dance, and party."[58]

Vicious attacks continued into the seventies. What students seemed to object to most vehemently were the weekly song and dance rituals on the Yard, ironically the most African-oriented social activity of all. Despite the barrage of criticism, Greeks bodaciously continued their rituals every Friday between 12:00 and 1:30. These public displays drew large crowds at

Howard between the fifties and late seventies, even though sororities and fraternities were routinely criticized during those years. Each organization could be identified by its style and a unique set of songs and movements that members passed on to pledges while they were on line.[59]

Campus sentiment began to soften by 1973 as the sororities and fraternities made their community service projects more public and fought back with articles about the legendary contributions of their national organizations.[60] During the late seventies, when the university started scheduling classes through the noon hour, yard stepping entered a slow period of decline, but Greek shows continued to grow in popularity. As a result, a group of Howard students decided to sponsor a competitive Greek show as one of the featured attractions of the 1976 homecoming week: "The first [competitive] one we had was held in Cramton Auditorium and it was packed. They were hanging from the ceiling. And it was a very good show. . . . Each one did an excellent job. The students liked it so well that ever since it has been a part of homecoming as one of the activities. In fact it was so well attended—Cramton holds 1,500—that we moved it to the gym, which could accommodate about 2,600, and we still didn't have enough room."[61]

Black sororities and fraternities made a dramatic comeback nationally during the early eighties, and as Howard Greek shows of the seventies evolved into step shows of the eighties, they gradually became some of the most popular social events on campus and *the* most widespread form of undergraduate Greek competition. Competitive stepping at Howard grew out of a long tradition of sorority and fraternity contests on campus. During their first few decades of existence, Howard's Greek-letter organizations vied for top scholastic ratings, campus offices, and athletic trophies. By the early thirties, Delta-sponsored "jabberwocks" (amateur vaudeville shows) provided an opportunity for sororities and fraternities to present competitive skits. During the latter part of 1950, competitive song fests were introduced to the campus by the Scroller Club of Kappa Alpha Psi fraternity.[62]

Viewed within a broad cultural and historical context, stepping is clearly a branch of the African American vernacular dance tree. Most step show performers at Howard, however, make a clear distinction between stepping and dancing. According to chapter step masters, dancing is a fluid form that does not have transitional stops and is usually done to music. Stepping, they say, is more precise, requires more energy, and is performed by producing sounds with the body.[63] It is also a complex, varied, and rapidly changing genre that defies generalizations. Styles, organizing principles, and terms vary geographically, from school to school within the same area, and even from chapter to chapter at a single college or university. Therefore, the organizing principles and definitions outlined in this study are limited to stepping practices at Howard University in the early nineties and based on *Hilltop* articles, interviews with Howard's step team leaders and college administrators, and observations made at campus step shows between 1991 and 1993.

Usually Howard step teams select their members through general consensus within a chapter. The Delta and Alpha step masters make announcements to their organizations that the first step show meeting will be held on a particular date. Those who choose to attend and stick it out win places on the team through dedication and hard work, even though they might not initially appear to be the best steppers. The Omegas and the Zetas, on the other hand, have cuts or audition sessions after a series of rehearsals. Those members who perform best make the team.[64] Andrew Johnstone, a Phi Beta Sigma step master, says that any frat brother "can be on the team if he has the capability, but it's a business; there's a lot of money at stake. . . . In just a two-month period, we won over three thousand dollars and you can put on a lot of programs with that. . . . So sometimes we have to be a little rough and cut people." While the Zetas have a specific competition team of six to eight members, the Deltas, according to Cedrice Davis, view stepping as a "chapter event" with floating team members: "Every show changes. . . . We don't have one team that does everything throughout the whole year. If we're doing a fall show we have a fall team or for a spring show we have a spring team . . . because with people's changing schedules and seniors trying to graduate, not everyone has the time to do a whole year's worth of stepping."[65]

Terms vary as much at Howard as organizational structures. The Ques of Omega Psi Phi use the term *marching* instead of *stepping* and their step masters are referred to as *show dogs*. The Alpha's term for the same position is *step freak*. In some chapters, the position of step master is handed down by the previous step master, but in others expert steppers become step masters through general consensus. These team leaders need to have a thorough understanding of how to put a winning show together, and in order to direct productive rehearsals they must be able to command the respect of the team members. They must also be persons who are precise in their movements and capable of picking new ones up quickly and teaching them effectively.[66]

Most of the step masters interviewed practice a teaching method which resembles that of African American tap dancers of the thirties and forties: rhythm articulation. Rather than using counts, they break down the movements into beats. Paul Woodruff, an Alpha step freak and a former drummer with Thunder Machine, the percussion section of Howard University's "soul stepping" marching band, describes his method: "I believe in breaking down every four beats. . . . When I was brought in they gave it to me all at once, but I could pick it up because I'm a drummer, beats stick with me. It's all a matter of learning a beat. It's not necessarily knowing the [movement]. If you know the beat, it's easy to pick up the [movement]. So you're concentrating on rhythm, not counts." "I step by sound," says Johnstone. "I step by listening to the beats and I'll just emulate the beats." Johnstone continues:

> Everything makes a distinct sound. Every stomp, every clap, even when you hit your thigh or hit your hands. So that's how I try to teach. . . . You just break everything into parts. You do two beats and then everybody goes through the two beats. Then you add on—it's a building process until you have the whole step. . . . We might not even finish one step in a week, not even a half of it. We just keep going through it until that one part is perfect and then we go to the next part because it doesn't make sense to move on until everybody has it.[67]

Before pledging was banned in 1990, initiates learned how to step on line, and just before the end of their probate period, they presented a public show on the Yard or in an auditorium on campus. Many sorority and fraternity members complain that the new intake process (usually a few days to a week) makes it impossible for candidates to learn how to step well before they officially join the group.

Preparation for the annual homecoming step show usually begins six to eight weeks in advance with two-hour rehearsals three to four times a week. As the show date approaches, rehearsals intensify; during the last couple of weeks, teams practice every day for two to three hours and longer if necessary. On weekday evenings rehearsals are usually between ten and one o'clock, after study hours and part time jobs end; on Saturday mornings they are held around ten or eleven. Woodruff explains: "Homecoming is the biggest show here so you want that to be a 'live' show and you want to win so you start far in advance. . . . You want to get your show together by the end of September so that by the first week of October you're doing nothing but polishing, deleting, working on form and technique, and making sure everything is precise."[68]

A good step show presentation has three parts: an introduction, a set of three to five or six steps, depending upon the time limit, and an exit. Most teams like to do something that will catch the audience off guard: A smoke-filled stage set up with three paper screens bearing the symbols of Omega Psi Phi held the crowd's attention at the Howard 1993 spring step show. One by one, as the smoke died down, three Ques exploded through the screens dressed in gold boots, khaki pants, purple gloves, head scarves, and sunglasses. As the barks and the cheers escalated, two more brothers strutted on stage to collect the sunglasses a minute before the performers broke into the first of the hard stomping "pump" steps for which the Ques are noted. "You want something that will leave the crowd struck with awe" says Damon Patterson, a show dog for Omega Psi Phi. "Amazingly, every time I've heard the Omegas announced, the audience will be in complete silence because they're expecting something like that. . . . So brothers are constantly putting more pressure on themselves to do something to shock the crowd."[69]

Zeta step master Valerie Holiday explains that her team usually dances on to music—something popular and easily recognizable by the crowd. "When it comes blasting over the system, the crowd will react and holler 'Ho!' And that's when you need the crowd. . . . So we always like to start with a song that's really hyped." Occasionally the Alphas enter with a "party walk," an organized line movement performed around the floor at a party. It is usually some form of stepping and is done to celebrate and give recognition to one's fraternity or sorority. Each organization has its own particular set of party walks that reflects its unique stepping style.[70]

The middle section, or body, of a step show presentation consists of choreographed sequences selected for the occasion. When putting this section together, teams shoot for accuracy, variety, originality, and smooth, flawless transitions that do not break the continuity of the performance because too many pauses detract from the overall impact of a show: "When you're competing for money," explains Patterson, "you really want to catch the eye of the judges and you want to get the audience involved at the same time. You want to be flashy and you constantly want to do something that hasn't been done before." Teams try to use "solid steps that you know will go over well."[71]

According to Johnstone, "your first step shouldn't be something that's into a lot of precision. It should be something that catches the crowd's attention quick and gets them involved. . . . You want to have a steady show and balance it out with some precision stuff, some pump stuff, and maybe something that gets them laughing."[72] The final step before the exit should definitely be something that leaves a lasting impression on the audience. Some teams exit by dancing off to music, others simply walk off, and many use party walks.

The idea is to get off quickly so that the judges will not delete points for exceeding the time limit. Teams are judged in several categories, including precision, creativity, complexity, appearance, showmanship, and performance. The panel of judges, which often consists of faculty and staff members, includes at least one representative from a graduate chapter of each organization.

Dress is always an important part of the planning process. At Howard the sororities are more likely to designate a particular person to select and purchase the outfits and shoes. Zeta Phi Beta has a "fashion coordinator," who shops for the clothes, makes alterations, and checks hair styles. Among the Ques, getting outfitted is more of a joint venture; they usually sit around and brainstorm until they come up with something that everyone likes. Sororities and fraternities pay close attention to the types of fabrics selected and the heaviness and sound quality of the shoes. Finding outfits that will allow for easy movement and flatter a range of body sizes and shapes is never an easy task.[73]

Because stepping has changed radically since the mideighties, performance apparel has changed, particularly for women. Undergraduate women at Howard no longer step in skirts and heels. Shorts, pants, and jumpsuits are better choices since innovations of the last few years have made female stepping more rigorous. Women hit the floor harder, incorporate more stunts or acrobatics, and tend to be more percussive than they were previously. But they still include more hand clapping and more singing than the fraternities. Johnstone, who has stepped in twenty to thirty shows up and down the East Coast concurs: "Women are throwing a lot harder than they used to. . . . I think to be more competitive and more interesting, they're switching to being more like fraternities. . . . Back in 1990 you could come sliding in late to the shows because they used to put the sororities on first. But now it's just not the same. . . . In a lot of places they put the women against the men in big open competitions. . . . Yeah, it's definitely going in that direction and it's a lot more fun to watch."[74]

Each sorority and fraternity has a characteristic movement style that varies depending on its regional location. At Howard, the Omegas are known for stepping hardest or doing what some step team members call "pump stomping"; the Sigmas also stomp, but they're more concerned with precise hand, leg, and foot movements meshed with complex rhythmical beats. According to Woodruff, Alphas combine more hard and fast stepping with some shuffling and hand clapping. The Kappas are noted for their flashy and skillful cane work.

Among the sororities, the women of Alpha Kappa Alpha do more dancing and hand clapping than other female teams. Although the Deltas claim that they do not have a signature style, the initiated eye and ear of any loyal Howard step show fan can easily recognize the Delta movement style and sound without being told the organization's name. Most fraternity step masters at Howard agree that the Deltas step harder than the other sorority teams and that they also have a reputation for being crowd-oriented show stoppers who are especially adept at performing the styles of other groups during salutes or cracks.[75]

Zeta Phi Beta's stepping style bears some resemblance to the Sigma style because of the close association between the two groups. According to Holiday, "each sorority tends to be influenced by another fraternity's style. I *know* our best source of steps is the Sigmas, so I'm not offended when that's pointed out. We'll take a Sigma step, make it feminine, and it'll be the exact same step."[76] The Sigmas and the Zetas are noted for their expert use of blindfolds, a technique that has been frequently adopted by other organizations.

Calls and signs or hand signals are used by sororities and fraternities as a way of bonding and identifying with each other and "a lot of non-Greeks know all the calls because they hear them everyday on the Yard." The Sigma's "Blue Phi" or the Alpha's "06" are all-too-familiar sounds at step shows, too, where chapter audience members use them as a way of supporting their brothers and sisters between steps or before and after their team's presentation. The Zetas sign, called the cat, is often used by their team at the end of a step: "It's used as a symbol to say that we're proud, we're Zetas, and we're here; we use it as an affirmation. We use the call 'ee-i-kee' to start and stop steps. . . . We generally try not to do anyone else's call because that's personal. They've earned a right to use it."[77]

Trade steps also serve as signatures for sororities and fraternities. These choreographed sequences are usually done on the Yard, although some teams occasionally use variations of them in competitive step shows. The Kappas "Yo, Baby, Yo," the Zeta's "Zeta Reggae," the AKA's "It's a Serious Matter," and the Sigma's "Nutcracker" are examples of trade steps that are performed nationally. When step teams salute or crack on other Greek-letter organizations they often do takeoffs on trade steps that are familiar to the audience.[78]

Howard's Alphas make a clear distinction between *show steps* and *yard steps*: "Yard steps are basic steps that boost morale and give spirit to your fraternity. A bunch of brothers will just happen to be on the Yard and we'll call the brothers around and just start stepping. It's a collective thing, it's a unifying thing, everybody's on the same course. . . . If old bros were to join us, they'd know them because they've come a long way—they're tradition. A show step has to be a lot flashier, a lot cleaner; the whole mind-set has to be different." The Yard is also the place where stepping fans are more likely to see "freaking." Most Howard step masters equate freaking with improvising, free-styling, or "doing your own thing." According to Holiday, the "Alphas are famous for freaking." One of the well-known trade steps that they do on the Yard, called the "Grandaddy," calls for collective freaking. Among the Alphas it is not just encouraged on the Yard; they occasionally use it in a step show, especially when their step freak starts a step.[79]

The Sigmas also use the term *freaking* to describe someone who is really "getting down": "You can say someone's freaking a step. That's like *working it* and that's what wins a lot of the time—if you have people like that on your team." According to Johnstone, most teams leave room for a little improvisation because it gets the crowd excited and involved:

> Usually you have somebody on your team who is "show-timish" and they'll do the step and it will look absolutely different from somebody else, although it might be the exact same step. I call it "stepping above the stage" because it's at a different level. It sounds the same but looks totally different. . . . So as a step master you don't discourage improvisation as long as they don't take it out too far and as long as it looks good. Too much improvisation can make you look unorganized. But the better you know the step, the easier it's gonna be for you to "freak it" or "work it" or "step above the stage."[80]

When undergraduates and graduates gather on the Yard after homecoming games, the emphasis is on songs and chants with incidental dance movements. For the most part, these ritual dances, songs, and chants are passed on orally; words are rarely written down.[81]

Steps done in competitive shows are usually preserved on videotape as future source material: "We try to get every show that we do videotaped. [First, so we can] ridicule each other as a joke, but it's also important to see how the show went, what got a good crowd response, what can be changed if necessary, and what can be kept the same."[82] Howard step masters say that music videos and tapes of shows from other areas of the country also provide new stepping ideas.

A few of Howard's teams travel extensively and exchange moves with their frat brothers or sorority sisters along the East Coast, especially Philadelphia and New York, where a lot of the newer steps originate. Johnstone, who steps competitively year round, describes this process: "So, we roadtrip to see our brothers other places and usually the first thing somebody talks about is 'What kind of steps you guys do up here?' or 'Have you seen this already?' And you just kind of trade and that's how it floats. . . . I personally feel that it floats from the East Coast to the West, because what I've seen groups do on the West Coast, I saw here years ago."[83]

Because styles vary so much geographically, "it's important to step according to where you are," says Woodruff. A winning presentation in Washington might lose further south, where dancing is more widely accepted in step shows. Winning an interfraternal stepping championship at the regional or national level depends almost as much on where the contest is held geographically and what particular style reigns there as it does on which team is really the most skillful. Having the time and money to enter on the district and state levels is another determining factor. Therefore, the acknowledged champions are not always necessarily the very best steppers in the organization. Johnstone points out that "being selected the best just means that you were the best among those teams that showed up."[84]

The same holds true for large privately sponsored open competitions that have become popular since the eighties. With the increased commercialization of stepping, winning has become more political and most teams do not step without contracts or other legal agreements. Even at Howard, where the homecoming step show is usually sold out early, participating teams are very conscious of how much money is being made and who receives the profit.

Howard's undergraduate chapters use the bulk of their award money to underwrite a host of community service projects that include tutorial and mentoring programs for children; assistance to the elderly; big brother and big sister programs; walk-a-thons; voluntary work in shelters, hospitals, and correctional facilities; and on-campus seminars, lectures, and conferences. The Zetas, who have grossed as much as $10,000 in one year, are occasionally able to award scholarships to high school students—something that is usually not possible for undergraduate chapters.[85]

On campus, step shows are not limited to the eight sororities and fraternities that make up the Panhellenic Council. Such groups as Kappa Kappa Psi and Tau Beta Sigma, national honorary band societies, also have step teams that compete periodically. According to Kappa Kappa Psi member Ron Paige, it is more difficult for his chapter to enter a Greek show at Howard than it is for frat brothers at colleges in the south, where Kappa Kappa Psi step teams regularly compete.[86]

Howard University step shows of the nineties have become more African in theme and there has been a concerted effort to promote unity among sororities and fraternities. University rules prohibit harsh cracking and profanity. The official 1990 homecoming step show opened the decade with the title "From Alpha to Omega: Stepping to Higher Ground." That was also the year that Paul Woodruff saw the quality of stepping skyrocket at Howard: "Stepping was brought to a whole new level—it was faster, things were more precise, more technical, and a lot more things were incorporated."[87]

When asked why they step or what they gain from stepping, most Howard step masters reply that it is, first of all, a way of expressing love for their organization. Second, it promotes spiritual unity and camaraderie within the chapter. And finally, on an individual level, it is an enjoyable way to learn discipline, organization, and time management. Woodruff says it taught him a lot about getting jobs done and not getting nervous in front of large groups. He sums up his experience with the Alpha team: "If I can do this, I can do anything."[88]

Stepping competitions furnish occasions to collectively celebrate and keep alive a cultural heritage that unites classic African and African American rituals of affirmation. Critics who dismiss this dance genre as undergraduate folly fail to recognize the cultural richness of the form and the vitally important role it plays as a carrier of black traditions in song, music, dance, and language. For its performers and loyal followers, stepping is a regenerative force and a way for black Americans to express who they are as Africans in the Western Hemisphere, bearers of such great ancient civilizations as Kongo, Yoruba, Akan, and Mande.

This dance genre should be seen within the context of a long tradition of African diasporic artistic forms that stage challenges and competitions as a way of keeping standards high while using rhythm, style, control, and dynamism to push genres forward. Stepping teams, like black American dancing vocal groups and black marching and dancing bands, provide multisensory experiences for audiences of eager and active participants. They serve as prominent repositories of black music and dance forms that have significantly shaped twentieth-century American culture. As we move toward the twenty-first century, African American body language has assumed center stage in this nation's evolving history of dance and sport, and in an ironic twist of historical fate "the formerly colonized now aesthetically colonize their former masters."[89]

Notes

Introduction

1. Ralph Ellison, *Going to the Territory* (New York: Random House, 1986), 139–41.

2. Zora Neale Hurston, "Characteristics of Negro Expression," in *The Sanctified Church: The Folklore Writings of Zora Neale Hurston* (Berkeley: Turtle Island, 1981), 55–56.

3. Robert C. Toll, *Blacking Up: The Minstrel Show in Nineteenth-Century America* (New York: Oxford University Press, 1977), 249.

4. John W. Roberts, "African American Diversity and the Study of Folklore," *Western Folklore* 52 (Apr. 1993): 157–71.

5. Michael J. Bell, *The World from Brown's Lounge: An Ethnography of Black Middle-Class Play* (Urbana: University of Illinois Press, 1983), 1–15.

6. Roberts, "African American Diversity," 168–69, emphasis added.

7. Roger D. Abrahams, *The Man-of-Words in the West Indies: Performance and the Emergence of Creole Culture* (Baltimore: Johns Hopkins University Press, 1983), xvii.

8. See Geneva Smitherman, *Black Talk: Words and Phrases from the Hood to the Amen Corner* (Boston: Houghton Mifflin, 1994).

9. Correspondence from Roger Abrahams, University of Pennsylvania, Mar. 1994.

10. Ibid.

11. Peter Abrahams, *Tell Freedom* (London: Faber and Faber, 1954; reprint, Harare, Zimbabwe: Zimbabwe Publishing House, 1982), 128–29.

12. Richard Price and Sally Price, *Two Evenings in Saramaka* (Chicago: University of Chicago Press, 1991), 1–37; Sally Price and Richard Price, *Afro-American Arts of the Suriname Rain Forest* (Los Angeles: Museum of Cultural History and the University of California Press, 1980), 183–85.

13. Albert Murray, *The Omni-Americans: Black Experience and American Cul-*

ture (New York: Outerbridge and Dienstfrey, 1970; reprint, New York: Vintage Books, 1983), 54.

Chapter 1: "*Gimme de Kneebone Bent*"

1. K. Kia Bunseki Fu-Kiau, "A Powerful Trio: Drumming-Singing-Dancing," ms.; John Miller Chernoff, *African Rhythm and African Sensibility: Aesthetics and Social Action in African Musical Idioms* (Chicago: University of Chicago Press, 1981), 167; John S. Mbiti, *African Religions and Philosophy*, 2d. ed. (London: Heinemann, 1989), 93.

2. Olly Wilson, "The Significance of the Relationship between Afro-American Music and West African Music," *Black Perspective in Music* 2, no. 1 (Spring 1974): 3–21; J. H. Kwabena Nketia, *The Music of Africa* (New York: W. W. Norton, 1974), 4.

3. Nketia, *The Music of Africa*, 31, 206–7; J. H. Kwabena Nketia, "The Interrelations of African Music and Dance," *Studia Musicologica* 7 (Budapest, Academiae Scientiarum Hungaricae) (1965): 91; Francis Bebey, *African Music: A People's Art* (New York: Lawrence Hill, 1975), 16.

4. Nketia, *The Music of Africa*, 32–33; Nketia, "Interrelations," 101.

5. Chernoff, *African Rhythm*, 160, emphasis added.

6. Ibid., 154; quotation from J. H. Kwabena Nketia, "Music in African Cultures: A Review of the Meaning and Significance of Traditional African Music," mimeographed (Legon, Accra, Ghana: Institute of African Studies, University of Ghana, 1966), 20, quoted in Chernoff, *African Rhythm*, 36.

7. Fu-Kiau, "A Powerful Trio."

8. Robert Farris Thompson, *African Art in Motion: Icon and Act* (Los Angeles: University of California Press, 1979), xii; Werner Gillon, *A Short History of African Art* (London: Viking, 1984; reprint, London: Penguin, 1988), 37.

9. Thompson, *African Art in Motion*, xiv, 44, 47, 112, quotations from 28 and 45; quotation from Peter H. Wood, "'Gimme de Kneebone Bent': African Body Language and the Evolution of American Dance Forms," in *The Black Tradition in American Modern Dance*, ed. Gerald E. Myers (American Dance Festival, 1988), 8.

10. Bebey, *African Music*, 120, 92, quotation from 122; Chernoff, *African Rhythm*, 75; Nketia, *The Music of Africa*, 4.

11. Chernoff, *African Rhythm*, 75, 79, 80–81, quotation from 81; Bebey, *African Music*, 119, 40.

12. Georges Balandier, *Daily Life in the Kingdom of the Kongo: From the Sixteenth to the Eighteenth Century* (New York: Pantheon, 1968), 232.

13. Nketia, *The Music of Africa*, 206–8, quotations from 208.

14. Ibid., 206; Nketia, "Interrelations," 92.

15. Nketia, "Interrelations," 91; Nketia, *The Music of Africa*, 209–10, 225;

Peggy Harper, "Dance in Nigeria," *Ethnomusicology* 13, no. 2 (May 1969): 289; Fu-Kiau, "A Powerful Trio."

16. Harper, "Dance in Nigeria," 293; Nketia, "Interrelations," 92.

17. Nketia, *The Music of Africa*, 210–13; Chernoff, *African Rhythm*, 146–51; Harper, "Dance in Nigeria," 290.

18. S. D. Cudjoe, "The Techniques of Ewe Drumming and the Social Importance of Music in Africa," *Phylon* 14, no. 3 (1953): 288.

19. Quotation from Robert Farris Thompson, "An Aesthetic of the Cool: West African Dance," *African Forum* 2, no. 2 (Fall 1966): 89; Ayo Bankole, Judith Bush, and Sadek H. Samaan, "The Yoruba Master Drummer," *African Arts* 8, no. 2 (Winter 1975): 54–55; Nketia, "Interrelations," 100.

20. J. H. Kwabena Nketia, "The Role of the Drummer in Akan Society," *African Music* 1, no. 1 (1954): 42.

21. Chernoff, *African Rhythm*, 143–47, quotation from 147.

22. W. C. Handy, *Father of the Blues: An Autobiography* (New York: Macmillan, 1941; reprint, New York: Collier Books, 1970), 5; Albert Murray, interview with author, New York, N.Y., 8 May 1993; Thompson, "An Aesthetic of the Cool: West African Dance," 88–95; Nketia, *The Music of Africa*, 209–10.

23. Harper, "Dance in Nigeria," 290; Thompson, "An Aesthetic of the Cool: West African Dance," 90.

24. Thompson, "An Aesthetic of the Cool: West African Dance," 93–94; Okot p'Bitek, *Song of Lawino, Song of Ocol* (London: Heinemann, 1984), 44, 47; Melville J. Herskovits, *The Myth of the Negro Past* (Boston: Beacon, 1990), 271.

25. Thompson, "An Aesthetic of the Cool: West African Dance," 93–94.

26. Ibid., 95.

27. Bebey, *African Music*, 115; Nketia, *The Music of Africa*, 177–78, 55–56.

28. Chernoff, *African Rhythm*, 71, quotation from 163; J. H. Kwabena Nketia, "Drums, Dance, and Song," *Atlantic Monthly*, Apr. 1959, 70.

29. Thompson, "An Aesthetic of the Cool: West African Dance," 95–96; Chernoff, *African Rhythm*, 71.

30. Marshall Stearns and Jean Stearns, *Jazz Dance: The Story of American Vernacular Dance* (New York: Macmillan, 1968), 123, quotations from 22; Thompson, "An Aesthetic of the Cool: West African Dance," 96.

31. Chernoff, *African Rhythm*, 149; Robert Farris Thompson, "An Aesthetic of the Cool," *African Arts* 7, no. 1 (Autumn 1973): 90–91, quotation from 41; Thompson, *African Art in Motion*, 43.

32. Chernoff, *African Rhythm*, 148–49, 65–67, 150, 141, quotation from 171; Thompson, *African Art in Motion*, 45; Nketia, *The Music of Africa*, 33.

33. Thompson, *African Art in Motion*, 45; Thompson, "An Aesthetic of the Cool," 41–43, 64–67.

34. J. H. Kwabena Nketia, "The Problem of Meaning in African Music," *Ethnomusicology* 6, no. 1 (Jan. 1962): 2; Thompson, *African Art in Motion*, 1.

35. Thompson, *African Art in Motion*, 1–5, quotations from 251–75.

36. Ibid., 274.

37. Nketia, *The Music of Africa*, 60; Bebey, *African Music*, 6–8; Chernoff, *African Rhythm*, 94.

38. Cudjoe, "Techniques of Ewe Drumming," 280–81; Bankole, Bush, and Samaan, "The Yoruba Master Drummer," 48.

39. Quotations from Nketia, *The Music of Africa*, 59–60, 61; Bankole, Bush, and Samaan, "The Yoruba Master Drummer," 48–52.

40. Nketia, *The Music of Africa*, 50.

Chapter 2: *"Keep to the Rhythm and You'll Keep to Life"*

1. Albert Murray, lecture, Center for Afro-American Studies, Wesleyan University, Middletown, Conn., spring 1985.

2. Kenneth Burke, *The Philosophy of Literary Form: Studies in Symbolic Action* (Baton Rouge: Louisiana State University Press, 1941; reprint, New York: Vintage Books, 1957), 253–62.

3. Bessie Jones and Bess Lomax Hawes, *Step It Down: Games, Plays, Songs, and Stories from the Afro-American Heritage* (New York: Harper and Row, 1972; reprint, Athens: University of Georgia Press, 1987), 124.

4. Herskovits, *Myth*, 76; John Michael Vlach, *The Afro-American Tradition in Decorative Arts* (Cleveland: Cleveland Museum of Art, 1978), 120, quotation from 148; Charles Joyner, *Down by the Riverside: A South Carolina Slave Community* (Urbana: University of Illinois Press, 1984), 237.

5. Olly Wilson, "The Influence of Jazz on the History and Development of Concert Music," in *New Perspectives on Jazz*, ed. David N. Baker (Washington, D.C.: Smithsonian Institution Press, 1990), 29; see also Wilson, "The Relationship between Afro-American Music and West African Music," 3–22; Olly Wilson, "The Association of Movement and Music as a Manifestation of a Black Conceptual Approach to Music-Making," in *More Than Dancing: Essays on Afro-American Music and Musicians*, ed. Irene V. Jackson (Westport, Conn.: Greenwood Press, 1985), 9–23.

6. Albert Murray, *Stomping the Blues* (New York: McGraw-Hill, 1976; reprint, New York: Vintage, 1982), 189.

7. Gerhard Kubik, *Angolan Traits in Black Music, Games, and Dances of Brazil: A Study of African Cultural Extensions Overseas*, Estudos de Anthropologia Cultural no. 10 (Lisboa: Centro de Estudos de Anthropologia Cultural, 1979), 20.

8. Wood, "'Gimme de Kneebone Bent,'" 7; Peter H. Wood, *Black Majority: Negroes in Colonial South Carolina from 1670 through the Stono Rebellion* (New York: Alfred A. Knopf, 1974; reprint, New York: W. W. Norton, 1975), 145, 335; Winifred Kellersberger Vass, *The Bantu Speaking Heritage of the United States*

(Los Angeles: Center for Afro-American Studies, University of California, 1979), 12.

9. Wood, "'Gimme de Kneebone Bent,'" 7; Robert Farris Thompson, *Flash of the Spirit: African and Afro-American Art and Philosophy* (New York: Random House, 1983), 103, quotation from 104.

10. C. Daniel Dawson, ed., *Dancing between Two Worlds: Kongo-Angola Culture and the Americas* (New York: Ragged Edge, 1991), iii; Balandier, *Daily Life*, 233; Kubik, *Angolan Traits*, 20.

11. Vass, *Bantu*, 3; Robert Farris Thompson and Joseph Cornet, *The Four Moments of the Sun: Kongo Art in Two Worlds* (Washington, D.C.: National Gallery of Art, 1981), 149; Philip D. Curtin, *The Atlantic Slave Trade: A Census* (Madison: University of Wisconsin Press, 1969), 222.

12. Vass, *Bantu*, 3.

13. Balandier, *Daily Life*, 153; Herskovits, *Myth*, 141, 297–98.

14. Lawrence W. Levine, *Black Culture and Black Consciousness: Afro-American Folk Thought from Slavery to Freedom* (New York: Oxford University Press, 1978), 5; Herskovits, *Myth*, 297–98.

15. Quotations from Murray, *Omni-Americans*, 184, Murray interview, and Murray, *Omni-Americans*, 185.

16. Robert Farris Thompson, lecture, New York University, New York, N.Y., spring 1991.

17. Quotations from Murray, *Omni-Americans*, 59, and Murray, *Stomping the Blues*, 254, 16.

18. I know this to be true because I grew up in a southern segregated environment where I was immersed in African American culture.

19. Gerald L. Davis, *The Performed Word* (Anthropology Film Center Foundation, 1982).

20. Ralph Ellison, "Remembering Richard Wright," in *Going to the Territory* (New York: Random House, 1986), 208.

21. Charles "Honi" Coles quoted in Jack Schiffman, *Harlem Heyday: A Pictorial History of Modern Black Show Business and the Apollo Theater* (Buffalo: Prometheus Books, 1984), 164–65; Murray, *Stomping the Blues*, 108.

22. James L. Smith, *Autobiography of James L. Smith* (Norwich, Conn., 1881), 27, quoted in John W. Blassingame, *The Slave Community: Plantation Life in the Antebellum South*, revised and enlarged (New York: Oxford University Press, 1979), 134; Herskovits, *Myth*, 265; Albert J. Raboteau, *Slave Religion: The "Invisible Institution" in the Antebellum South* (New York: Oxford University Press, 1980), 245; see also Sterling Stuckey, *Slave Culture: Nationalist Theory and the Foundations of Black America* (New York: Oxford University Press, 1988), 3–97.

23. See Eileen Southern, *The Music of Black Americans*, 2d ed. (New York: W. W. Norton, 1983), and Dena Epstein, *Sinful Tunes and Spirituals: Black Folk Music to the Civil War* (Urbana: University of Illinois Press, 1981).

24. Mahalia Jackson with Evan McLeod Wylie, *Movin' on Up* (New York: Hawthorn Books, 1966), 66; Thomas A. Dorsey, "Gospel Music," in *Reflections on Afro-American Music*, ed. Dominique-René de Lerma (Kent, Ohio: Kent State University Press, 1973), 190–91, quoted in Levine, *Black Culture*, 184.

25. Quotation from Sidney Bechet, *Treat It Gentle* (London: Cassell, 1960; reprint, New York: Da Capo Press, 1978), 66; Lazarus E. N. Ekwueme, "African-Music Retentions in the New World," *Black Perspective in Music* 2, no. 2 (Fall 1974): 137–39.

26. Douglas Henry Daniels, "Lester Young: Master of Jive," *American Music* 3, no. 3 (Fall 1985): 317.

27. Ralph Ellison, *Shadow and Act* (New York: Random House, 1964; reprint, New York: Vintage Books, 1972), xvii; Murray, *Omni-Americans*, 54–55.

28. Balandier, *Daily Life*, 166–69, quotation from 169.

29. Gillon, *Short History*, 236, 152, 156, 34, quotation from 87. See Angela Fisher, *Africa Adorned* (New York: Harry N. Abrams, 1984).

30. Gustavus Vassa quoted in Arna Bontemps, ed., *Great Slave Narratives* (Boston: Beacon, 1969), 100.

31. Richard Newman, "The Brightest Star: Aida Overton Walker in the Age of Ragtime and Cakewalk," ms., 5.

32. Honi Coles, "The Dance," in *The Apollo Theater Story* (New York: Apollo Operations, 1966), 9.

33. Phyllis Ashinger, "Dress and Adornment of African American Entertainers," in *African American Dress and Adornment: A Cultural Perspective*, ed. Barbara M. Starke, Lillian O. Holloman, and Barbara K. Nordquist (Dubuque, Iowa: Kendall/Hunt, 1990), 179–87.

34. Duke Ellington, *Music Is My Mistress* (Garden City, N.J.: Doubleday, 1973; reprint, New York: Da Capo Press, 1976), 81.

35. Willie "the Lion" Smith with George Hoefer, *Music on My Mind: The Memoirs of an American Pianist* (New York: Doubleday, 1964; reprint, New York: Da Capo Press, 1978), 52–53, 155.

36. Tom Davin, "Conversation with James P. Johnson," in *Jazz Panorama: From the Pages of the Jazz Review*, ed. Martin Williams (New York: Crowell-Collier, 1962; reprint, New York: Da Capo Press, 1979), 56, 59–60.

37. Rex Stewart quoted in Nat Shapiro and Nat Hentoff, eds., *Hear Me Talkin' to Ya: The Story of Jazz as Told by the Men Who Made It* (New York: Rinehart, 1955; reprint, New York: Dover, 1966), 206.

38. Thomas Dorsey quoted in Sandra R. Lieb, *Mother of the Blues: A Study of Ma Rainey* (Amherst: University of Massachusetts Press, 1981), 28–30.

39. Frank C. Taylor with Gerald Cook, *Alberta Hunter: A Celebration in Blues* (New York: McGraw-Hill, 1987), 84, 41.

40. Léopold Sédar Senghor, "L'esprit de la civilisation ou les lois de la culture négro-africaine," *Présence Africaine* (Paris) 8–10 (1956): 60, quoted in Janheinz Jahn, *Muntu: African Culture and the Western World* (New York: Grove Press, 1961; reprint, New York: Grove Weidenfeld, 1990), 164. Millicent Hod-

son, "How She Began Her Beguine: Dunham's Dance Literacy," in *Kaiso!: Katherine Dunham, An Anthology of Writings*, ed. Vèvè A. Clark and Margaret B. Wilkerson (Berkeley: CCEW Women's Center, Institute for the Study of Social Change, University of California, 1978), 197–98.

41. James Berry with Mura Dehn, "Jazz Profound," *Dance Scope* 11, no. 1 (Fall–Winter 1976–77): 24.

42. Duke Ellington quoted in Stanley Dance, *The World of Earl Hines* (New York: Scribner, 1977; reprint, New York: Da Capo Press, 1983), 3; Ellison, *Shadow and Act*, 234; Vlach, *Afro-American Tradition*, 150.

43. Robert Farris Thompson, "Coming down the Body Line: Kongo Atlantic Gestures and Sports," in *Dancing between Two Worlds: Kongo-Angola Culture and the Americas*, ed. C. Daniel Dawson (New York: Ragged Edge, 1991), 8; Judith Bettelheim, "Jonkonnu and Other Christmas Masquerades," in *Caribbean Festival Arts*, ed. John W. Nunley and Judith Bettelheim (Seattle: University of Washington Press, 1988), 64.

44. Murray, *Stomping the Blues*, 50, 90, 126.

45. Rex Stewart, *Jazz Masters of the 30s* (New York: Macmillan, 1972; reprint, New York: Da Capo Press, 1982), 40; Hurston, "Characteristics," 54; Robert Farris Thompson, "Kongo Influences on African-American Artistic Culture," in *Africanisms in American Culture*, ed. Joseph E. Holloway (Bloomington: Indiana University Press, 1990), 157–64; see also Benjamin G. Cooke, "Nonverbal Communication among Afro-Americans: An Initial Classification," in *Rappin' and Stylin' Out: Communication in Urban Black America*, ed. Thomas Kochman (Urbana: University of Illinois Press, 1972), 32–64.

46. Hurston, "Characteristics," 55.

47. Quotation from Portia Maultsby, "Africanisms in African American Music," in *Africanisms in American Culture*, ed. Joseph E. Holloway (Bloomington: Indiana University Press, 1990), 195; Gerald L. Davis, *I Got the Word in Me and I Can Sing It, You Know: A Study of the Performed African-American Sermon* (Philadelphia: University of Pennsylvania Press, 1985), 26–27.

48. G. Davis, *I Got the Word*, 26–31.

49. Paul Carter Harrison, *The Drama of Nommo: Black Theater in the African Continuum* (New York: Grove Press, 1972), 72–73; John Michael Vlach, "Afro-American Aesthetic," in *Encyclopedia of Southern Culture*, ed. Charles Reagan Wilson and William Ferris (Chapel Hill: University of North Carolina Press, 1989), 457–58; Stuckey, *Slave Culture*, 88.

50. Ralph Ellison, "Juneteenth," *Quarterly Review of Literature* 13, nos. 3–4 (1965): 274–76.

Chapter 3: Mocking and Celebrating

1. David Dalby, "Jazz, Jitter, and Jam," *New York Times*, 10 Nov. 1970; Thompson, "An Aesthetic of the Cool: West African Dance," 85.

2. Ralph Ellison, lecture, Harvard University, Cambridge, Mass., 1 Dec. 1973.

3. John Playford, *The English Dancing Master* (1650), ed. Leslie Bridgewater and Hugh Mellor (London: Hugh Mellor, 1933), iii, quoted in Joseph E. Marks III, *America Learns to Dance: A Historical Study of Dance Education in America before 1900* (New York: Exposition Press, 1957; reprint, New York: Dance Horizons, 1976), 18; Southern, *Music*, 26; Marks, *America Learns*, 18–20.

4. Richard Kraus, *History of the Dance: In Art and Education* (Englewood Cliffs, N.J.: Prentice-Hall, 1969), 98–99; Marks, *America Learns*, 14, 15, 18, 20.

5. Marks, *America Learns*, 22–23, 25; Mary Newton Stanard, *Colonial Virginia: Its People and Customs* (Philadelphia: J. B. Lippincott, 1917), 140–42, 146.

6. Marks, *America Learns*, 25, 27; Richard Nevell, *A Time to Dance: American Country Dancing from Hornpipes to Hot Hash* (New York: St. Martin's Press, 1977), 32.

7. Southern, *Music*, 45; "Memoirs of a Monticello Slave," in *Jefferson at Monticello*, ed. James A. Bear Jr. (Charlottesville: University of Virginia, c. 1967), quoted in Epstein, *Sinful Tunes*, 122; Epstein, *Sinful Tunes*, 120–22.

8. Pierre Rameau, *The Dancing Master* (1725), translated by C. W. Beaumont (London: C. W. Beaumont, 1931), 1–2, quoted in Marks, *America Learns*, 49; Marks, *America Learns*, 27.

9. Marks, *America Learns*, 41–47.

10. *Sentimental Beauties, and Moral Delineations from the Celebrated Dr. Blair, and much Admired Authors; Selected with a View to Refine the Taste, Rectify the Judgement; and mould the Heart to Virtue*, 4th ed. (Philadelphia: F. Baily, 1792), quoted in ibid., 47.

11. Kraus, *History*, 108; Marks, *America Learns*, 63–65.

12. Frederick Law Olmstead, *The Cotton Kingdom: A Traveller's Observations on Cotton and Slavery in the American Slave States* (New York: Alfred A. Knopf, 1953), 350.

13. Kraus, *History*, 108; Samuel A. Floyd Jr. and Marsha J. Reisser, "Social Dance Music of Black Composers in the Nineteenth Century and the Emergence of Classic Ragtime," *Black Perspective in Music* 8, no. 2 (Fall 1980): 161–64.

14. Epstein, *Sinful Tunes*, 7–9, 21–76.

15. John F. Szwed and Morton Marks, "The Afro-American Transformation of European Set Dances and Dance Suites," *Dance Research Journal* 20, no. 1 (Summer 1988): 29.

16. Willis Lawrence James, "The Romance of the Negro Folk Cry in America," *Phylon* 16, no. 1 (1955): 18; Szwed and Marks, "Transformation," 32.

17. Thomas L. Riis, *Just before Jazz: Black Musical Theater in New York, 1890 to 1915* (Washington, D.C.: Smithsonian Institution Press, 1989), 3.

18. Isaac Williams, *Sunshine and Shadow of Slave Life* (East Saginaw, Mich., 1885), 61, quoted in Southern, *Music*, 185; Robert Russa Moton, *Finding a Way Out: An Autobiography* (New York: Doubleday, Page, 1920; reprint, College Park,

Md.: McGrath, 1969), 18–19, quoted in Lynne Fauley Emery, *Black Dance in the United States from 1619 to 1970* (Palo Alto, Calif.: National Press Books, 1972), 87–89; Tom Fletcher, *One Hundred Years of the Negro in Show Business* (New York: Burdge, 1954; reprint, New York: Da Capo Press, 1984), 19; Emery, *Black Dance*, 87–99.

19. Joseph Boskin, *Sambo: The Rise and Demise of an American Jester* (New York: Oxford University Press, 1986), 50; Work Projects Administration, *The Negro in Virginia* (New York: Hastings House, 1940), 89; Emery, *Black Dance*, 89, 119.

20. B. A. Botkin, ed., *Lay My Burden Down: A Folk History of Slavery* (Chicago: University of Chicago Press, 1945; reprint, Athens: University of Georgia Press, 1989), 56–57.

21. Roger D. Abrahams, *Singing the Master: The Emergence of African American Culture in the Plantation South* (New York: Pantheon, 1992), 130, xxii, xxvi, 85, 27, xviii-xix.

22. Herskovits, *Myth*, 138.

23. Works Projects Administration, *Negro in Virginia*, 93.

24. Blassingame, *Slave Community*, 107.

25. Raboteau, *Slave Religion*, 225.

26. Eugene D. Genovese, *Roll, Jordan, Roll: The World the Slaves Made* (New York: Pantheon, 1974; reprint, New York: Vintage Books, 1976), 570–71; Charlie Grandy quoted in Work Projects Administration, *Negro in Virginia*, 95.

27. Joyner, *Down by the Riverside*, 139, quotation from 134.

28. J. R. Creecy, *Scenes in the South and Other Miscellaneous Pieces* (Philadelphia: J. B. Lippincott, 1860), 21–23. Many thanks to Charmaine Warren for bringing this book to my attention.

29. Ira De A. Reid, "The John Canoe Festival," *Phylon* 3, no. 4 (Fourth Quarter, 1942): 349–50, 353–54, 357–60, quotation from 360; Bettelheim, "Jonkonnu," 39–83.

30. Southern, *Music*, 122; Stuckey, *Slave Culture*, 73–74.

31. William D. Piersen, *Black Yankees: The Development of an Afro-American Subculture in Eighteenth-Century New England* (Amherst: University of Massachusetts Press, 1988), 117–28.

32. Southern, *Music*, 54.

33. Melvin Wade, "Shining in Borrowed Plumage: Affirmation of Community in the Black Coronation Festivals of New England (c.1750–c.1850)," *Western Folklore* 40, no. 3 (July 1981): 211–31, quotation from 218.

34. Ibid., 218; Piersen, *Black Yankees*, 122.

35. A. A. Opoku, *Festivals of Ghana* (Accra, Ghana: Ghana Publishing, 1970), 4–6; Wade, "Shining," 218–25; see also Joseph P. Reidy, "'Negro Election Day' and Black Community Life in New England, 1750–1860," *Marxist Perspectives* 1, no. 3 (Fall 1978): 106–10.

36. Southern, *Music*, 54–57; A. J. Williams-Myers, "Pinkster Carnival: Africanisms in the Hudson River Valley," *Afro-Americans in New York Life and History* 9, no. 1 (Jan. 1985): 7–17; Sterling Stuckey, "The Skies of Consciousness: African Dance at Pinkster in New York, 1750–1840," in *Going through the Storm: The Influence of African American Art in History* (New York: Oxford University Press, 1994), 53–80; Shane White, "Pinkster in Albany, 1803: A Contemporary Description," *New York History* 70, no. 2 (Apr. 1989): 191–99.

37. Southern, *Music*, 56.

38. White, "Pinkster in Albany," 198; Williams-Myers, "Pinkster Carnival," 11–13; Shane White, "Pinkster: Afro-Dutch Syncretization in New York City and the Hudson Valley," *Journal of American Folklore* 102, no. 403 (Jan.–Mar. 1989): 68–69.

39. James Fenimore Cooper, *Satanstoe* (New York: G. P. Putnam's Sons, 1845), 66–67, quoted in Epstein, *Sinful Tunes*, 67.

40. Thomas F. Devoe, *The Market Book*, vol. 1 (New York: printed for the author, 1862), 322, 344–45, quotation from 344; Williams-Myers, "Pinkster Carnival," 9–13.

41. John F. Watson, *Annals of Philadelphia*, 2d ed., rev. (Philadelphia: A. Hart, J. W. Moore, J. Penington, U. Hunt, and H. F. Anners, 1850), 2:265, quoted in Southern, *Music*, 57.

42. Blassingame, *Slave Community*, 106.

43. Wood, *Black Majority*, 299, 316.

44. Levine, *Black Culture*, 297.

45. Jones and Hawes, *Step It Down*, 24.

46. Fletcher, *One Hundred Years*, VII.

Chapter 4: Black Dance on the Road

1. Southern, *Music*, 89.

2. Stearns and Stearns, *Jazz Dance*, 42–44; Southern, *Music*, 90–91.

3. Toll, *Blacking Up*, 43–44, quotation from 43; Southern, *Music*, 90–91.

4. Constance Rourke, *American Humor: A Study of the National Character* (New York: Harcourt, Brace, 1931), 86; Toll, *Blacking Up*, 46–47.

5. Henry A. Kmen, "Old Corn Meal: A Forgotten Urban Negro Folksinger," *Journal of American Folklore* 75 (Jan.–Mar. 1962): 29–34; T. Allston Brown, "The Origin of Negro Minstrelsy," in *Fun in Black; or, Sketches of Minstrel Life* by Charles H. Day (New York: Robert M. DeWitt, 1874), quoted in Eileen Southern, "In Retrospect: Black Musicians and Early Ethiopian Minstrelsy," *Black Perspective in Music* 3, no. 1 (Spring 1975): 77–78.

6. Toll, *Blacking Up*, 52–57.

7. Hans Nathan, *Dan Emmett and the Rise of Early Negro Minstrelsy* (Norman: University of Oklahoma Press, 1977), 83, 85, 90–93, quotations from 73, 90, 75.

8. Marian Hannah Winter, "Juba and American Minstrelsy," in *Chronicles of the American Dance: From the Shakers to Martha Graham*, ed. Paul Magriel (New York: Dance Index, 1948; reprint, New York: Da Capo Press, 1978), 39, 42; Charles Dickens, *American Notes* (1842), quoted in ibid., 48.

9. Winter, "Juba," 47–50.

10. Ibid., 50, quotation from 39.

11. Toll, *Blacking Up*, 195, 198, 200, 211–12, 228; Southern, *Music*, 233; James Weldon Johnson, *Black Manhattan* (New York: Alfred A. Knopf, 1930; reprint, New York: Atheneum, 1977), 93.

12. During slavery the pigeon wing and the buck dance were widely performed by African Americans. When these dances were appropriated for the minstrel stage, they were billed together and called the buck and wing. As the term evolved, it included new kinds of movements; by 1900, *buck and wing* was used as a generic term for *tap dance* as well. Twentieth-century tap dancers have described buck dancing as flat-footed tap, performed close to the floor. The buck resembled a time step and the wing, which continued to evolve through the teens and twenties, was initially a hop and sideward thrust of one foot. During the thirties, the wing became a highly technical tap step with many variations. Stearns and Stearns, *Jazz Dance*, 176, 191; Emery, *Black Dance*, 89–90.

13. Johnson, *Black Manhattan*, 89; Winter, "Juba," 57–58; Alain Locke, "The Age of Minstrelsy," in *The Afro-American in Music and Art*, ed. Lindsay Patterson (Cornwells Heights, Penn.: Publishers Agency, under the auspices of the Association for the Study of Afro-American Life and History, 1978), 33–34.

14. Arthur Marshall quoted in Stearns and Stearns, *Jazz Dance*, 50–51.

15. Quotations from Winter, "Juba," 58, 61; Johnson, *Black Manhattan*, 89–90, 93; Fletcher, *One Hundred Years*, 103; Southern, *Music*, 234.

16. Fletcher, *One Hundred Years*, 53; Southern, *Music*, 233; Ike Simond, *Old Slack's Reminiscence and Pocket History of the Colored Profession from 1865 to 1891* (by the author, 1891; reprint, Bowling Green, Ohio: Bowling Green University Popular Press, 1974), 18.

17. Robert C. Toll, *On with the Show: The First Century of Show Business in America* (New York: Oxford University Press, 1976), 115; Fletcher, *One Hundred Years*, 41; Simond, *Old Slack's*, xxiii; Johnson, *Black Manhattan*, 93.

18. Riis, *Just before Jazz*, 5–7; Simond, *Old Slack's*, xvii, xxiv-xxv; Johnson, *Black Manhattan*, 93; Toll, *Blacking Up*, 245–48.

19. Simond, *Old Slack's*, xix.

20. Toll, *Blacking Up*, 243; Simond, *Old Slack's*, xxiv-xxv; Winter, "Juba," 42.

21. Southern, *Music*, 293–94; Stearns and Stearns, *Jazz Dance*, 59.

22. Lawrence W. Levine, *Highbrow Lowbrow: The Emergence of Cultural Hierarchy in America* (Cambridge, Mass.: Harvard University Press, 1990), 21–23, quotation from 9; Robert C. Allen, *Horrible Prettiness: Burlesque and American Culture* (Chapel Hill: University of North Carolina Press, 1991), 178, 87–88.

23. Robert Bogdan, *Freak Show: Presenting Human Oddities for Amusement and Profit* (Chicago: University of Chicago Press, 1990), 25–68; Allen, *Horrible Prettiness*, 29, 178–93; Neil Harris, *Humbug: The Art of P. T. Barnum* (Boston: Little, Brown, 1973; reprint, Chicago: University of Chicago Press, 1981), 235–76.

24. Quotation from Riis, *Just before Jazz*, 14; Johnson, *Black Manhattan*, 59–60.

25. Southern, *Music*, 240, 250–51, quotation from Eileen Southern, *The Music of Black Americans in History* (New York: W. W. Norton, 1971), 254.

26. Southern, *Music*, 251; Thomas Riis, "Blacks on the Musical Stage," in *Images of Blacks in American Culture: A Reference Guide to Information Sources*, ed. Jessie Carney Smith (New York: Greenwood Press, 1988), 32–33; Thomas L. Riis, "The Music and Musicians in Nineteenth-Century Productions of *Uncle Tom's Cabin*," *American Music* 4, no. 3 (Fall 1986): 268.

27. Fletcher, *One Hundred Years*, 287; Riis, "Blacks on the Musical Stage," 33.

28. Allen Woll, *Black Musical Theater: From Coontown to Dreamgirls* (Baton Rouge: Louisiana State University Press, 1989; reprint, New York: Da Capo Press, 1991), 4; Johnson, *Black Manhattan*, 95–96; Southern, *Music*, 295–96; Stearns and Stearns, *Jazz Dance*, 118, 123; Riis, *Just before Jazz*, 12, 13.

29. Southern, *Music*, 251; Stearns and Stearns, *Jazz Dance*, 75–76, 181, Willie Covan quoted on 76.

30. Southern, *Music*, 252; Johnson, *Black Manhattan*, 96; Fletcher, *One Hundred Years*, 41–42.

31. Review, *New York Times*, 26 May 1895, sect. 2, p. 16, quoted in Riis, *Just before Jazz*, 24; Riis, *Just before Jazz*, 22–24, Fletcher, *One Hundred Years*, 91, 94; Southern, *Music*, 253–54.

32. Johnson, *Black Manhattan*, 96–97, quotation from 96; Riis, *Just before Jazz*, 19–20, 22; Southern, *Music*, 296.

33. Stearns and Stearns, *Jazz Dance*, 78, Ida Forsyne quoted on 251; Johnson, *Black Manhattan*, 99–101; Riis, *Just before Jazz*, 24–25.

34. Johnson, *Black Manhattan*, 100–101; Southern, *Music*, 296; Riis, *Just before Jazz*, 24–26; Stearns and Stearns, *Jazz Dance*, 77–78.

35. Stearns and Stearns, *Jazz Dance*, 85, quotation from 91.

36. Ibid., 85–88, quotation from 88; Jeni LeGon, interview with Rusty Frank, Vancouver, B.C., Canada, 17 Aug. 1989, in *Tap!: The Greatest Tap Dance Stars and Their Stories, 1900–1955*, ed. Rusty E. Frank (New York: William Morrow, 1990), 122.

37. Stearns and Stearns, *Jazz Dance*, 89; Count Basie and Albert Murray, *Good Morning Blues: The Autobiography of Count Basie* (New York: Random House, 1985), 135.

38. Dewey "Pigmeat" Markham with Bill Levinson, *Here Comes the Judge!* (New York: Popular Library, 1969), 103; Stearns and Stearns, *Jazz Dance*, 89.

39. Quotation from John E. Rousseau and Tom Price, "Zulu—Its History," in *Farewell to the 80s, Welcome the 90s*, Official 1990 Program, Zulu Social Aid and Pleasure Club, New Orleans, La., 29; Southern, *Music*, 294–95; Stearns and Stearns, *Jazz Dance*, 77.

40. Southern, *Music*, 294–95.

41. Southern, *Music*, 294; Lieb, *Mother of the Blues*, 7–8.

42. Eleanor J. Baker, "Silas Green Show," in *Encyclopedia of Southern Culture*, ed. Charles Reagan Wilson and William Ferris (Chapel Hill: University of North Carolina Press, 1989), 223–24; Southern, *Music*, 294.

43. Charles Reagan Wilson, "Traveling Shows," in *Encyclopedia of Southern Culture*, ed. Charles Reagan Wilson and William Ferris (Chapel Hill: University of North Carolina Press, 1989), 1247–49, quotation from 1248.

44. Pigmeat Markham quoted in Stearns and Stearns, *Jazz Dance*, 73.

45. Stearns and Stearns, *Jazz Dance*, 63.

46. Bogdan, *Freak Show*, 40–41, quotation from 44; Wilson, "Traveling Shows," 1247.

47. Southern, *Music*, 295.

48. Fletcher, *One Hundred Years*, 149.

49. Garvin Bushell with Mark Tucker, *Jazz from the Beginning* (Ann Arbor: University of Michigan Press, 1990), 11–12.

50. Buster Bailey quoted in Shapiro and Hentoff, *Hear Me Talkin' to Ya*, 77.

51. Nettie Compton quoted in Stearns and Stearns, *Jazz Dance*, 71.

52. Brooks McNamara, *Step Right Up* (Garden City, N.Y.: Doubleday, 1976), 45–51, 170.

53. Ulysses "Slow Kid" Thompson quoted in Stearns and Stearns, *Jazz Dance*, 64–65, "crazy quilt blend," 65; Woll, *Black Musical Theater*, 32–33.

54. Helen Oakley Dance, *Stormy Monday: The T-Bone Walker Story* (Baton Rouge: Louisiana State University Press, 1987; reprint, New York: Da Capo Press, 1990), 17–18; Al Rose, *Eubie Blake* (New York: Schirmer Books, 1983), 28–29; Wilson, "Traveling Shows," 1248; Bruce Bastin, "From the Medicine Show to the Stage: Some Influences upon the Development of a Blues Tradition in the Southeastern United States," *American Music* 2, no. 1 (Spring 1984): 31.

55. Walter Fuller quoted in Dance, *Earl Hines*, 166; Buster Smith quoted in Ross Russell, *Jazz Style in Kansas City and the Southwest* (Berkeley: University of California Press, 1983), 76.

56. Wilson, "Traveling Shows," 1247; Bogdan, *Freak Show*, 58–60.

57. Stearns and Stearns, *Jazz Dance*, 65–70; Joe McKennon, *A Pictorial History of the American Carnival*, vol. 2 (Sarasota, Fla.: Carnival, 1972), 81.

58. Shapiro and Hentoff, *Hear Me Talkin' to Ya*, 285, 307, Jo Jones quoted on 306; Stanley Dance, *The World of Count Basie* (New York: Charles Scribner's Sons, 1980; reprint, New York: Da Capo Press, 1985), 299; Bechet, *Treat It Gentle*, 96; Buck Clayton and Nancy Miller Elliott, *Buck Clayton's Jazz World* (New York: Oxford University Press, 1989), 85.

59. Pigmeat Markham quoted in Stearns and Stearns, *Jazz Dance*, 63.

60. Willie Covan, interview with Rusty Frank, Los Angeles, Calif., 9 June 1988, in Frank, ed., *Tap!* 25; Leonard Reed, interview with Rusty Frank, Hollywood, Calif., 8 June 1988, in ibid., 40–41; Peg Leg Bates, interview with Rusty Frank, Kerhonskon, New York, 13 Nov. 1988, in ibid., 49; Stearns and Stearns, *Jazz Dance*, 74, 83.

Chapter 5: Dancing Singers and Singing Dancers

1. Riis, *Just before Jazz*, xxii.

2. Ibid., 28; Johnson, *Black Manhattan*, 98; unidentified review, Feb. 6, 1900, *A Trip to Coontown* Folder, Clipping Files of the Theater Collection of Houghton Library, Harvard University, quoted in Riis, *Just before Jazz*, 77–78; Henry T. Sampson, *Blacks in Blackface: A Source Book on Early Black Musical Shows* (Metuchen, N.J.: Scarecrow Press, 1980), 321; Southern, *Music*, 297; Woll, *Black Musical Theater*, 12–13.

3. Southern, *Music*, 268–69, 298.

4. Will Marion Cook, "Clorindy; or, The Origin of the Cakewalk," *Theater Arts* (Sept. 1947), quoted in Southern, *Music*, 298; James Weldon Johnson, *Along This Way: The Autobiography of James Weldon Johnson* (New York: Viking, 1933; reprint, London: Penguin, 1990), 151–52.

5. Ann Charters, *Nobody: The Story of Bert Williams* (New York: Macmillan, 1970), 21, 31, 36–37; Stearns and Stearns, *Jazz Dance*, 121.

6. Fletcher, *One Hundred Years*, 105.

7. Ibid., 107; Stearns and Stearns, *Jazz Dance*, 123–24; Johnson, *Black Manhattan*, 106.

8. Fletcher, *One Hundred Years*, 181; Stearns and Stearns, *Jazz Dance*, 117, 122; Newman, "Brightest Star."

9. Southern, *Music*, 299–300; Stearns and Stearns, *Jazz Dance*, 119–20; Riis, *Just before Jazz*, 45–46.

10. Riis, *Just before Jazz*, 178–82, quotation from 178; Woll, *Black Musical Theater*, 50, 53, 54; Southern, *Music*, 292.

11. Stearns and Stearns, *Jazz Dance*, 127–30, Ethel Williams quoted on 125.

12. Johnson, *Black Manhattan*, 174; Riis, *Just before Jazz*, 179–80; Stearns and Stearns, *Jazz Dance*, 130.

13. B. Kellner, ed., *"Keep A-Inchin' Along": Selected Writings of Carl Van Vechten about Black Arts and Letters* (Westport, Conn.: Greenwood Press, 1979), 21, 25, quoted in Riis, *Just before Jazz*, 182.

14. Johnson, *Black Manhattan*, 170–74.

15. Bobbi King, "Conversation with . . . Eubie Blake (Continued): A Legend in His Own Lifetime," *Black Perspective in Music* 1, no. 2 (Fall 1973): 151–53.

16. Johnson, *Black Manhattan*, 186–88; Southern, *Music*, 427–28; Stearns and Stearns, *Jazz Dance*, 132–33; Woll, *Black Musical Theater*, 60–62.

17. *New York American*, 22 May 1922, quoted in Woll, *Black Musical Theater*, 71; Stearns and Stearns, *Jazz Dance*, 134–35, quotation from 139.

18. Southern, *Music*, 428.

19. Stearns and Stearns, *Jazz Dance*, 140–44.

20. Woll, *Black Musical Theater*, 98, 95, quotations from 98, 94; Stearns and Stearns, *Jazz Dance*, 142.

21. Johnson, *Black Manhattan*, 190; Stearns and Stearns, *Jazz Dance*, 145, quotation from 134.

22. Stearns and Stearns, *Jazz Dance*, 144, 146–47; Johnson, *Black Manhattan*, 190.

23. Woll, *Black Musical Theater*, 95–97, 154; Stearns and Stearns, *Jazz Dance*, 146, 148.

24. *Philadelphia Public Ledger*, n.d., in Florence Mills File, Theater Collection, Philadelphia Free Library, Philadelphia, Penn., quoted in Woll, *Black Musical Theater*, 104, 106.

25. Stearns and Stearns, *Jazz Dance*, 147–48; Woll, *Black Musical Theater*, 117.

26. Stearns and Stears, *Jazz Dance*, 151–54, quotation from 153; Woll, *Black Musical Theater*, 121.

27. Stearns and Stearns, *Jazz Dance*, 153–54; Woll, *Black Musical Theater*, 131–32.

28. Archie Ware quoted in Stearns and Stearns, *Jazz Dance*, 265.

29. Stearns and Stearns, *Jazz Dance*, 154–59.

30. Southern, *Music*, 291

31. Quotation from Riis, *Just before Jazz*, 169; Southern, *Music*, 291–92.

32. Riis, *Just before Jazz*, 160–62, 166–68.

33. Southern, *Music*, 292–93.

34. Riis, "Blacks on the Musical Stage," 39.

35. Stearns and Stearns, *Jazz Dance*, 85, Pete Nugent quoted on 79; Riis, "Blacks on the Musical Stage," 40; Riis, *Just before Jazz*, 18.

36. Clarence Muse and Ernest "Baby" Seals quoted in Stearns and Stearns, *Jazz Dance*, 79.

37. Stearns and Stearns, *Jazz Dance*, 79–81, quotation from 80.

38. Ibid., 80, 82, 87, 90, Tiny Ray quoted on 81, Henry "Rubberlegs" Williams quoted on 83.

39. Fletcher, *One Hundred Years*, 173; Riis, "Blacks on the Musical Stage," 40; Riis, *Just before Jazz*, 166–68.

40. Riis, "Blacks on the Musical Stage," 39; Southern, *Music*, 293.

41. William Howland Kenney III, "The Influence of Black Vaudeville on Early Jazz," *Black Perspective in Music* 14, no. 3 (Fall 1986): 234–35; William H. Kenney, "James Scott and the Culture of Classic Ragtime," *American Music* 9, no. 2 (Summer 1991): 173, 174; Ed Kirkeby, *Ain't Misbehavin': The Story of Fats Waller* (New York: Dodd, Mead, 1966; reprint, Da Capo Press, 1975), 23–25; Dance, *Earl Hines*, 206; Basie and Murray, *Good Morning Blues*, 32, 69–70.

42. Riis, "Blacks on the Musical Stage," 40–41; Stearns and Stearns, *Jazz Dance*, 80; Riis, *Just before Jazz*, 170.

43. Smith, *Music on My Mind*, 170.

44. Lewis Allan Erenberg, "Urban Night Life and the Decline of Victorianism: New York City's Restaurants and Cabarets, 1890–1918" (Ph.D. diss., University of Michigan, 1974), 2–140, 326–39.

45. Perry Bradford, *Born with the Blues* (New York: Oak Publications, 1965), 163–64; Erenberg, "Urban Night Life," 134–40.

46. James Weldon Johnson, *The Autobiography of an Ex-Coloured Man* (New York: Alfred A. Knopf, 1927), quoted in Johnson, *Black Manhattan*, 75–76; Erenberg, "Urban Night Life," 140–41; Johnson, *Black Manhattan*, 59, 74–75; George Hoefer, "Jazz Odyssey, Vol. 3: The Sound of Harlem," accompanying booklet to *Jazz Odyssey*, vol. 3: *The Sound of Harlem* (Columbia Records, Jazz Archive Series, Mono-C3L 33, 1964).

47. Johnson, *Black Manhattan*, 74–78, quotation from 74; David Levering Lewis, *When Harlem Was in Vogue* (New York: Alfred A. Knopf, 1981; reprint, New York: Oxford University Press, 1989), 29.

48. Smith, *Music on My Mind*, 91–93, 94; Hoefer, "Jazz Odyssey."

49. Smith, *Music on My Mind*, 94, 96–97.

50. Bushell, *Jazz*, 28–29.

51. Jervis Anderson, *This Was Harlem: A Cultural Portrait, 1900–1950* (New York: Farrar Straus Giroux, 1982), 71, 171; Hoefer, "Jazz Odyssey."

52. Johnson, *Black Manhattan*, 180; Robert Sylvester, *No Cover Charge: A Backward Look at the Night Clubs* (New York: Dial Press, 1956), 42–68.

53. Anderson, *This Was Harlem*, 171; Hoefer, "Jazz Odyssey"; Lewis, *When Harlem Was in Vogue*, 106.

54. Hoefer, "Jazz Odyssey."

55. Albert Murray quoted in Stanley Crouch, "The Rotten Club," *Village Voice*, 5 Feb. 1985, 59; Hoefer, "Jazz Odyssey."

56. Cab Calloway and Bryant Rollins, *Of Minnie the Moocher and Me* (New York: Thomas Y. Crowell, 1976), 99–100, quotation from 88.

57. Lena Horne and Richard Schickel, *Lena* (New York: Doubleday, 1965), 51.

58. Ibid., 57, 52; Murray interview.

59. Calloway and Rollins, *Minnie*, 93, 96; Bessie Dudley, interview with author and Robert G. O'Meally, New York, N.Y., 23, 29 June 1992; Jim Haskins, *The Cotton Club: A Pictorial and Social History of the Most Famous Symbol of the Jazz Era* (New York: Random House, 1977); Thomas J. Clark, "Cotton Club," accompanying booklet to *The Original Cotton Club Orchestras* (Audiofidelity Enterprises, AFE-3-13, 1985).

60. Lewis, *When Harlem Was in Vogue*, 105; Hoefer, "Jazz Odyssey"; Stanley Dance, *The World of Duke Ellington* (New York: Charles Scribner's Sons, 1970; reprint, Da Capo Press, 1981), 68.

61. Smith, *Music on My Mind*, 158–59, 166–68, quotation from 158; Sylvester, *No Cover Charge*, 56.

62. Bushell, *Jazz*, 49–50; Samuel B. Charters and Leonard Kunstadt, *Jazz: A History of the New York Scene* (Garden City, N.Y.: Doubleday, 1962; reprint, New York: Da Capo Press, 1984), 196; Hoefer, "Jazz Odyssey."

63. Sonny Greer quoted in Dance, *Duke Ellington*, 69.

64. Dicky Wells, interview with Linda Kuehl, New York, N.Y., 3 Aug. 1971, from the files of Robert G. O'Meally; Smith, *Music on My Mind*, 159–61; Hoefer, "Jazz Odyssey."

65. Crouch, "Rotten Club," 57.

Chapter 6: Jazz Music in Motion

1. Bushell, *Jazz*, 23, 26–27, quotation from 27; Kenney, "Influence of Black Vaudeville," 235.

2. Bushell, *Jazz*, 54–57, quotation from 57; Clark, "Cotton Club," 9.

3. Dance, *Earl Hines*, 71.

4. Gunther Schuller and Martin Williams, "Big Band Jazz: From the Beginnings to the Fifties," accompanying booklet to *Big Band Jazz: From the Beginnings to the Fifties* (RCA, the Smithsonian Collection of Recordings, DMM 6–0610 LP Edition R 030, 1983).

5. Cholly Atkins, telephone interview with author, 15 May 1992; LeRoy Myers and Marion Coles, interview with author, New York, N.Y., 8 Nov. 1994.

6. Coles, "The Dance," 8–9, first two quotations from 8; Ted Fox, *Showtime at the Apollo* (New York: Holt, Rinehart, and Winston, 1985), 97–98, quotation from 98.

7. Brenda Dixon-Stowell, "Between Two Eras: 'Norton and Margot' in the Afro-American Entertainment World," *Dance Research Journal* 15, no. 2 (Spring 1983): 11–20.

8. Coles, "The Dance," 8; Marion Coles, telephone interview with author, 15 May 1995; Atkins interview, 15 May 1992.

9. Stearns and Stearns, *Jazz Dance*, 231–36, quotation from 231–32.

10. Ibid., 244–46; Cholly Atkins, telephone interview with author, 25 July 1992.

11. Stearns and Stearns, *Jazz Dance*, 282.

12. Baby Laurence quoted in ibid., 337; Whitney Balliett, *New York Notes: A Journal of Jazz, 1972–75* (Boston: Houghton Mifflin, 1976), 142; Sally Sommer, "Tap and How It Got That Way: Feet, Talk to Me!" *Dance Magazine*, Sept. 1988, 59–60.

13. Quotations from Louis Bellson, interview with Robert G. O'Meally, San Jose, Calif., 8 June 1992, from the files of Robert G. O'Meally; Jane Goldberg, "A Drum Is a Tapdancer," in "The Village Voice Jazz Special," a special section

of *Village Voice*, 30 Aug. 1988, 11–13; Stanley Dance, *The World of Swing* (New York: Charles Scribner's Sons, 1974; reprint, New York: Da Capo Press, 1979), 184; Leroy Williams, telephone interview with author, 1 May 1992.

14. Max Roach quoted in Goldberg, "A Drum Is a Tapdancer," 12; Dannie Richmond quoted in ibid., 12; Philly Joe Jones quoted in ibid., 11–12.

15. Ellison, *Shadow and Act*, 208–9; Ellington, *Music Is My Mistress*, 161–62; Myers interview.

16. Jimmy Crawford quoted in Dance, *Swing*, 124.

17. Stearns and Stearns, *Jazz Dance*, 337–38; Hoefer, "Jazz Odyssey."

18. Leonard Reed, interview with Rusty Frank, Hollywood, Calif., 8 June 1988, in *Tap!* ed. Rusty Frank (New York: William Morrow, 1990), 42.

19. Vlach, "Afro-American Aesthetic," 457; Baby Laurence quoted in Stearns and Stearns, *Jazz Dance*, 341.

20. Dance, *Swing*, 399, 402.

21. Honi Coles quoted in Melba Huber, "Tap Talk," *Dance Pages* 9, no. 4 (Spring 1992): 18.

22. This information was taken from various interviews with Cholly Atkins and Honi Coles; Stearns and Stearns, *Jazz Dance*, 351–52, 339; Frank, *Tap!* 259.

23. Hoefer, "Jazz Odyssey."

24. Fox, *Showtime*, 74–75, 80–81, 98, 100, Andy Kirk quoted on 81, Sandman Sims quoted on 98, 100.

25. Coles, "The Dance," 9; Fox, *Showtime*, 75–77.

26. Dicky Wells and Stanley Dance, *The Night People: Reminiscences of a Jazzman* (Boston: Crescendo, 1971), 53, 113.

27. Romare Bearden quoted in Anderson, *This Was Harlem*, 241; Fox, *Showtime*, 82.

28. *The Savoy Story*, Twenty-Fifth Anniversary of the Savoy Ballroom Brochure, 1951; Hoefer, "Jazz Odyssey."

29. Quotation from Lewis, *When Harlem Was in Vogue*, 170; Hoefer, "Jazz Odyssey"; *The Savoy Story*.

30. *The Savoy Story*.

31. Stearns and Stearns, *Jazz Dance*, 322–23; Murray, *Stomping the Blues*, 23–42; Frankie Manning, interview with Robert P. Crease, New York, N.Y., 22–23 July 1992, Jazz Oral History Program, Smithsonian Institution.

32. Barbara Engelbrecht, "Swinging at the Savoy," *Dance Research Journal* 15, no. 2 (Spring 1983): 7; Stearns and Stearns, *Jazz Dance*, 322–25, 329.

33. Ellison, *Shadow and Act*, 206–7; Nat Hentoff, liner notes to *Big Band at the Savoy Ballroom* (Radio Corporation of America, LPM/LSP-2543, 1958); Stearns and Stearns, *Jazz Dance*, 324; Wells and Dance, *Night People*, 59.

34. Wells and Dance, *Night People*, 77.

35. William "Cat" Anderson quoted in Dance, *Duke Ellington*, 153.

36. Dance, *Duke Ellington*, 13.

37. Pops Foster and Tom Stoddard, *Pops Foster: The Autobiography of a New Orleans Jazzman* (Berkeley: University of California Press, 1973), 166.

38. Lester Young quoted in Nat Shapiro and Nat Hentoff, eds., *The Jazz Makers: Essays on the Greats of Jazz* (New York: Rinehart, 1957; reprint, New York: Da Capo Press, 1979), 267.

39. Baby Dodds and Larry Gara, *The Baby Dodds Story*, rev. ed. (Baton Rouge: Louisiana State University Press, 1992), 88.

40. Jimmy Crawford quoted in Dance, *Swing*, 124.

41. Stearns and Stearns, *Jazz Dance*, 325.

42. Manning interview.

43. *The Savoy Story*; Alice Irene Pifer, "Back into Swing," *20/20*, 28 July 1989, transcript; *Duke Ellington and His Orchestra, 1929–1941* (Jazz Classics, Amvest Video, Rahway, N.J., 1987); Manning interview; Norma Miller, interview with Ernie Smith, Bolton Landing, N.Y., 23–24 Sept. 1992, Jazz Oral History Program, Smithsonian Institution; Robert Crease, "Last of the Lindy Hoppers," *Village Voice*, 25 Aug. 1987, 27–32; Norma Miller, telephone interview with author, 14 Dec. 1992; Robert P. Crease, "The Lindy Hop," *Research Forum Papers: The 1988 International Early Dance Institute* (June 1988): 1–11.

44. Dance, *Swing*, 71; Wells and Dance, *Night People*, 62; Philip W. Payne, ed. "The Swing Era 1938–39: Where Swing Came From," accompanying booklet to *The Swing Era 1938–39: Where Swing Came From* (Time-Life Records, New York, STL 343, 1971), 55.

45. Charters and Kundstadt, *Jazz*, 257–59, quotation from 259.

46. Ellington, *Music Is My Mistress*, 100; Barry Ulanov, *A History of Jazz in America* (New York: Viking Press, 1952), 166–73.

47. Ellison, *Shadow and Act*, 243–44; Albert Murray and Wynton Marsalis, "Good Evening Blues," lecture, Alice Tully Hall, Lincoln Center for the Performing Arts, New York, N.Y., 12 May 1992.

48. Ralph Ellison, "Harlem's America," from the U.S. Senate Investigation of the Crisis in our Cities, *New Leader* 49, no. 19 (26 Sept. 1966): 22–35, quotation from 23.

49. Murray and Marsalis, "Good Evening Blues."

50. Dance, *Duke Ellington*, 13; Ellington, *Music Is My Mistress*, 264, 281; Ellison, *Shadow and Act*, 268; Murray interview; Buster Brown, interview with author, New York, N.Y., 31 Oct. 1994.

51. Wynton Marsalis, interview with Robert G. O'Meally, New York, N.Y., July 1992, from the files of Robert G. O'Meally; Murray interview.

52. Tom Davin, "Conversation with James P. Johnson," in *Jazz Panorama*, ed. Martin Williams (New York: Crowell-Collier, 1962; reprint, New York: Da Capo Press, 1979), 44–61, quotation from 56; Louis Armstrong quoted in Shapiro and Hentoff, *Hear Me Talkin' to Ya*, 111.

53. Dizzy Gillespie with Al Fraser, *To Be or Not to Bop: Memoirs* (New York:

Doubleday, 1979; reprint, New York: Da Capo Press, 1985), 26–27, 223, Sarah Vaughan quoted on 179, Ella Fitzgerald quoted on 273, and Dizzy Gillespie quoted on 42.

54. Randy Weston and Ben Riley quoted in Toby Byron and Richard Saylor, *Thelonious Monk, American Composer* (Masters of American Music Series, Toby Byron/Multiprises in association with Taurus Film, Munich, and Videoarts, Japan, 1991).

55. Murray, *Good Morning Blues*, 85–86.

56. Eddie Durham quoted in Dance, *Count Basie*, 65; Stanley Dance, "The Complete Jimmy Lunceford, 1939–40," accompanying booklet to *The Complete Jimmy Lunceford, 1939–40* (CBS Disques, France, CBS 66421, 1981).

57. Nat Pierce quoted in Dance, *Swing*, 342; Dance, "The Complete Jimmy Lunceford."

58. Murray, *Stomping the Blues*, 138.

59. Frederic Ramsey Jr., "Jazz Odyssey, Vol. 1: The Sound of New Orleans, 1917–1947," accompanying booklet to *Jazz Odyssey, Vol. 1: The Sound of New Orleans, 1917–1947* (Columbia Records, Mono-C3L 30, 1964).

60. Max Roach quoted in Goldberg, "A Drum Is a Tapdancer," 12.

61. Max Roach quoted in Gillespie, *To Be or Not to Bop*, 232–33.

62. Dudley interview; Cholly Atkins interviews, 1988–92.

63. Dance, *Duke Ellington*, 14.

Chapter 7: "Let the Punishment Fit the Crime"

1. Danielle Masterson, "From the Roaring '20s to the Space Age," *Rhythm and Business* 1, no. 4 (June 1987): 18; Stearns and Stearns, *Jazz Dance*, 307; Cholly Atkins, telephone interview with author, 25 Jan. 1988.

2. Quotation from Stearns and Stearns, *Jazz Dance*, 307; Nelson George, *Where Did Our Love Go?: The Rise and Fall of the Motown Sound* (New York: St. Martin's Press, 1985), 90–91; Atkins interview, 25 Jan. 1988; Cholly Atkins, interview with author, East Elmhurst, N.Y., 17 July 1988.

3. Deanne Stillman, "Cholly Atkins, Dancing Machine," *Rolling Stone*, 20 Oct. 1977, 38; Stearns and Stearns, *Jazz Dance*, 307.

4. Atkins interview, 17 July 1988; Atkins interview, 25 Jan. 1988.

5. Charles "Honi" Coles, interview with author, East Elmhurst, N.Y., 17 July 1988.

6. Stearns and Stearns, *Jazz Dance*, 305–7, quotation from 305; LaVaughn Robinson, interview with author, Boulder, Colo., 23 June 1987; Charles "Honi" Coles, interview with author, East Elmhurst, N.Y., 9 Jan. 1988.

7. Dan Gallagher, *Over the Top to Bebop* (Camera Three, WCBS-TV, New York, 1965); Coles interview, 9 Jan. 1988; Atkins interview, 25 Jan. 1988.

8. Quotation from Effie Mihopoulus, "Interview with Honi Coles," *Salome: A Literary Dance Magazine*, nos. 44–46 (1986): 17; Atkins interview, 25 Jan. 1988; Coles interview, 9 Jan. 1988.

9. Ramsey, "Jazz Odyssey."

10. Stearns and Stearns, *Jazz Dance*, 141, 146, 148.

11. Ibid., 159, Buddy Bradley quoted on 168.

12. Katie Maria Doitch, "Tap Dancing—A Re-Definition," *New Dance* (London), no. 29 (Summer 1984): 10.

13. Sally R. Sommer, "Hearing Dance, Watching Film," *Dance Scope* 14, no. 3 (1980): 52. Even though Fred Astaire became an international idol, he was not a jazz tapper, as such, but a stylist who fused tap and ballroom dance.

14. Doitch, "Tap Dancing," 10.

15. Ellison, *Shadow and Act*, 199; Martin Williams, "The Smithsonian Collection of Classic Jazz," 3d ed., accompanying booklet to *The Smithsonian Collection of Classic Jazz* (Smithsonian Insitution, produced in association with Columbia Special Products, P6 11891, 1973), 9; Southern, *Music*, 474–75, 479.

16. Southern, *Music*, 477; Coles interview, 9 Jan. 1988; Brown interview.

17. Ellison, *Shadow and Act*, 206–7; Southern, *Music*, 479; Stearns and Stearns, *Jazz Dance*, 1.

18. Stearns and Stearns, *Jazz Dance*, 307, quotation from 305; Fox, *Showtime*, 133; Coles, "The Dance," 8.

19. Coles interview, 9 Jan. 1988; Patrick Montgomery, *Rock and Roll: The Early Days* (RCA/Columbia Pictures Home Video, 1985).

20. Coles interview, 17 July 1988; Masterson, "Roaring '20s," 18.

21. Atkins interview, 25 Jan. 1988; Stearns and Stearns, *Jazz Dance*, 359–60; George, *Where Did Our Love Go?* 91.

22. Melvin Franklin quoted in Gerri Hirshey, *Nowhere to Run: The Story of Soul Music* (New York: Times Books, 1984), 206; Gladys Knight quoted in Fox, *Showtime*, 261; Atkins interview, 25 Jan. 1988.

23. Masterson, "Roaring '20s," 19.

24. George, *Where Did Our Love Go?* 9, 10, 15–28.

25. Ibid., 31; Smokey Robinson quoted in Hirshey, *Nowhere to Run*, 133–34; Ed Ward, Geoffrey Stokes, and Ken Tucker, *Rock of Ages: The Rolling Stone History of Rock and Roll* (New York: Summit Books, 1986), 297.

26. George, *Where Did Our Love Go?* 88; Hirshey, *Nowhere to Run*, 125, 194–95; Mary Wilson, *Dreamgirl: My Life as a Supreme* (New York: St. Martin's Press, 1986), 169.

27. George, *Where Did Our Love Go?* 87.

28. Ibid., 87–89.

29. Atkins interview, 18 July 1988; Hirshey, *Nowhere to Run*, 165–66, 205; Masterson, "Roaring '20s," 19.

30. Wilson, *Dreamgirl*, 170; Stephanie Bennett and Steve Alpert, *Girl Groups*

(MGM/UA Home Entertainment Group, 1983); George, *Where Did Our Love Go?* 93.

31. Atkins interview, 25 Jan. 1988.

32. Hirshey, *Nowhere to Run*, 205, quotation from 200.

33. Atkins interview, 25 Jan. 1988.

34. Art Cromwell, *Watch Me Move!* (KCET, Los Angeles, 1986).

35. Atkins quoted in Stillman, "Cholly Atkins," 38; Cholly Atkins, interview with author, New York, N.Y., 8 Nov. 1994.

36. Atkins quoted in George, *Where Did Our Love Go?* 92.

37. Atkins interview, 25 Jan. 1988.

38. Atkins quoted in George, *Where Did Our Love Go?* 92; Atkins quoted in Stillman, "Cholly Atkins," 38.

39. Quotation from Stearns and Stearns, *Jazz Dance*, 360; Cromwell, *Watch Me Move!*; Arnold Shaw, *The Rockin' 50's* (New York: Hawthorn Books, 1974; reprint, New York: Da Capo Press, 1987), 176.

40. The Flamingos in Alan Freed, *Go Johnny Go* (Hal Roach Releases, 1958); Frankie Lymon and the Teenagers in *Rock! Rock! Rock!* (Directors Corporation of America, 1957); Ronettes in Lee Savin and Phil Spector, *That Was Rock: The T.A.M.I./T.N.T. Show* (Media Home Entertainment, 1984); Gladys Knight and the Pips in Neal Marshal, Susan Solomon, and Marty Callner, *Gladys Knight and the Pips and Ray Charles* (Home Box Office/Televisa International Production, Vestron Video, 1984); Temptations in *The Sounds of Motown* (Dave Clark International Productions, Sony Video LP, 1985); Jackson 5 in Don Mischer and Buz Kohan, *Motown 25: Yesterday—Today—Forever* (MGM/UA Home Video, 1983).

41. Richard Street quoted in Masterson, "Roaring '20s," 36; Atkins interviews, 1988–94.

Chapter 8: "W'en de Colo'ed Ban' Comes Ma'chin' down de Street"

1. Florida A&M Office of Public Relations, "The Florida A&M University 215 Piece Marching Band: Notable Quotes" (1987), 1.

2. Southern, *Music*, 7–10.

3. Edward Bowdich, *Mission from Cape Coast Castle to Ashantee* (London, 1819), quoted in ibid., 8.

4. Southern, *Music*, 44–45.

5. Epstein, *Sinful Tunes*, 147–48; Southern, *Music*, 27, 50–52; Paul A. Cimbala, "Fortunate Bondsmen: Black 'Musicianers' and Their Role as an Antebellum Southern Plantation Slave Elite," *Southern Studies* 18, no. 3 (Fall 1979): 295–98, 302–3.

6. Cimbala, "Fortunate Bondsmen," 297–300, quotations from 299, 297–98.

7. Raoul F. Camus, *Military Music of the American Revolution* (Chapel Hill: University of North Carolina Press, 1976), 41–42. For a detailed account of Train-

ing Day in New England, see H. Telfer Mook, "Training Day in New England," *New England Quarterly* 11, no. 4 (Dec. 1938): 675–97.

8. Raoul Camus, "Military Music," in *The New Grove Dictionary of American Music*, vol. 3, ed. H. Wiley Hitchcock and Stanley Sadie (London: Macmillan, 1986), 228–30; Henry George Farmer, *Handel's Kettledrums and Other Papers on Military Music* (London: Hinrichsen Edition, 1965), 44–46, 103; Eileen Southern, "In Retrospect: Early African Musicians in Europe," *Black Perspective in Music*, 1, no. 2 (Fall 1973): 166–67.

9. Farmer, *Handel's Kettledrums*, 41–46, 103–4, quotation from 45; Southern, "In Retrospect," 166–67, quotation from 166. Henry George Farmer, *The Rise and Development of Military Music* (London: W. Reeves, 1912; reprint, Freeport, N.Y.: Books for Libraries Press, 1970), 71–78; Henry George Farmer and James Blades, "Janissary Music," in *The New Grove Dictionary of Music and Musicians*, vol. 9, ed. Stanley Sadie (London: Macmillan, 1980), 496–98.

10. Farmer, *Handel's Kettledrums*, 46.

11. Quotations from Southern, "In Retrospect," 166–67; Camus, *Military Music*, 43–45; Farmer, *Rise and Development*, 77.

12. Stewart, *Jazz Masters*, 161; Whitney Balliett, *The Sound of Surprise: Forty-six Pieces on Jazz* (New York: E. P. Dutton, 1959), 147. See also Johnson, *Black Manhattan*, 122; Lionel Hampton and James Haskins, *Hamp: An Autobiography* (New York: Warner Books, 1989), 26; Dodds and Gara, *Baby Dodds*, 31; Dance, *Swing*, 119.

13. Southern, *Music*, 64, quotation from 65; Margaret Hindle Hazen and Robert M. Hazen, *The Music Men: An Illustrated History of Brass Bands in America, 1800–1920* (Washington, D.C.: Smithsonian Institution Press, 1987), 6.

14. Southern, *Music*, 66–67.

15. Floyd and Reisser, "Social Dance Music," 162–63; Southern, *Music*, 107.

16. Eileen Southern, "Frank Johnson of Philadelphia and His Promenade Concerts," *Black Perspective in Music*, 5, no. 1 (Spring 1977): 3–18, quotation from 4; Floyd and Reisser, "Social Dance Music," 162–63.

17. Southern, *Music*, 107–10.

18. James M. Trotter, *Music and Some Highly Musical People* (Boston: Lee and Shepard, 1878; New York: Charles T. Dillingham, 1878; reprint, New York: Johnson Reprint Corporation, 1968), 307.

19. Historical Society of Pennsylvania and the Historical Society of Saratoga Springs, "One Hundred and Sixty Years of the Music of Francis (Frank) Johnson (1792–1844)," program notes, July 20, 1978; Southern, *Music*, 110.

20. Hazen, *Music Men*, 2; Southern, *Music*, 207–11.

21. Thomas Wentworth Higginson, *Army Life in a Black Regiment* (Boston: Lee and Shepard, 1869; reprint, New York: W. W. Norton, 1984), 136–37. I am grateful to John Szwed for bringing this source to my attention. Southern, *Music*, 206.

22. Southern, *Music*, 208, 205, 255.

23. Handy, *Father of the Blues*, 35–38, quotations from 36, 35–36, 37–38.

24. Trotter, *Music*, 275–76, quotation from 280; Southern, *Music*, 229.

25. Toll, *Blacking Up*, 119–20, 124.

26. Ibid., 248–49, quotation from 249; Fletcher, *One Hundred Years*, 61.

27. Toll, *Blacking Up*, 249–51; William J. Schafer, *Brass Bands and New Orleans Jazz* (Baton Rouge: Louisiana State University Press, 1977), 15.

28. Piersen, *Black Yankees*, 136–40, quotations from 136, 138, 139.

29. William Cullen Bryant, *Letters of a Traveller; or, Notes of Things Seen in Europe and America* (New York: George P. Putnam, 1850), 86–87, quoted in Lynne Fauley Emery, *Black Dance from 1619 to Today*, 2d rev. ed. (Princeton: Princeton Book Company, 1988), 114–15; Susan G. Davis, *Parades and Power: Street Theater in Nineteenth-Century Philadelphia* (Philadelphia: Temple University Press, 1986; reprint, Berkeley: University of California Press, 1988), 84–101.

30. Quotation from Abrahams correspondence; Allen, *Horrible Prettiness*, 107; Fletcher, *One Hundred Years*, 94.

31. For a discussion of black drill team competitions in Philadelphia, see Jerrilyn M. McGregory, "'There Are Other Ways to Get Happy': African-American Urban Folklore" (Ph.D. diss., University of Pennsylvania, 1992), 278–81.

32. Fletcher, *One Hundred Years*, 20–22, quotations from 21, 20.

33. Ibid., 22; John Chilton, *A Jazz Nursery: The Story of the Jenkins' Orphanage Bands of Charleston, South Carolina* (London: Bloomsbury Book Shop, 1980), 2–3.

34. Chilton, *Jazz Nursery*, 2–3, 25, quotation from 13; Dance, *Duke Ellington*, 145; "Jenkins Bands," *Time*, 26 Aug. 1935, 25.

35. Wells and Dance, *Night People*, 6; Leonard De Paur quoted in Chilton, *Jazz Nursery*, 31.

36. Chilton, *Jazz Nursery*, 14, 38, 52, 56, 58; "Jenkins Bands," 25.

37. Russell, *Jazz Style*, 45–46; Hazen, *Music Men*, 5.

38. Hazen, *Music Men*, 1, 4, 5, 8, 11–12, quotation from 12.

39. Ibid., 1, 11–13, quotation from 12.

40. Bechet, *Treat It Gentle*, 215; Schafer, *Brass Bands*, 10; Southern, *Music*, 340.

41. Paul Eduard Miller, "Fifty Years of New Orleans Jazz," *Esquire's Jazz Book, 1945* (New York: A. S. Barnes, 1945), 1, 3, 5; Luke Fontana, *New Orleans and Her Jazz Funeral Marching Bands* (New Orleans: Distribution, Jazz, 1980), 1, 7; Southern, *Music*, 340–41; Mark C. Gridley, *Jazz Styles: History and Analysis*, 3d ed. (Englewood Cliffs, N.J.: Prentice Hall, 1988), 40–42.

42. Fontana, *New Orleans*, 1, 7; Southern, *Music*, 341; Gridley, *Jazz Styles*, 40–42.

43. Schafer, *Brass Bands*, 13–15.

44. Ibid., 12.

45. Karl Koenig, "The Plantation Belt Brass Band and Musicians," *Second Line* 33 (Fall 1981): 24–25, quotation from 34.

46. Quotation from Schafer, *Brass Bands,* 22; Koenig, "Plantation," 24–38.

47. Schafer, *Brass Bands,* 66–68, 28, 29, 33; Koenig, "Plantation," 35.

48. Bechet, *Treat It Gentle,* 62; Frederic Ramsey Jr., "Music from the South, Vol. 1: Country Brass Bands," accompanying booklet to *Music from the South,* vol. 1, *Country Brass Bands* (Folkways LP, FA 2650, 1961); Al Rose and Edmond Souchon, *New Orleans' Jazz: A Family Album* (Baton Rouge: Louisiana State University Press, 1967), 182.

49. Schafer, *Brass Bands,* 30, 32.

50. Smith, *Music on my Mind,* 74–75; Southern, *Music,* 349–50.

51. Robert Kimball and William Bolcom, *Reminiscing with Sissle and Blake* (New York: Viking, 1973), 58, 59; Gunther Schuller, "James Reese Europe," in *Dictionary of American Negro Biography,* ed. Rayford W. Logan and Michael R. Winston (New York: W. W. Norton, 1982), 214.

52. Johnson, *Black Manhattan,* 118–22.

53. Ibid., 120–21; R. Reid Badger, "James Reese Europe and the Prehistory of Jazz," *American Music* 7, no. 1 (Spring 1989): 48–49; Southern, *Music,* 344.

54. Johnson, *Black Manhattan,* 122.

55. Ibid., 122–23; Southern, *Music,* 343–45; Badger, "James Reese Europe," 49–51.

56. Johnson, *Black Manhattan,* 123–24.

57. Badger, "James Reese Europe," 48; Lewis A. Erenberg, "Everybody's Doin' It: The Pre-World War I Dance Craze, the Castles, and the Modern American Girl," *Feminist Studies* 3, nos. 1–2 (Fall 1975): 155–57, quotation from 156; Ron Welburn, "James Reese Europe and the Infancy of Jazz Criticism," *Black Music Research Journal* 7 (1987): 35–39.

58. Badger, "James Reese Europe," 48–52, 55; Schuller, "James Reese Europe," 214; Johnson, *Black Manhattan,* 124; Southern, *Music,* 344–45.

59. James Reese Europe quoted in Kimball and Bolcom, *Reminiscing,* 64.

60. James Reese Europe quoted in *Readings in Black American Music,* ed. Eileen Southern, 2d ed. (New York: W. W. Norton, 1983), 240; Southern, *Music,* 350; Schuller, "James Reese Europe," 214.

61. Noble Sissle quoted in Kimball and Bolcom, *Reminiscing,* 68.

62. Editorial in *New York Times,* 12 May 1919, quoted in Southern, *Music,* 352; Schuller, "James Reese Europe," 214; Lewis, *When Harlem Was in Vogue,* 3.

63. Schuller, "James Reese Europe," 215.

64. Handy, *Father of the Blues,* 69.

65. See, for example, Dance, *Earl Hines,* 188; Russell, *Jazz Style,* 172; Dance, *Duke Ellington,* 134; Hampton and Haskins, *Hamp,* 20–23.

66. Southern, *Music,* 284–85, 301; Handy, *Father of the Blues,* 69; Ron Wel-

burn, "Ralph Ellison's Territorial Vantage," *Grackle* 4 (1977–78): 8–9; Hampton and Haskins, *Hamp*, 21.

67. Hampton and Haskins, *Hamp*, 20–21.

68. Southern, *Music*, 281–83.

69. Ralph Ellison quoted in Welburn, "Ralph Ellison," 9; Dance, *Count Basie*, 146; Julian C. Adderley Sr., interview with author, Tallahassee, Fla., 9 May 1988; Robert G. O'Meally, interview with author, New York, N.Y., 1 Aug. 1993.

70. Ellison, *Shadow and Act*, 10–11.

Chapter 9: The FAMU Marching 100

1. Szwed and Marks, "Transformation," 32.

2. Leonard C. Bowie, "History of the Florida A&M University Band," *Band Day Souvenir Program*, 2 Oct. 1965, 8–10, quotation from 10.

3. Hurston, "Characteristics," 55–56, emphasis added.

4. Julian C. Adderley Sr. interview.

5. Frank E. Pinder II, *Pinder: From Little Acorns* (Tallahassee, Fla.: Florida Agricultural and Mechanical University Foundation, 1986), 27.

6. Dwight Oliver Wendell Holmes, *The Evolution of the Negro College* (Bureau of Publications, Teachers College, Columbia University, 1934; reprint, New York: Arno Press and the New York Times, 1969), 150–52; Bureau of Education, Department of the Interior, *Survey of Negro Colleges* (Washington, D.C.: GPO, 1929; reprint, New York: Negro Universities Press, 1969), 212; Florida A&M Office of Public Relations, "Florida A&M—The University" (1987); Pinder, *Pinder*, 28.

7. Leander Kirksey, telephone interview with author, 25 May 1988.

8. Leedall W. Neyland and John W. Riley, *The History of Florida Agricultural and Mechanical University* (Gainesville: University of Florida Press, 1963), 119.

9. "Founder's Day Brings N.B. Young and Memories," *FAMU Alumni News* (Mar.–Apr. 1971): 5, 10, quotation from 5; Cassandra Watson, "Adderleys Contribute to FAMU Musical History," *Voice of the Archivist* 3, no. 1 (Fall 1983): 4.

10. Nathan B. Young, telephone interview with author, 23 Oct. 1988.

11. James D. Anderson, *The Education of Blacks in the South, 1860–1935* (Chapel Hill: University of North Carolina Press, 1988), 197; Julian C. Adderley Sr. interview; Nat Adderley, telephone interview with author, 15 May 1988.

12. Julian C. Adderley Sr. interview; Pinder, *Pinder*, 28; Leander Kirksey, interview with author, New Haven, Conn., 25 June 1988.

13. Julian C. Adderley Sr. interview.

14. Quotation from Gerald Burke, "Some Reflections on a Life of Accomplishments in Music" (1988), ms., 2; Kirksey interview, 25 May 1988.

15. Quotation from Nat Adderley interview, 15 May 1988; Kirksey interview, 25 June 1988.

16. Nat Adderley interview, 15 May 1988; Kirksey interview.

17. William Patrick Foster, interview with author, Tallahassee, Fla., 5 May 1988.

18. Nat Adderley, telephone interview with author, 9 May 1988.

19. William Patrick Foster, telephone interview, 1 August 1995; Nat Adderley interview, 9 May 1988.

20. Clifford Edward Watkins, "The Works of Three Selected Band Directors in Predominantly Black American Colleges and Universities" (Ph.D. diss., Southern Illinois University, 1975), 100, 102.

21. Julian White, interview with author, Tallahassee, Fla., 8 May 1988; Thomas Lyle, telephone interview with author, 11 May 1988.

22. Beverly Barber, interview with author, Tallahassee, Fla., 6 May 1988; Lyle interview.

23. Lyle interview; "FAMU's Incomparable Marching 100," *Courier*, undated article from the files of Julian White.

24. Julian White interview; "Band Faculty Members—'The Nuts and Bolts Team,'" *A&M: Florida A&M University Bulletin for Faculty, Staff, and Friends* 3, no. 1 (Oct. 1989): 18–19.

25. Julian White interview.

26. Ibid.

27. Jean Wardlow, "Rattlers Go: Sisssssss . . . Boom-Bah!" *Miami Herald*, 5 Dec. 1964, B1; Watkins, "Band Directors," 90.

28. Lyle interview; Julian White interview.

29. Foster interview.

30. "The Roots and Flowering of a Fine Musical Tradition," *School Musician, Director, and Teacher*, 49, no. 3 (Nov. 1977): 53.

31. Julian White interview.

32. Robert L. Allen, "The Rattlers Roll On," *Black Collegian*, 4, no. 3 (1974): 55; Watkins, "Band Directors," 96.

33. William P. Foster, "My Best Half-Time Show," *Instrumentalist* (Oct. 1964): 33–34.

34. Julian White interview; Foster interview.

35. Transcription of videotape of Circle City Classic, Indianapolis, Ind., 1986.

36. Thompson, "Kongo Influences," 161–63.

37. Ibid., 161–62.

38. Ibid., 162; Roger D. Abrahams and John F. Szwed, *After Africa* (New Haven: Yale University Press, 1983), 1–2.

39. Thompson, *African Art in Motion*, 9; Fletcher, *One Hundred Years*, 67, 292, 105.

40. Thompson, *African Art in Motion*, 13–14.

41. Barbara Wynn quoted in Barrington Salmon, "It's FAMU's Family Get-

Together," *Tallahassee Democrat*, 3 Nov. 1991, 1C; Julian White interview; Frank E. Pinder II, interview with author, Chevy Chase, Md., 27 Nov. 1988.

42. Author's notes from FAMU performance at "Homecoming '90—Rattler Venom More Potent Than Ever," homecoming preconcert show at Florida A&M University, Tallahassee, Fla., 19 Oct. 1990.

43. Julian White interview.

44. Ibid.

45. Col. Bernard D. Hendricks quoted in Michael Rachlin, "FAMU's Bill Foster Takes Marching 100 to New Fame," *Miami Times*, 27 Dec. 1985; William Foster quoted in Charles S. Farrell, "The Greatest Half-Time Show in America," *Chronicle of Higher Education* (14 Nov. 1984): 32; Julian White interview.

46. Quotation from Julian White interview; "The Best Band in the Land," *Ebony*, Nov. 1963, 172–78.

47. Farrell, "Greatest," 34.

48. Julian White interview.

49. "William P. Foster: A Fabled Director and His Band," *Ebony*, Dec. 1984, 30; Julian White interview.

50. Lake-Sumpter Community College Lyceum Series, "The Florida A&M University Symphonic Band in Concert," program notes, 26 Feb. 1988; Peter Slevin, "Blue, White, and Red Parade," *Miami Herald*, 15 July 1989, 1A, 20A; Gail Schmoller, "FAMU Marching Band: The Marching 100 in Paris," *Center for Black Music Research Digest* 2, no. 2 (Fall 1989): 1, 13; Bill Cotterell, "Marching 100 Is the Very Best, French Director Says," *Tallahassee Democrat*, 15 June 1989; Alvin Hollins Jr., "Florida A&M's 'Marching 100' Moonwalks during French Bicentennial," *Strike* (homecoming booklet, Oct. 1989), 44, 56; Julian White interview.

51. Jean Paul Goude quoted in Sharon Perry Saunders, "FAMU Marching 100, the Hottest Act in Paris" (Office of Public Relations, Florida A&M University, July 23, 1989), 6; Gary Fineout, "FAMU Band Plans Paris Step Show," *Florida Flambeau*, 15 June 1989, 2; Peter Slevin, "Florida Soul Storms Bastille," *Miami Herald*, 13 July 1989, 1A, 20A.

52. "The 'Marching 100,' the Hottest Thing in Paris—Bastille Day '89," *A&M: Florida A&M University Bulletin for Faculty, Staff, and Friends* 3, no. 1 (Oct. 1989): 12–14.

53. Slevin, "Blue, White, and Red Parade," 20A.

54. Quotation from James M. Markham, "A Made-for-TV French Bicentennial and Summit," *New York Times*, International Sunday, 16 July 1989; Saunders, "FAMU Marching 100," 1.

55. Mike Ewen, "The Band That Can't Be Beat," *Florida* (Sunday magazine of the *Orlando Sentinel*), 24 Sept. 1989, 45.

56. Arienne Wallace, "FAMU's 'Music Man,'" *Tallahassee Magazine*, Fall 1987, 17; Julian White interview.

57. Julian White quoted in "Band Faculty Members," 18.

Chapter 10: African American Mutual Aid Societies

1. Carter G. Woodson, *The African Background Outlined* (Washington, D.C.: Association for the Study of Negro Life and History, 1936; reprint, New York: Negro Universities Press, 1968), 168–71.

2. Edward N. Palmer, "Negro Secret Societies," *Social Forces* 23, no. 2 (Dec. 1944): 207–12; August Meier, *Negro Thought in America, 1880–1915: Racial Ideologies in the Age of Booker T. Washington* (Ann Arbor: University of Michigan Press, 1988), 8–16, 24, 42–58, 121–57; Walter Weare, "Fraternal Orders, Black," in *Encyclopedia of Southern Culture,* ed. Charles Reagan Wilson and William Ferris (Chapel Hill: University of North Carolina Press, 1989), 158–59.

3. W. E. B. Du Bois, ed., *Economic Co-operation among Negro Americans* (Atlanta: Atlanta University Press, 1907), 96.

4. "Sororities and Fraternities: In Step with Giving," *UPSCALE* 3, no. 5 (Apr.–May 1992): 46–49; "Black Fraternities and Sororities: Sigma Gamma Rho," *Ebony,* Feb. 1991, 80–82; "Black Fraternities and Sororities: Delta Sigma Theta," *Ebony,* Feb. 1990, 92–94; "Black Fraternities and Sororities: Kappa Alpha Psi," *Ebony,* May 1990, 174–76; "Black Fraternities and Sororities: Omega Psi Phi," *Ebony,* Sept. 1993, 112–14; "Alpha Phi Alpha Fraternity," *Ebony,* Nov. 1989, 128–30; "Alpha Kappa Alpha Sorority: Eighty Years of Service and Sisterhood," *Ebony,* Oct. 1988, 38–40; "Black Fraternities and Sororities: Zeta Phi Beta," *Ebony,* May 1991, 58–60.

5. Melville J. Herskovits, *Dahomey: An Ancient West African Kingdom,* vol. 1 (New York: J. J. Augustin, 1938; reprint, Evanston, Ill.: Northwestern University Press, 1967), 242–44, 250–53; Herskovits, *Myth,* 82, 140, 160–62, 166–67, 197–203; Captain F. W. Butt-Thompson, *West African Secret Societies: Their Organizations, Officials, and Teaching* (London: H. F. & G. Witherby, 1929; reprint, New York: Argosy-Antiquarian, 1969), 12–15, 86. See also Yaya Diallo and Mitchell Hall, *The Healing Drum: African Wisdom Teachings* (Rochester, Ver.: Destiny Books, 1989).

6. Basil Davidson, *The African Genius: An Introduction to African Cultural and Social History* (Boston: Little, Brown, 1970), 91–106, quotations from 95, 100–101; Margaret Washington Creel, "Gullah Attitudes toward Life and Death," in *Africanisms in American Culture,* ed. Joseph E. Holloway (Bloomington: Indiana University Press, 1990), 77.

7. Thompson, *African Art in Motion,* 173–81, quotation from 180.

8. Balandier, *Daily Life,* 170–71, 215–16, 220, quotation from 233; Creel, "Gullah Attitudes," 78.

9. Herskovits, *Myth,* 82–83, 140–41, 160–63, quotation from 161.

10. Joyner, *Down by the Riverside,* 58–59.

11. William R. Bascom, "Acculturation among the Gullah Negroes," *American Anthropologist* 43, no. 1 (1941): 43–50, reprinted in August Meier and Elliott Rudwick, eds. *The Making of Black America* (New York: Atheneum, 1969), 37.

12. Judith Bettelheim, "Festivals in Cuba, Haiti, and New Orleans," in *Car-*

ibbean Festival Arts, ed. John W. Nunley and Judith Bettelheim (Seattle: University of Washington Press, 1988), 137–42, quotation from 140.

13. Daniel J. Crowley, "American Institutions of Yoruba Type," *Man* 53 (May 1953): 80. For similar organizations in Bermuda, see Frank E. Manning, *Black Clubs in Bermuda: Ethnography of a Play World* (Ithaca: Cornell University Press, 1973), 32–34.

14. Robert L. Harris Jr., "Early Black Benevolent Societies, 1780–1830," *Massachusetts Review* 20 (Autumn 1979): 603, 609–16, 619.

15. Ibid., 612–13, quotation from 613.

16. Ibid., 611, 612, 614–17.

17. Ibid., 611, 617–20.

18. Quotation from Monroe N. Work, "Secret Societies as Factors in the Social and Economical Life of the Negro," in *Democracy in Earnest: Southern Sociological Congress, 1916–1918*, ed. James E. McCulloch (Washington, D.C.: Southern Sociological Congress, 1918; reprint, New York: Negro Universities Press, 1969), 344–45; John Sibley Butler, *Entrepreneurship and Self-Help among Black Americans: A Reconsideration of Race and Economics* (Albany: State University of New York Press, 1991), 80–81; Palmer, "Negro Secret Societies," 209.

19. Vincent Harding, "Religion and Resistance among Antebellum Negroes, 1800–1860," in *The Making of Black America*, ed. August Meier and Elliott Rudwick (New York: Atheneum, 1969), 194–95; Work, "Secret Societies," 343–45.

20. Walter B. Weare, *Black Business in the New South: A Social History of the North Carolina Mutual Life Insurance Company* (Urbana: University of Illinois Press, 1973), 9; Harris, "Early Black Societies," 612, 617.

21. Work, "Secret Societies," 344.

22. Robert L. Harris Jr., "Charleston's Free Afro-American Elite: The Brown Fellowship Society and the Humane Brotherhood," *South Carolina Historical Magazine* 82, no. 4 (1981): 291, 296, 289, quotation from 298.

23. Quotation from John Hope Franklin, *From Slavery to Freedom: A History of Negro Americans*, 6th ed. (New York: McGraw-Hill, 1988), 146; Meier, *Negro Thought*, 15; Harris, "Early Black Societies," 617; Butler, *Entrepreneurship*, 99; Jeffrey R. Brackett, "Notes on the Progress of the Colored People of Maryland since the War," ed. Herbert B. Adams, *Johns Hopkins University Studies in Historical and Political Science* (July–Sept. 1890): 48.

24. Butler, *Entrepreneurship*, 100–101, 102–3; Franklin, *Slavery*, 95; Rayford W. Logan, "Prince Hall," in *Dictionary of American Negro Biography*, ed. Rayford W. Logan and Michael Winston (New York: W. W. Norton, 1982), 279–80.

25. Weare, *Black Business*, 10–12, quotation from 11; Franklin, *Slavery*, 259–60; Du Bois, *Economic Cooperation*, 126, 93; Brackett, "Notes," 52–53.

26. W. H. Gibson Sr., *History of the United Brothers of Friendship and Sisters of the Mysterious Ten, in Two Parts: A Negro Order* (Louisville, Ky.: Bradley and Gilbert, 1897; reprint, Freeport, N.Y.: Books for Libraries Press, 1971), iii, v, 113; Du Bois, *Economic Cooperation*, 124–25.

27. Wendell P. Dabney, *Maggie L. Walker and the I. O. of Saint Luke: The Woman and Her Work* (Cincinnati: Dabney Publishing, 1927), 12–13, 37–38, 40, 66; Margaret Duckworth, "Maggie L. Walker," in *Notable Black American Women*, ed. Jessie Carney Smith (Detroit: Gale Research, 1992), 1188–93.

28. A. E. Bush and P. L. Dorman, *History of the Mosaic Templars of America: Its Founders and Officials* (Little Rock: Central, 1924), 81–83, 139, 153–54, 174–75, 195–98, 208, 209, 211, 213, 220, 221, quotation from 153.

29. William Taylor Thom, *The True Reformers* (Washington, D.C.: GPO, 1902), 807–14, quotation from 807; Du Bois, *Economic Co-operation*, 101–4.

30. Brackett, "Notes," 50.

31. Quotation from Du Bois, *Economic Co-operation*, 98; Butler, *Entrepreneurship*, 100; Howard W. Odum, *Social and Mental Traits of the Negro: Research into the Conditions of the Negro Race in Southern Towns; a Study in Race Traits, Tendencies, and Prospects* (New York: Columbia University, 1910; reprint, New York: AMS Press, 1968), 129.

32. Weare, *Black Business*, 12–13; Brackett, "Notes," 54.

33. Odum, *Social and Mental Traits*, 129.

34. Ibid., 109; Bush and Dorman, *History*, 197, 198.

35. Edward Franklin Frazier, *The Negro in the United States* (New York: Macmillan, 1949), 380; Gibson, *United Brothers*, 101–2.

36. Johnson, *Black Manhattan*, 167–69, quotation from 168–69.

37. Handy, *Father of the Blues*, 76; Dance, *Swing*, 46.

38. Stewart, *Jazz Masters*, 82; Dance, *Duke Ellington*, 55.

39. Harry Carney quoted in Dance, *Duke Ellington*, 71; Gillespie, *To Be or Not to Bop*, 32, 121, 197; Bushell, *Jazz*, 115; Smith, *Music on My Mind*, 47; Marion Coles interview.

40. Jackson, *Movin' on Up*, 37; Russell, *Jazz Style*, 191; Murray, *Stomping the Blues*, 136.

41. Henry A. Kmen, *Music in New Orleans: The Formative Years, 1791–1841* (Baton Rouge: Louisiana State University Press, 1966), 3–5, quotation from 4.

42. Ibid., 6–17, 43–54, 204, 227–30, quotation from 43; John Blassingame, *Black New Orleans, 1860–1880* (Chicago: University of Chicago Press, 1973), 145–46.

43. Schafer, *Brass Bands*, 10, P. B. S. Pinchback quoted on 12.

44. Claude F. Jacobs, "Benevolent Societies of New Orleans Blacks during the Late Nineteenth and Early Twentieth Centuries," *Louisiana History* 29, no. 1 (Winter 1988): 22; Blassingame, *Black New Orleans*, 147.

45. Blassingame, *Black New Orleans*, 144–47, quotation from 145.

46. Ibid., 143–48; Jacobs, "Benevolent Societies," 21–23.

47. Charles Edward Smith, liner notes to *Jazz Begins: Sounds of New Orleans Streets—Funeral and Parade Music by the Young Tuxedo Brass Band* (Atlantic LP 1297, 1958); Donald M. Marquis, *In Search of Buddy Bolden: First Man of Jazz* (Baton Rouge: Louisiana State University Press, 1978; reprint, New York: Da Capo

Press, 1980), 32; Robert C. Reinders, "Sound of the Mournful Dirge," *Jazz: A Quarterly of American Music*, no. 4 (Fall 1959): 296; New Orleans Jazz Club, "Matters of Life and Death," *Second Line* 31 (Fall 1979): 44.

48. New Orleans Jazz Club, "Matters of Life and Death," 44; Reinders, "Sound of the Mournful Dirge," 298.

49. Zutty Singleton quoted in Smith, "Jazz Begins"; Fontana, *New Orleans*, 13.

50. Kathleen Chase, "Syncopated Dirges, Ragtime Parades," *Americas* 16, no. 3 (Mar. 1964): 20.

51. Schafer, *Brass Bands*, 43.

52. Michael White, "The New Orleans Brass Band in the Twentieth Century: Nature, Style, and Social Significance," *Xavier Review* 4, nos. 1–2 (1984): 23.

53. Michael White, interview with author, New Orleans, La., 22 July 1990.

54. Quotation from White, "New Orleans Brass Band," 26; Michael White interview; Danny Barker, interview with author, New Orleans, La., 22 July 1990; Gregory Stafford, interview with author, New Orleans, La., 24 July 1990.

55. Michael White interview.

56. Thompson and Cornet, *Four Moments*, 148–49, quotation from 149; Kmen, *Music in New Orleans*, 10–12.

57. Robert Farris Thompson, "Recapturing Heaven's Glamour: Afro-Caribbean Festivalizing Arts," in *Caribbean Festival Arts*, ed. John W. Nunley and Judith Bettelheim (Seattle: University of Washington Press, 1988), 20, 28, quotation from 20. Many thanks to Robert Farris Thompson for bringing this source to my attention.

58. Rex Nettleford, "Implications for Caribbean Development," in *Caribbean Festival Arts*, ed. John W. Nunley and Judith Bettelheim (Seattle: University of Washington Press, 1988), 183–97, quotation from 186; Abrahams and Szwed, *After Africa*, 28–31. See also John W. Nunley and Judith Bettelheim, eds. *Caribbean Festival Arts* (Seattle: University of Washington Press, 1988).

59. Michael White quoted in St. Clair Bourne, *New Orleans Brass* (National Geographic Explorer, 1989); Michael White interview.

60. Michael White quoted in Bourne, *New Orleans*; Michael White interview.

61. K. Kia Bunseki Fu-Kiau quoted in Thompson, "Recapturing," 23.

62. Louis Armstrong, *Satchmo: My Life in New Orleans* (New York: Prentice-Hall, 1954; reprint, New York: Da Capo Press, 1986), 225; White, "New Orleans Brass Band," 30; Michael White interview.

63. William R. Jankowiak, "Black Social Aid and Pleasure Clubs: Marching Associations in New Orleans" (Jean Lafitte National Historical Park and Preserve and the National Park Service, sponsored by the Department of Anthropology at Tulane University, 1989), 26, 42–48; Nathaniel Gray and Norman Dixon, interview with author, New Orleans, La., 29 July 1990.

Chapter 11: Stepping

1. Transcription of videotape of "Stepping in Sequence," homecoming step show at Howard University, Washington, D.C., 30 Oct. 1991.

2. Ibid.

3. Sally Sommer, "Stepp Up the Heat," *Village Voice*, 2 Feb. 1988, 33.

4. "Gumboot" dancing, South Africa's oldest township dance, started at the end of the nineteenth century in the mining compounds, where group dancing was the primary source of recreation. Between the 1970s and 1980s, it was introduced in North American urban areas and showcased by many of the dance companies that performed styles of traditional African dances. Just how this genre was picked up by black fraternities and sororities requires further study, but I am fairly certain that the percussive "thigh-slapping" style executed by Phi Beta Sigma stepping teams is inspired by gumboot dancing. See Anne Beresford, *We Jive like This* (A Cinecontact/Kinoki Production for the Arts Council of Great Britain, 1991); Veit Erlmann, *African Stars: Studies in Black South African Performance* (Chicago: University of Chicago Press, 1991), 100.

5. Abrahams, *Singing the Master*, 83.

6. Bebey, *African Music*, 92.

7. K. Kia Bunseki Fu-Kiau, telephone interview with author, 23 Jan. 1994.

8. Ibid.; Robert Farris Thompson, *Face of the Gods: Art and Altars of Africa and the African Americas* (New York: Museum for African Art, 1993), 56.

9. Thompson, *Face of the Gods*, 56.

10. Kubik, *Angolan Traits*, 49–50. Many thanks to Danny Dawson for introducing me to Kubik's writings. Abrahams, *Singing the Master*, xx; Epstein, *Sinful Tunes*, 141–44; Blassingame, *Slave Community*, 125.

11. Solomon Northup, *Twelve Years a Slave: Narrative of Solomon Northup* (Auburn, N.Y.: Derby and Miller, 1853), reprinted in *Puttin' on Ole Massa: The Slave Narratives of Henry Bibb, William Wells Brown, and Solomon Northup*, ed. Gilbert Osofsky (New York: Harper and Row, 1969), 346.

12. Quotation from Fu-Kiau interview; Herskovits, *Dahomey*, 255.

13. Abrahams, *Singing the Master*, 93–94.

14. Nketia, *The Music of Africa*, 67; Fu-Kiau interview. Many thanks to C. Daniel Dawson for bringing the information about Zambia and Mozambique to my attention.

15. Epstein, *Sinful Tunes*, 144; Arthur Freed, *Panama Hattie* (Turner Entertainment, 1942; MGM/UA Home Video 1990); Cholly Atkins, telephone interview with author, 26 June 1993.

16. Transcription of step show videotape.

17. Ibid.

18. Davis, *I Got the Word*, 30–31.

19. Abrahams, *Man-of-Words*, 21–39. See also Balandier, *Daily Life*; John C.

Messenger Jr., "The Role of Proverbs in a Nigerian Judicial System," *Southwestern Journal of Anthropology* 15, no. 1 (Spring 1959): 64–73; Kofi Awoonor, *Guardians of the Sacred Word* (New York: Nok, 1974).

20. Ethel M. Albert, "'Rhetoric,' 'Logic,' and 'Poetics' in Burundi: Culture Patterning of Speech Behavior," *American Anthropologist*, vol. 66, no. 6, part 2 (Dec. 1964): 35, quoted in Abrahams, *Man-of-Words*, 22; Abrahams, *Man-of-Words*, 29.

21. Abrahams, *Singing the Master*, 107–10, quotation from 112; Abrahams, *Man-of-Words*, 27–29.

22. Roger D. Abrahams, *Talking Black* (Rowley, Mass.: Newbury House, 1976), 39, 45–57, quotation from 45; Geneva Smitherman, *Talkin and Testifyin: The Language of Black America* (Boston: Houghton Mifflin, 1977; reprint, Detroit: Wayne State University Press, 1985), 108.

23. Roger D. Abrahams, *Deep Down in the Jungle: Negro Narrative Folklore from the Streets of Philadelphia* (Hatboro, Penn.: Folklore Associates, 1964), 267; Claudia Mitchell-Kernan, "Signifying, Loud-Talking, and Marking," in *Rappin' and Stylin' Out: Communication in Urban Black America*, ed. Thomas Kochman (Urbana: University of Illinois Press, 1972), 316, 332–33; Smitherman, *Black Talk*, 86–87, 94.

24. Smitherman, *Talkin and Testifyin*, 119.

25. Transcription of step show videotape.

26. Ibid.

27. Ibid.

28. Rayford W. Logan, *Howard University: The First Hundred Years, 1867–1967* (New York: New York University Press, 1969), 18, 20, 25–26; C. Eric Lincoln, "The Negro Colleges and Cultural Change," *Daedalus* 100, no. 3 (Summer 1971): 619–20; St. Clair Drake, "The Black University in the American Social Order," *Daedalus* 100, no. 3 (Summer 1971): 838–39.

29. Lincoln, "Negro Colleges," 612, quotation from 611; Drake, "Black University," 839.

30. Logan, *Howard University*, 102; Lincoln, "Negro Colleges," 611–12.

31. Monroe H. Little, "The Extra-Curricular Activities of Black College Students, 1868–1940," *Journal of Negro History* 65, no. 2 (Spring 1980): 139.

32. Ibid., 136–38; Logan, *Howard University*, 124–26; Bernard Wayne Franklin, "Deeds and Dreams: The Extracurriculum in Selected Afro-American Colleges, 1915–1930" (Ed.D. diss., Teachers College, Columbia University, 1983), 26–29.

33. John Robson, ed., *Baird's Manual of American College Fraternities*, 17th ed. (Menasha, Wisc.: George Banta, 1963), 7–9; Oscar M. Voorhees, *The History of Phi Beta Kappa* (New York: Crown, 1945), 3–17.

34. Charles H. Wesley, *The History of Alpha Phi Alpha: A Development in College Life*, rev. ed. (Chicago: Foundation, 1981), x-16.

35. Ibid., 15–27, 54–55, quotation from xii.

36. Quotations from Little, "Extra-Curricular Activities," 140; André McKenzie, "Fraters: Black Greek-Letter Fraternities at Four Historically Black Colleges, 1920–1960" (Ed.D. diss., Teachers College, Columbia University, 1986), 140–41.

37. Raymond Wolters, *The New Negro on Campus: Black College Rebellions of the 1920s* (Princeton: Princeton University Press, 1975), 70–73, 135; Wesley, *Alpha Phi Alpha*, 40–44.

38. Norma E. Boyd, *A Love That Equals My Labors: The Life Story of Norma E. Boyd* (Washington, D.C.: Alpha Kappa Alpha Sorority, 1980), 33–34, 42, quotation from 71.

39. Marjorie H. Parker, *Alpha Kappa Alpha through the Years, 1908–1988* (Chicago: Mobium, 1990), 9–12, quotation from 254; Boyd, *Love*, 71–72.

40. Robert L. Gill, *The Omega Psi Phi Fraternity and the Men Who Made Its History: A Concise History* (Washington, D.C.: Omega Psi Phi Fraternity, 1963), vi, 1–4.

41. Herman Dreer, *The History of the Omega Psi Phi Fraternity, 1911–1939: A Brotherhood of Negro College Men* (Washington, D.C.: Omega Psi Phi Fraternity, 1940), 1–24, quotation from 24.

42. Paula Giddings, *In Search of Sisterhood: Delta Sigma Theta and the Challenge of the Black Sorority Movement* (New York: William Morrow, 1988), 46–50, quotation from 46.

43. Ibid., 46–58; Mary Elizabeth Vroman, *Shaped to Its Purpose: Delta Sigma Theta—the First Fifty Years* (New York: Random House, 1965), 11–13; Parker, *Alpha Kappa Alpha*, 36–37.

44. W. Sherman Savage and L. D. Reddick, *Our Cause Speeds On: An Informal History of the Phi Beta Sigma Fraternity* (Atlanta: Fuller, 1957), 23, 14–15, A. Langston Taylor quoted on 14, originally quoted in *Crescent* 33, no. 1 (Spring 1949).

45. Arizona Cleaver Stemons quoted in Ola Adams, *Zeta Phi Beta Sorority, 1920–1965* (Washington, D.C.: Zeta Phi Beta Sorority, 1965), 7–8.

46. William L. Crump, *The Story of Kappa Alpha Psi: A History of the Beginning and Development of a College Greek Letter Organization, 1911–1983*, 3d ed. (Philadelphia: Kappa Alpha Psi Fraternity, 1983), xxi, 49, quotation from 3.

47. Ibid., xx–xxi, 1–5, 24–27.

48. Pearl Schwartz White, *Behind These Doors—A Legacy: The History of Sigma Gamma Rho Sorority* (Chicago: Sigma Gamma Rho Sorority, 1974), 1–10, 209, 314.

49. "Secret Societies Losing Their Hold on Students," *Hilltop*, 12 Apr. 1924, 4; "Howard University Center of Negro Collegiate Fraternal Activities," *Hilltop*, 31 Oct. 1924, 1; "Inter-Fraternal Games," *Hilltop*, 28 Mar. 1928, 2; "Phi Beta Sigma Holds Thanksgiving Forum," *Hilltop*, 12 Dec. 1929, 3; "Fraternities Have Launched into Their Various National Campaign Movements," *Hilltop*, 25 Apr. 1928, 1; "Omega Psi Phi Observe Negro Achievement," *Hilltop*, 21 Nov. 1929,

1, 4; "Among the Greeks," *Hilltop*, 15 Oct. 1931, 2; "The Inter-Fraternity Council," *Hilltop*, 16 Oct. 1930, 2; "Sigma Gamma Rho Sponsors Panel Discussion," *Hilltop*, 20 Apr. 1941, 1; "Omegas Hold Conference," *Hilltop*, 8 Feb. 1946, 1; "Alphas Pace Inter-fraternity Games," *Hilltop*, 26 Feb. 1948, 2; "Kappas Sponsor Essay Contest," *Hilltop*, 5 Apr. 1950, 2.

50. "Omega Psi Phi Fraternity to Celebrate 'Negro Achievement,'" *Hilltop*, 7 Nov. 1929, 1; "Phi Beta Sigma Fraternity Observes Bigger and Better Negro Business Week," *Hilltop*, 10 Apr. 1930, 1; "Marcus Garvey Speaks," 22 Jan. 1924, 2; "Dr. W. E. B. Du Bois to Deliver Commencement Address," *Hilltop*, 29 May 1930, 1; "Mary McCloud Bethune Visits Howard University," *Hilltop*, 21 Dec. 1936, 1; "African Ghandi Speaks on World Peace," *Hilltop*, 17 Apr. 1950, 1.

51. Savage and Reddick, *Our Cause Speeds On*, 21; Gill, *Omega Psi Phi*, 3.

52. "The Color Question at Howard University or 'Much Ado about Nothing,'" *Hilltop*, 22 May 1929, 6; "Interfraternity Council Holds Men's Mass Meeting," *Hilltop*, 22 May 1929, 5; "Fraternities and Elections," *Hilltop*, 29 May 1930, 2; "Free-Swinging Student Council Takes Over May, Grid, Hilltop Voting: Greeks Go Underground," *Hilltop*, 17 Mar. 1953, 3.

53. See, for example, "Kappa Alpha Psi Gives Dance," *Hilltop*, 22 Feb. 1928, 4; "Among the Greeks," *Hilltop*, 11 Dec. 1930, 2; "Among the Greeks," *Hilltop*, 28 Apr. 1933, 2; "Alpha Phi Alpha News," *Hilltop*, 11 Feb. 1942, 5; "The Mardi Gras," *Hilltop*, 25 May 1956, 5.

54. "King 'Jazz,'" *Hilltop*, 15 Feb. 1924, 4.

55. "Initial 'Frat' Dance Scores Huge Success," *Hilltop*, 13 Nov. 1935, 1.

56. "All Fraternities and Sororities Coincide in Initiation Periods for Probationers," *Hilltop*, 8 Dec. 1937, 1.

57. Vincent Johns, interview with author, Washington, D.C., 8 Apr. 1993.

58. Ibid. See, for example, "Greeks Killing Themselves," *Hilltop*, 13 Apr. 1962, 2; "Pledging Is Here," *Hilltop*, 18 Feb. 1966, 2; "Hypocrisy of Black Greekdom," *Hilltop*, 12 Jan. 1968, 4; "Reply to Greek Challenge," *Hilltop*, 22 Nov. 1968, 8, 9; "Greek Mythology Explored," *Hilltop*, 10 Oct. 1969, 6, 8, 10.

59. See, for example, "The Greeks: Here We Go Again," *Hilltop*, 30 Oct. 1970, 6; "Greeks Called Pathetic," *Hilltop*, 23 Oct. 1970, 6, 8; "Campus Speak Out," *Hilltop*, 13 Nov. 1970, 12.

60. See, for example, "It's Greek Time Again," *Hilltop*, 9 Feb. 1973, 6; "Campus Speak Out," *Hilltop*, 8 Mar. 1974, 10; "The Alphas Respond," *Hilltop*, 28 Feb. 1975, 1; "Tell Greeks What You Want and Want What You Ask For," *Hilltop*, 16 Mar. 1979, 5.

61. Quotation from Johns interview; Raymond Archer, interview with author, Washington, D.C., 8 Apr. 1993; "Howard University Homecoming Official Calendar of Events, *Hilltop*, 8 Oct. 1976, 10.

62. "Fraternities and Sororities: A Dramatic Comeback on Campus," *Ebony*, Dec. 1983, 93–94, 96, 98; "Secret Societies Losing Their Hold," 4; "Omega Psi

Phi Leads in Fraternity Scholarship," *Hilltop*, 7 Apr. 1932, 1; "Scrollers Hold Song Contest," *Hilltop*, 26 Nov. 1951, 3.

63. Damon Patterson, interview with author, Washington, D.C., 8 Apr. 1993; Valerie Holiday, interview with author, Washington, D.C., 9 Apr. 1993; Paul Woodruff, interview with author, Washington, D.C., 9 Apr. 1993; Andrew Johnstone, interview with author, Washington, D.C., 9 Apr. 1993; Cedrice Davis, interview with author, Washington, D.C., 10 Apr. 1993.

64. Ibid.

65. Johnstone interview; Davis interview; Holiday interview.

66. Patterson interview; Holiday interview; Woodruff interview; Johnstone interview; Davis interview.

67. Woodruff interview; Johnstone interview.

68. Woodruff interview; Johnstone interview; Patterson interview; Holiday interview; Davis interview.

69. Patterson interview.

70. Holiday interview; Woodruff interview.

71. Quotation from Patterson interview; Holiday interview; Woodruff interview; Johnstone interview; Davis interview.

72. Johnstone interview.

73. Ibid.; Patterson interview; Holiday interview; Woodruff interview; Davis interview.

74. Quotation from Johnstone interview; Holiday interview; Davis interview.

75. Johnstone interview; Patterson interview; Holiday interview; Woodruff interview.

76. Holiday interview.

77. Ibid.

78. Ibid.; Johnstone interview; Woodruff interview.

79. Quotation from Woodruff interview; Holiday interview; Johnstone interview.

80. Johnstone interview.

81. Ibid.; Holiday interview; Woodruff interview.

82. Johnstone interview.

83. Ibid.

84. Woodruff interview; Johnstone interview.

85. Johnstone interview; Patterson interview; Holiday interview; Woodruff interview; Davis interview.

86. Ron Paige, interview with author, Washington, D.C, 1 May 1992.

87. Woodruff interview; Patterson interview; Holiday interview; "Homecoming '90 Promises History, Tradition, Diversity," *Hilltop*, 12 Oct. 1990, A2, A6.

88. Woodruff interview; Patterson interview; Holiday interview; Johnstone interview.

89. Robert Farris Thompson, "Recapturing," 17–29, quotation from 19; Wood, "Gimme de Kneebone Bent,'" 7–8.

Index

JACQUI MALONE is an associate professor of drama, theater, and dance at Queens College and a former member of the Eleo Pomare Dance Company.

Books in the Series Folklore and Society

George Magoon and the Down East Game War: History, Folklore, and the Law
Edward D. Ives

Diversities of Gifts: Field Studies in Southern Religion
Edited by Ruel W. Tyson, Jr., James L. Peacock, and Daniel W. Patterson

Days from a Dream Almanac   *Dennis Tedlock*

Nowhere in America: The Big Rock Candy Mountain and Other Comic
Utopias   *Hal Rammel*

The Lost World of the Craft Printer   *Maggie Holtzberg-Call*

Listening to Old Voices: Folklore in the Lives of Nine Elderly People
Patrick B. Mullen

Wobblies, Pile Butts, and Other Heroes: Laborlore Explorations   *Archie Green*

Transforming Tradition: Folk Music Revivals Examined
Edited by Neil V. Rosenberg

Morning Dew and Roses: Nuance, Metaphor, and Meaning in Folksongs
Barre Toelken

The World Observed: Reflections on the Fieldwork Process
Edited by Bruce Jackson and Edward D. Ives

Last Cavalier: The Life and Times of John A. Lomax, 1867–1948
Nolan Porterfield

Steppin' on the Blues: The Visible Rhythms of African American Dance
Jacqui Malone